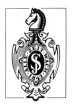

Since 1973 the Royal College of Obstetricians and Gynaecologists has regularly convened Study Groups to address important growth areas within obstetrics and gynaecology. An international group of eminent scientists and clinicians from various disciplines is invited to present the results of recent research and take part in in-depth discussion. The resulting volume, containing the papers presented and also edited transcripts of the discussions, is published within a few months of the meeting and provides a summary of the subject that is both authoritative and up to date.

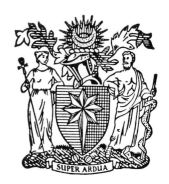

Previous RCOG Study Group publications available from Springer-Verlag:

Early Pregnancy Loss
Edited by R. W. Beard and F. Sharp

AIDS in Obstetrics and Gynaecology
Edited by C. N. Hudson and F. Sharp

Fetal Growth
Edited by F. Sharp, R. B. Fraser and
R. D. G. Milner

The Royal College of Obstetricians and Gynaecologists gratefully acknowledges the sponsorship of the Micturition Study Group by Aspen Medical Limited, Dantec Electronics Limited, KabiVitrium Limited and Ormed Limited

Micturition

Edited by
J. O. Drife, P. Hilton and S. L. Stanton

With 101 Figures

Springer-Verlag
London Berlin Heidelberg New York
Paris Tokyo Hong Kong

James O. Drife, FRCS, MRCOG
Consultant Obstetrician and Gynaecologist, Department of Obstetrics
and Gynaecology, Clinical Sciences Building, Leicester Royal Infirmary, LE2 7LX, UK

Paul Hilton, MD, BS, MRCOG
Senior Lecturer, Department of Obstetrics and Gynaecology, Univer-
sity of Newcastle upon Tyne, Princess Mary Maternity Hospital, Great
North Road, Newcastle upon Tyne, NE2 3BD, UK

Stuart L. Stanton, FRCS, FRCOG
Consultant Obstetrician and Gynaecologist, Urodynamic Unit,
Department of Obstetrics and Gynaecology, St George's Hospital
Medical School, Cranmer Terrace, London SW17 0RE, UK

ISBN 3–540–19614–5 Springer-Verlag Berlin Heidelberg New York
ISBN 0–387–19614–5 Springer-Verlag New York Berlin Heidelberg

British Library Cataloguing in Publication data
Drife, J. O. (James Owen), *1947–*
Micturition.
1. Man. Urination.
I. Title. II. Hilton, Paul, *1950–* III. Stanton, Stuart L. *1938–*
612.461
ISBN 3–540–19614–5

Typeset, printed and bound by The Bath Press, Avon
2128/3916–543210   Printed on acid-free paper

Preface

Urinary incontinence is a humiliating disability and a common problem in gynaecological clinics. In some centres specialised facilities are available for its investigation and treatment but in most hospitals the general gynaecologist has to manage this difficult condition. For both generalist and subspecialist it is timely to summarise advances in our knowledge of normal and abnormal micturition.

Since 1973 the Royal College of Obstetricians and Gynaecologists, through its Scientific Advisory Committee, has convened Study Groups on important growth areas in our specialty. The College invites an international panel of leading researchers to participate in a workshop, allowing time for in-depth discussion as well as the presentation of papers. It is hoped that this will produce not only an up-to-date summary of current knowledge but also a useful interaction between individuals and between specialties.

This book is the result of the 21st Study Group, which was held in October 1989. The participants included urological and colorectal surgeons and a neurologist, as well as scientists and gynaecologists. The meeting began with sessions on basic science and advances in the investigation of the lower urinary tract, then covered voiding difficulties, genuine stress incontinence and detrusor instability, before a final session on the relationship between urinary incontinence and alimentary tract problems. The discussions formed an essential part of the meeting, and it is hoped that the lightly edited versions reproduced here will convey to the reader the stimulating atmosphere of the Study Group.

The editors are very grateful to Miss Sally Barber, Postgraduate Education Secretary of the RCOG, for her work in ensuring that this volume was produced on schedule, and to the participants who so generously gave their time and expertise to discussing this important subject.

December 1989

J. O. Drife
P. Hilton
S. L. Stanton

Contents

SECTION VI: PROLAPSE AND ALIMENTARY TRACT

Participants

Professor K.-E. Andersson
Department of Clinical Pharmacology, Lund University Hospital, S-221 85 Lund, Sweden

Ms L. D. Cardozo
Consultant Obstetrician & Gynaecologist, King's College Hospital, Denmark Hill, London SE5 9RS, UK

Dr J. O. L. DeLancey
Assistant Professor of Obstetrics & Gynaecology, University of Michigan Medical Center, Medical Professional Building D2202, 1500 E. Medical Center Drive, Box 0718, Ann Arbor, Michigan 48109–0718, USA

Dr J. O. Drife
Convener of Study Groups, RCOG, Senior Lecturer & Honorary Consultant, Department of Obstetrics & Gynaecology, Leicester Royal Infirmary, Leicester LE2 7LX, UK

Mr M. M. Henry
Consultant Surgeon, Central Middlesex Hospital, Acton Lane, London NW10, UK

Mr P. Hilton
Senior Lecturer in Obstetrics & Gynaecology (Honorary Consultant), Department of Obstetrics & Gynaecology, University of Newcastle upon Tyne, Princess Mary Maternity Hospital, Great North Road, Newcastle upon Tyne, NE2 3BD, UK

Mr C. N. Hudson
Consultant Gynaecologist, St Bartholomew's Hospital, West Smithfield, London EC1A 7BE, UK

Mr R. S. Kirby
Consultant Urologist, St Bartholomew's Hospital, West Smithfield, London EC1A 7BE, UK

Dr S. Kulseng-Hanssen
Consultant, Department of Obstetrics & Gynaecology, Baerum Hospital, 1316 Baerum Sykehus, Norway

Mr A. R. Mundy
Senior Lecturer in Urology, Institute of Urology and the United Medical and Dental Schools and Consultant Urological Surgeon, Guy's Hospital at the St Peter's Hospitals, St Thomas Street, London SE1 9RT, UK

Mr K. Murray
Consultant Urological Surgeon, Department of Urology, Kent & Canterbury Hospital, Ethelbert Road, Canterbury, Kent, UK

Dr A. B. Peattie
Lecturer in Obstetrics & Gynaecology, St George's Hospital Medical School, Cranmer Terrace, Tooting, London SW17, UK

Dr S. Plevnik
Honorary Research Fellow at St George's Hospital Medical School, London, Dragomer Na Grivi 20, 61351 Brezovica pri Ljubljana, Yugoslavia

Dr M. J. Quinn
Registrar in Obstetrics & Gynaecology, Royal United Hospital, Combe Park, Bath BA1 3NG, UK

Mr P. J. R. Shah
Senior Lecturer in Urology and Consultant Urologist, Institute of Urology, 172 Shaftesbury Avenue, London WC2H 8JE, UK

Dr A. M. Shepherd
Associate Specialist in Urogynaecology, Ham Green Hospital, Pill, Bristol BS20 0HW, UK

Mr S. L. Stanton
Consultant Obstetrician & Gynaecologist, Urodynamic Unit Department of Obstetrics & Gynaecology, St George's Hospital Medical School, Lanesborough Wing, Cranmer Terrace, London SW17 0RE, UK

Dr J. R. Sutherst
Consultant Obstetrician & Gynaecologist, Arrowe Park Hospital, Arrowe Park Road, Upton, Wirral, Liverpool L49 5LN, UK

Dr M. Swash
Consultant Neurologist, The London Hospital, Whitechapel, London
E1 1BB, UK

Dr ir R. van Mastrigt
Division of Urodynamics, Erasmus University, Rotterdam, PO Box
1738, 3000 DR Rotterdam, The Netherlands

Mr E. Versi
Senior Registrar, Department of Obstetrics & Gynaecology, The London
Hospital, Whitechapel, London E1 1BB, UK

Dr D. W. Warrell
Consultant Urological Gynaecologist, St Mary's Hospital, Hathersage
Road, Manchester M13 0JH, UK

Additional Contributors

Mr I. Eardley
Research Registrar in Urology, St Bartholomew's Hospital,
West Smithfield, London EC1A 7BE, UK

Professor B. Klevmark
Department of Surgery, Section of Urology, Rikshospitalet, Oslo 1,
Norway

Mr C. Spence-Jones
Senior Registrar, Department of Obstetrics & Gynaecology,
St Bartholomew's Hospital, West Smithfield, London EC1A 7BE, UK

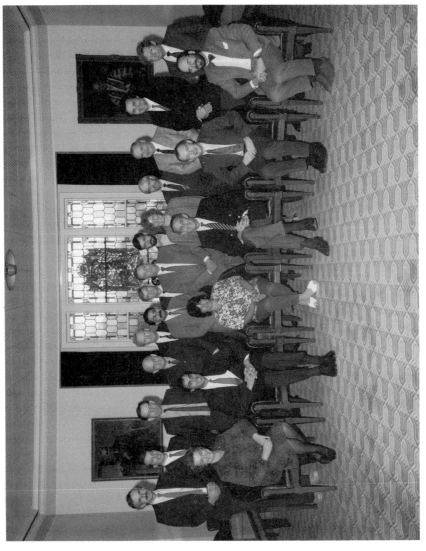

Back row: Dr ir R. van Mastrigt, Mr C. Spence-Jones, Dr M. J. Quinn, Mr C. N. Hudson, Dr S. Kulseng-Hanssen, Mr E. Versi, Professor K.-E. Andersson, Dr D. W. Warrell, Dr J. O. L. DeLancey, Dr A. B. Peattie, Mr K. H. A. Murray, Dr J. R. Sutherst, Dr S. P. Plevnik, Mr M. M. Henry.
Front row: Dr A. M. Shepherd, Mr P. J. R. Shah, Ms L. D. Cardozo, Mr S. L. Stanton, Mr P. Hilton, Dr J. O. Drife.

Section I

Basic Science

Chapter 1

Anatomy of the Urethral Sphincters and Supports

J. O. L. DeLancey

Introduction

When a woman coughs, pressure in the urethra rises simultaneously with intra-abdominal pressure, preventing urine from leaving the bladder. When she increases her intra-abdominal pressure during voiding, however, urine flow can increase, and many women are able to evacuate their bladders without a detrusor contraction, simply by abdominal straining. This apparent paradox where an increase in abdominal pressure prevents urine loss in one situation, and causes it in another illustrates the multifaceted nature of the urinary control mechanism. It must allow for both continence during stress, and also spontaneous voiding. The anatomical model and theoretical concepts we use to help us understand our observations about the lower urinary tract must cover both of these aspects of *urinary control*.

Understanding the nature of this control has important implications. Current concepts such as "pressure transmission" which suggest that the proximal urethra is in an abdominal position where it is compressed by intra-abdominal pressure are useful in explaining some aspects of continence, but may not adequately cover all observations of voiding. In fact, it mirrors some of the clinical problems related to the treatment of patients with stress incontinence. Although we are able to cure stress incontinence in almost all women, many have postoperative voiding dysfunction, and some have detrusor instability, which persist as problems of urinary control despite stress continence.

At present there is a plethora of physiological measurements of lower urinary tract function. Technology has provided us with an almost overwhelming amount of data concerning the function of the sphincteric mechanism. These give an indirect view of the continence mechanism but offer no theoretical framework to tie them together. Trying to understand the urinary control mechanism from these indirect observations is like trying to understand the inner workings of a watch by observing its hands, and listening to it tick. From these "functional" findings we can form many theories about its mechanism, but it is only by opening it up to examine its inner construction that we will understand its true workings.

The Continence Mechanism [1]

Evolution has placed a number of structures in and around the lower urinary tract to provide for urinary control. Examination of their structure often suggests the logic which gave rise to their development. Their arrangement, like other structural aspects of the human body, is not random and their anatomy reflects the function which these structures have evolved to accomplish. This report describes the composition of the continence mechanism as it relates to the function of the lower urinary tract.

Table 1.1.   Structures potentially involved in continence

Structures intrinsic to the lower urinary tract
   Detrusor loop of the bladder base musculature
   Trigonal ring
   Circular smooth muscle of the urethra
   Striated urogenital sphincter (sphincter urethrae)
   Urethral connective tissue
   Urethral submucous vascular plexus
   Urethral mucosa

Structures extrinsic to the lower urinary tract
   Connective tissue supports (endopelvic fasciae)
   Muscular supports (levator ani)
   Striated urogenital sphincter (compressor urethrae and urethrovaginal sphincter)

Subdivisions of the Continence Mechanism

A list of structures which might influence continence is presented in Table 1.1. Clinical observations suggest that these structures can be grouped into two different systems: one which has to do with normal lower urinary tract support and one which determines normal sphincteric function. Problems with sphincteric function can be further divided into: (a) those that involve the proximal or internal sphincter (in the vesical neck), and (b) those that involve the external sphincter (primarily the striated urogenital sphincter, but to some extent the other urethral structures as well). A functional classification would therefore divide these structures as follows:

1. Urethral supports
2. Sphincteric mechanism
    Internal sphincter (vesical neck)
    External sphincter

The internal sphincter lies at the level of the vesical neck and in patients with myelodysplasia or previous surgery it can be open, resulting in the occurrence of stress incontinence despite normal support. The distal urethral sphincter lies below the vesical neck and is capable of voluntary contraction. When urine gets past the vesical neck, as it does in many continent women [2], this mechanism acts to ensure continence. Therefore, contrary to previous thoughts, damage to the external sphincter in patients who have previously depended upon it for stress continence, can be associated with the development of stress incontinence [3].

Location of Structures Involved in Continence

In order to correlate our functional observations with the anatomy of these structures, some way of comparing anatomy and observed physiology is needed. The spatial relationships of the elements in the sphincteric mechanism provide one way to do this and are illustrated in Fig. 1.1. Before beginning a description of the structures, the following overall relationships will help in the understanding of their organisation.

The internal sphincter mechanism lies in the region where the urethral lumen traverses the bladder wall. This region is often referred to as the vesical neck. It extends for approximately the first 20% of the urethral lumen. From 20%–80% of its luminal length the urethra forms the distal sphincteric mechanism. Its bulkiest component is the striated urogenital sphincter. The important structures which

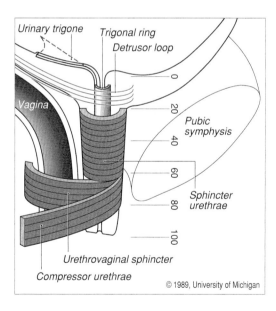

Fig. 1.1. Diagrammatic representation showing the component parts of the internal and external sphincteric mechanisms and their locations. The sphincter urethrae, urethrovaginal sphincter and compressor urethrae are all parts of the striated urogenital sphincter muscle. (© University of Michigan.)

support the urethra and vesical neck have their attachments to the paraurethral tissues in the area from approximately 20%–60% of urethral length, but may influence the urethra and vesical neck beyond this region.

The Supportive Mechanism [1,4]

Nature of Support

Problems with support of the proximal urethra and vesical neck are by far the most common cause of stress incontinence. Early clinical studies of this region involved static bead-chain cystourethrograms and described the relationship between the urethra and pubic bones. Anatomic investigations performed to explain this support describe dense bands of connective tissue which attach the paraurethral tissues of the distal two-thirds of the urethra to the lower portion of the pubic bones, called the pubourethral ligaments [5]. These were said to lie just lateral to the midline and blend with the perineal membrane (=urogenital diaphragm) [6].

Since the time of static bead-chain studies, dynamic examinations of this area have expanded our knowledge of urethral support. The following findings reveal that there must be structures in addition to the pubourethral ligaments which are involved in support.

1. In the normal standing woman, the vesical neck lies above the attachment of pubourethral ligaments to the pubic bones [7].
2. The positions of the proximal urethra and vesical neck are mobile and under voluntary control [8].

Fluoroscopy shows that contraction of the levator ani muscles can elevate the vesical neck [8], and also, that relaxation of these muscles at the time of urination may obliterate the posterior urethrovesical angle [9] (Fig. 1.2). This indicates that the levator ani have a role in controlling vesical neck support. Furthermore, the normal location of the vesical neck at a level 2–3 cm above the insertion of the pubourethral ligaments [7] can be explained by the origin and insertion of the levator muscles. Clinically the junction of this mobile upper portion of the urethra which is influenced by the levators and the lower fixed portion of the urethra occurs at 56% urethral length and has been termed the "knee of the urethra" [10]. This is the region where the urethra enters the perineal membrane [11] and reflects its firm fixation by this structure.

Structure of the Supportive Mechanism [4]

From these observations one would expect that the support of the urethra involves both voluntary muscle and connective tissue elements, and this is indeed the case. The anterior vaginal wall and urethra arise from the urogenital sinus, and are intimately connected. The support of the urethra depends, not on attachments of the urethra itself to adjacent structures, but upon the connection of the vagina and periurethral tissues to the muscles and fascia of the pelvic wall.

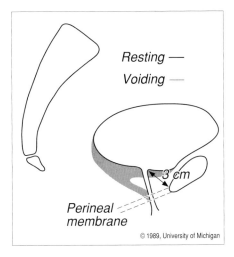

Fig. 1.2. Topography and mobility of the normal proximal urethra and vesical neck based upon resting and voiding in normal women [7,9]. (© University of Michigan.)

Table 1.2. Structure/function hypotheses

Structure	Hypothetical function
Levator ani (through muscular attachment of urethral supports	Tonic contraction helps maintain high position of vesical neck and may contract during cough to support vesical neck. Relaxes to change position of vesical neck relative to pubovesical muscles to facilitate micturition.
Fascial connection to arcus tendineus	Assists levators in support and limits the downward excursion of the vesical neck when the levators are relaxed, or overcome during cough.
Pubovesical muscles and ligaments	May facilitate vesical neck opening by pulling on vesical neck when levators relax and may contribute to closure when they are contracted.
Internal sphincteric mechanism	Maintains vesical neck closure at rest and is necessary in addition to normal support for continence during cough.
External sphincteric mechanism	Resting tone contributes to resting urethral pressure, and contraction prevents incontinence when proximal mechanism leaks.

Some review of the anatomy of the space of Retzius is helpful in understanding urethral support (Fig. 1.3). On each side of the pelvis, there is a band of fibres which is attached at one end to the lower sixth of the pubic bone, 1 cm from the midline, and at the other to the ischial spine. This is the arcus tendineus fasciae pelvis (ATFP). In its anterior portion this band lies on the inner surface of the levator ani muscle which arises some 3 cm above the ATFP. Posteriorly, the levator ani arises from a second fibrous arch, the arcus tendineus levator ani, which fuses with the ATFP near the spine.

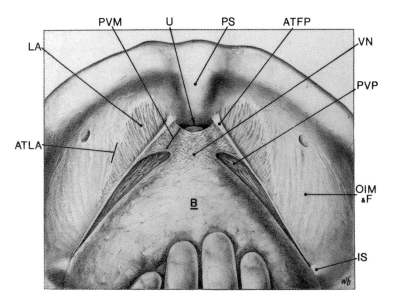

Fig. 1.3. Space of Retzius (drawn from cadaver dissection). Pubovesical muscle (PVM) can be seen going from vesical neck (VN) to arcus tendineus fasciae pelvis (ATFP) and running over the paraurethral vascular plexus (PVP). ATLA = arcus tendineus levator ani, B = bladder, IS = ischial spine, LA = levator ani muscles, OIM&F = obturator internus muscle and fascia, PS = pubic symphysis, and U = urethra. Reprinted with permission Alan R. Liss [16].

The tissues which provide urethral support have two lateral attachments, a fascial attachment and a muscular attachment (Figs. 1.4 and 1.5). The fascial attachment of the urethral supports connects the periurethral tissues and anterior vaginal wall to the ATFP and have been called the paravaginal fascial attachments by Richardson [12]. The muscular attachment connects these same periurethral tissues to the medial border of the levator ani muscle [13,14] and has also been referred to as the vaginolevator attachment in the author's previous work [11]. These attachments allow the normal resting tone of the levator ani muscle [15], along with the fascial attachments, to maintain the position of the vesical neck. When the muscle relaxes at the onset of micturition, it allows the vesical neck to rotate downward to the limit of the elasticity of the fascial attachments, and then contraction at the end of urination allows it to resume its normal position.

Also within this region are the pubovesical muscles (Figs. 1.3 and 1.4) which are extensions of the detrusor [16,17]. They lie within connective tissue, and when both muscular and fibrous elements are considered together, they are called the pubovesical ligaments in much the same way that the smooth muscle and connective tissue of the ligamentum teres uteri are referred to as the round ligaments of the uterus. Although sometimes the *terms* pubovesical ligament and pubourethral ligament have been considered to be synonymous, the pubovesical ligaments are different structures from the urethral supportive tissues [16]. The former run in front of the vesical neck rather than underneath it, where one would expect

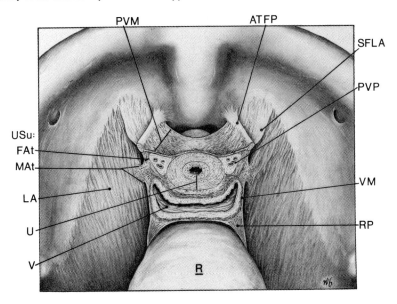

Fig. 1.4. Cross-section of the urethra (U), vagina (V), arcus tendineus fasciae pelvis (ATFP), and superior fascia of levator ani (SFLA) just below the vesical neck (drawn from cadaver dissection). Pubovesical muscles (PVM) lie anterior to urethra and anterior and superior to paraurethral vascular plexus (PVP). The urethral supports (USu) ("the pubourethral ligaments") attach the vagina and vaginal surface of the urethra to the levator ani muscles (LA) (MAt = muscular attachment) and to the superior fascia of the levator ani (FAt = fascial attachment). Additional abbreviations: R, rectum; RP, rectal pillar; and VM, vaginal wall muscularis. Reprinted with permission Alan R. Liss [16].

supportive tissues to be found. It is not surprising, therefore, that these detrusor fibres are histologically similar in stress incontinent patients, and continent women [18]. The actual supportive tissues of the urethra, as described above, are separated from the pubovesical ligament by a prominent vascular plexus [16]. Rather than supporting the urethra, the pubovesical muscles may be responsible for assisting in active vesical neck opening as some have observed [19,20].

The relationship between urethral support and sphincteric function is a complex one. Miniaturised pressure transducers have permitted the recording of the rapid sequence of events that occur during a cough and reveal a significant increase in intraurethral pressure. These urethral pressure changes have been ascribed to the "transmission" of abdominal pressure to the "intra-abdominal" portion of the urethra. Anatomically, it is not clear what separates the abdominal from the extra-abdominal urethra. Examination of sagittal sections of the urethra [Fig. 1.6] reveals no single structure which the urethra pierces to exit the abdomen, and the entire length of the urethra is separated from the lumen of the vagina only by the vaginal wall. Rather than the urethra piercing a single specific layer between the pelvic and extrapelvic cavities, it is incorporated into the pelvic floor.

The complex series of events which occur during a cough suggests that the several pelvic floor structures which surround the urethra and attach it to its adjacent bony and muscular supports are the things which influence its pressure. If passive pressure transmission were the only factor involved in continence, then

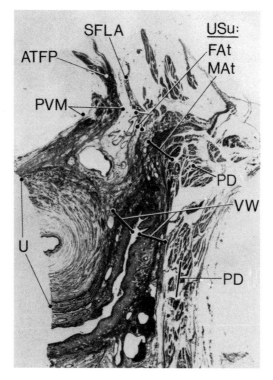

Fig. 1.5. Cross-section of the urethra (U), vaginal wall (VW), and pelvic diaphragm (PD) (levator ani) from the right half of the pelvis taken just below the vesical neck at approximately the same level shown in Fig. 1.4. The pubovesical muscles (PVM) can be seen anterior to the urethra, and attach to the arcus tendineus fasciae pelvis (ATFP). Urethral supports (USu) run underneath (dorsal to) the urethra and vessels. Some of its fibres (MAt) attach to the muscle of the levator ani (LA) while others (FAt) are derived from the vaginal wall (VW) and vaginal surface of the urethra (U) and attach to the superior fascia of the levator ani (SFLA). Reprinted with permission Alan R. Liss [16].

pressures during a cough would be maximum in the proximal urethra. Measurements, however, reveal that the distal urethra has the highest pressure elevations [21,22]. This occurs from 60%–80% of urethral length in the region where the compressor urethrae and urethrovaginal sphincter are found suggesting that these muscles augment urethral pressure in this region. These pressures frequently exceed the increase in intravesical pressure, revealing a contribution of factors other than the influence of abdominal pressure. In addition, these pressure rises precede the rise in abdominal pressure, an observation which suggests contraction of the pelvic floor muscles preparing for the cough [21]. This does not imply that abdominal pressure is an unimportant influence on urethral pressure during a cough, but does raise the question of whether this is the only factor involved and how this occurs. The fact that some patients persist in having stress incontinence despite adequate suspension of the urethra further supports the need to expand our concept of the urethra's response during a cough. Furthermore, recent studies have demonstrated the importance of denervation of the pelvic floor to the problem of stress urinary incontinence and genital prolapse [23,24]. This new area of investi-

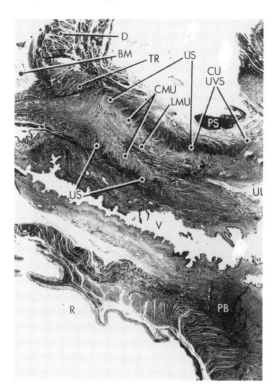

Fig. 1.6. Sagittal section from a 29-year-old cadaver. Cut just lateral to the midline and not quite parallel to it. The section contains tissue nearer the midline in the distal urethra where the lumen can be seen than at the vesical neck. BM, bladder mucosa; CMU, circular smooth muscle of the urethra; CU, compressor urethrae; D, detrusor muscle; LMU, longitudinal smooth muscles of the urethra; PB, perineal body; PS, pubic symphysis; R, rectum; TR, trigonal ring; UL, urethral lumen; US, urethral sphincter; UVS, urethrovaginal sphincter; V, vagina. Reprinted with permission from the American College of Obstetricians and Gynecologists, Obstet Gynecol 1986; 68:91.

gation may prove helpful in further understanding the relationship of structure and function in the mechanism of urinary continence.

Mobility and its Role in Voiding

The normal mobility of the upper urethra is an aspect of lower urinary tract function which has been noted for a number of years, yet its relationship to the supportive mechanism of the urethra has received relatively little attention. The downward descent of the vesical neck often seen at the onset of micturition may alter the arrangement of the tissues around the vesical neck and this change in configuration could be responsible for the difference in urethral function during voiding. Relaxation of the levator ani with micturition might place the tissues around the urethra in an arrangement where increases in intra-abdominal pressure would no longer increase intraurethral pressure, thereby explaining increases in urinary flow with valsalva during micturition. Conversely, when the levators are tonically contracted, as is usually the case, these tissues may be disposed in such a way that an increase in urethral pressure occurs during a cough. These issues deserve further scrutiny.

Sphincters

Internal Sphincter [25]

Observation of an open vesical neck in patients with stress incontinence was made by Howard Kelly in his original description of this condition. Documentation of the clinical importance of this phenomenon as differentiated from other types of stress incontinence caused by poor support was made McGuire [26] and termed Type III stress incontinence. In these individuals the proximal centimetre of the urethral lumen has poor intrinsic closure. This can occur either because of defective innervation to the region, or surgical trauma.

Lying in this region are two tissues which surround the proximal centimetre of the urethra. These are the detrusor loop, and the trigonal ring. The first of these is a localised band of detrusor muscle which forms a U-shaped loop, open posteriorly, and running anterior to the vesical neck. A localised innervation of the base of the bladder may allow this to function in a different way from the muscle of the dome [27]. In addition, the trigonal ring is also found in this region [28]. Woodburne [29], has further reported a high concentration of elastin here which may contribute to closure. Finally, as discussed previously, mechanical factors may favour compression of the vesical neck here.

Some authors have felt that the mechanical arrangement of these tissues influences vesical neck closure. Most of these concepts have contained the idea that there are two opposing loops which pull in opposite directions rather than a circular sphincter at this level. Olesen [30] has described an anterior suspension mechanism attached bilaterally to the ATFP which forms one loop creating the anterior angulation between the bladder and urethra. This would oppose the traditionally considered loop of supportive tissue which is responsible for the posterior urethrovesical angle. In this model, the opposing tension of the two loops would act to close the vesical neck by exerting equal and opposite forces as the urethra descended during a cough. Radiographically, Olesen was able to demonstrate a loss of the anterior angulation between the bladder and urethra, and surgical repair of the anterior suspension mechanism was effective in curing incontinence in these patients. A better understanding of the relationship between vesical neck closure and these mechanical arrangements may prove helpful to our understanding of continence.

External Sphincter [1]

Urethral support and the proximal sphincter both act to prevent urine from entering the proximal urethra. In young healthy nulliparous women, this may be the level of continence, but this may not be true for all continent women. In fact, 50% of women *proven* to be continent have urine enter the urethra during a cough [2]. In these individuals, the function of the distal urethra makes the difference between continence and incontinence. The importance of this mechanism is illustrated by the occurrence of stress incontinence in patients in whom the distal urethra is excised during radical vulvectomy. These patients develop incontinence despite a lack of change in urethral support or resting sphincteric function [3].

A lack of appreciation for the role of the extrinsic continence mechanism has come, perhaps, from inaccurate descriptions in the older anatomic literature. This is a difficult area to dissect, and microscopic examination of the urethra in situ has been hampered by difficulties in sectioning the pubic bones. Most authors have therefore removed the urethra in order to study it microscopically, and have, therefore, missed the extensions of its striated muscle outside of its walls. Recent descriptions by Oelrich [31], however, have corrected much of this confusion, and correlate well with functional observations.

Closure of the urethra comes from a number of different tissue elements. Smooth muscle, striated muscle, and vascular elements each contribute between a quarter and a third of the urethra's closing pressure at rest [32]. The outer layer of the urethra is formed by the muscle of the striated urogenital sphincter which is located from about 20%–80% of urethral luminal length [11]. In its upper two-thirds the sphincter fibres lie in a circular orientation, whereas distally, they leave the confines of the urethra and insert either into the vaginal wall as the urethrovaginal sphincter, or into the region just above the perineal membrane as the compressor urethrae [31] (Figs. 1.1 and 1.7). This muscle is composed largely of slow twitch muscle fibres [33] which are well suited to maintaining the constant tone which this muscle exhibits, as well as allowing voluntary increases in activity as a back-up continence mechanism during times when the need for increased closure pressure arises. In the distal urethra, this striated muscle compresses the urethra from above, and proximally, it constricts the lumen. It is also possible that the striated urogenital sphincter muscle plays a role in stress continence beyond its resting and conscious voluntary contraction. As previously mentioned, measurements of urethral pressure during a cough have shown that the rise in pressure is highest in the distal area of the urethra, around 60% of urethral length [34] in the region where the considerable bulk of muscle of the compressor urethrae and urethrovaginal sphincter are found [11].

The smooth muscle of the urethra has an inner longitudinal layer, and a thin outer circular layer, with the former being by far the more prominent of the two. They lie inside the striated urogenital sphincter muscle, and are present throughout the upper four-fifths of the urethra. The configuration of the circular muscle suggests a role in constricting the lumen. This layer, however, is thin, and much less prominent than the striated urogenital sphincter muscle. The longitudinal smooth muscle contracts during micturition, assisting in funnelling the urethra, and shortening it.

Lying within the urethra is a surprisingly well developed vascular plexus which is more prominent than one would expect for the ordinary demands of so small an organ. These vessels have several specialised types of arteriovenous anastomoses [28] which could assist in forming a watertight closure of the mucosal surfaces. They may also fill during a cough from the pressure on the intra-abdominal vessels which supply them. Occlusion of the arterial inflow in these venous reservoirs has been shown to influence urethral closure pressure [32].

The lower portion of the urethra is lined by non-keratinising squamous epithelium similar to that in the vagina. In the bladder transitional epithelium is found. The junction between these two tissues may occur in the upper urethra or bladder base. As is true in the vagina, the squamous epithelium of the urethra

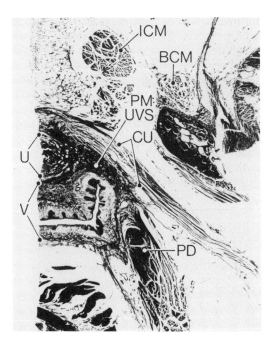

Fig. 1.7. Cross-section taken just above the level of the perineal membrane (PM) showing the compressor urethrae (CU) and urethrovaginal sphincter (UVS) portions of the striated urogenital sphincter. BCM, bulbocavernosus muscle; ICM, ischiocavernosus muscle; PD, pelvic diaphragm (levator ani); U, urethra; V, vagina. Reprinted with permission from the American College of Obstetricians and Gynecologists, Obstet Gynecol 1988; 72:296–301.

is hormonally sensitive, and undergoes significant change depending on its state of oestrogen stimulation.

In addition to the contractile and vascular tissue of the urethra, there is a considerable quantity of connective tissue interspersed within the muscle, and the submucosa. This tissue has both collagenous and elastin fibres. It is difficult, however, to study the function of these tissues specifically, because there is no specific way to block their action either pharmacologically or surgically.

Conclusions

Our current success in treating stress urinary incontinence has been reached without knowledge of much of this anatomical information. What then is the role of this detailed analysis? The vesical neck, urethra, and their surrounding tissues function not only to maintain continence during increases in abdominal pressure, but they also participate in the normal process of micturition. Despite descriptions of over 100 operations for stress urinary incontinence and considerable urodynamic literature, our overall surgical success with this condition has not changed since the advent of retropubic operations. During this time, also, problems with voiding dysfunction, and to some extent postoperative bladder instability have persisted as unsolved dilemmas.

At the present time, there are not specific ways to analyse the function of each of the structures and determine what their role is in continence and voiding. Yet, with the spectacular progress in bioengineering, ultrasonography, and computerised remote position sensing, we may soon have the capability to change this. We may finally be able to study the actual activities of these individual parts of the continence mechanism in continent and incontinent women to determine the exact nature of its dysfunction, and design therapy for that specific problem. This approach could hold the potential to return normal urinary control to individuals rather than simply restoring continence during stress.

Acknowledgements

Portions of this chapter have been borrowed and modified from recent reviews by the author as indicated by the citations made in the section headings and reference list.

References

1. DeLancey JOL. Anatomy and physiology of urinary continence. Clin Obstet Gynecol (in press).
2. Versi E, Cardozo LD, Studd JWW, Brincat M, O'Dowd TM, Cooper DJ. Internal urinary sphincter in maintenance of female continence. Br Med J 1986; 292:166–7.
3. Reid GC, DeLancey JOL, Hopkins MP, Roberts JA, Morley GW. Urinary incontinence following radical vulvectomy. Obstet Gynecol, 1989; (in press).
4. DeLancey JOL. Anatomy and embryology of the lower urinary tract. In: Clinics in Obstetrics and Gynecology. Philadelphia: W.B. Saunders (in press).
5. Zacharin RF. The anatomic supports of the female urethra. Obstet Gynecol 1968; 32:754–9.
6. Milley PS, Nichols DH. The relationship between the pubo-urethral ligaments and the urogenital diaphragm in the human female. Anat Rec 1971; 170:281–3.
7. Noll LE, Hutch JA. The SCIPP line: an aid in interpreting the voiding lateral cystourethrogram. Obstet Gynecol 1969; 33:680–9.
8. Muellner SR. Physiology of micturition. J Urol 1951; 65:805–10.
9. Jeffcoate TNA, Roberts H. Observations on stress incontinence of urine. Am J Obstet Gynecol 1952; 64:721–38.
10. Westby M, Asmussen M, Ulmsten U. Location of maximum intraurethral pressure related to urogenital diaphragm in the female subject as studied by simultaneous urethrocystometry and voiding urethrocystography. Am J Obstet Gynecol 1982; 144:408–12.
11. DeLancey JOL. Correlative study of paraurethral anatomy. Obstet Gynecol 1986; 68:91–7.
12. Richardson AC, Edmonds PB, Williams NL. Treatment of stress urinary incontinence due to paravaginal fascial defect. Obstet Gynecol 1981; 57:357–62.
13. DeLancey JOL, Starr RA. The histology of the connection between the vaginal and levator ani muscles. J Reprod Med (in press).
14. DeLancey JOL. Structural aspects of the extrinsic continence mechanism. Obstet Gynecol 1988; 72:296–301.
15. Parks AG, Porter NH, Melzak J. Experimental study of the reflex mechanism controlling muscles of the pelvic floor. Dis Colon Rectum 1962; 5:407–14.
16. DeLancey JOL. Pubovesical ligament: a separate structure from the urethral supports (pubo-urethral ligaments). Neurourol Urodynam 1989; 8:53–61.
17. Gil Vernet S. Morphology and function of the vesico-prostato-urethral musculature. Treviso, Italy: Edizioni Canova 1968; 39–40.
18. Wilson PD, Dixon JS, Brown ADG, Gosling JA. Posterior pubo-urethral ligaments in normal and genuine stress incontinent women. J Urol 1983; 130:802–5.

19. McGuire E. Urethral sphincter mechanisms. Urol Clin North Am 1979; 6:39–49.
20. Power RMH. An anatomical contribution to the problem of continence and incontinence in the female. Am J Obstet Gynecol 1954; 67:302–14.
21. Constantinou CE. Resting and stress urethral pressures as a clinical guide to the mechanism of continence in the female patient. Urol Clin North Am 1985; 12:247–58.
22. Hilton P, Stanton SL. Urethral pressure measurement by microtransducer: the results in symptom-free women and in those with genuine stress incontinence. Br J Obstet Gynaecol 1983; 90:919–33.
23. Smith ARB, Hosker GL, Warrell DW. The role of partial denervation of the pelvic floor in the aetiology of genitourinary prolapse and stress incontinence of urine: a neurophysiological study. Br J Obstet Gynaecol 1989; 96:24–8.
24. Snooks SJ, Badenoch DF,Tiptaft RC et al. Perineal nerve damage in genuine stress urinary incontinence: an electrophysiological study. Br J Urol 1985; 57:422–6.
25. DeLancey JOL. Functional anatomy of the female lower urinary tract and pelvic floor. In: Neurobiology of continence. Chichester: Wiley (in press).
26. McGuire EJ. Urodynamic findings in patients after failure of stress incontinence operations. Prog Clin Biol Res 1981; 78:351–60.
27. Elbadawi A. Neuromuscular mechanisms of micturition. In: Yalla SV, McGuire EJ, Elbadawi A, Blaivas JG, eds. Neurourology and urodynamics. New York: Macmillan, 1988; 3–35.
28. Huisman AB. Aspects on the anatomy of the female urethra with special relation to urinary continence. Contrib Gynecol Obstet 1983; 10:1–31.
29. Woodburne RT. Anatomy of the bladder and bladder outlet. J Urol 1968; 100:474–87.
30. Olesen KP, Walter S, Hald T. Anterior bladder suspension defects in the female: radiological classification with urodynamic evaluation. Anatomically corrective operations. Acta Obstet Gynecol Scand 1980; 59:535–42.
31. Oelrich TM. The striated urogenital sphincter muscle in the female. Anat Rec 1983; 205:223–32.
32. Rud T, Anderson KE, Asmussen M, Hunting A, Ulmsten U. Factors maintaining the intraurethral pressure in women. Invest Urol 1980; 17:343–7.
33. Gosling JA, Dixon JS, Critchley HOD, Thompson SA. A comparative study of the human external sphincter and periurethral levator ani muscles. Br J Urol 1981; 53:35–41.
34. Constantinou CE, Govan DE. Spatial distribution and timing of transmitted and reflexly generated urethral pressures in healthy women. J Urol 1982; 127:964–9.

Chapter 2

Innervation of the Bladder, Urethra and Pelvic Floor

M. Swash

The innervation of the bladder and urethra is complex. There are components from the autonomic and from the somatic nervous systems. The pelvic floor, on the other hand, is innervated only by somatic efferent and afferent nerve fibres. The normal functioning of the urethral sphincter depends on co-ordinated action of the sphincter mechanism, consisting of a smooth, non-striated internal urinary sphincter and striated voluntary periurethral sphincter muscles, with appropriate relaxation and contraction of the detrusor musculature of the bladder wall. Thus, the autonomic and somatic nervous systems must be co-ordinated for appropriate function. The synthesis of activity necessary to produce this effect is a function of the central nervous system, both at spinal and brainstem levels. The act of micturition is under voluntary control, from cortically derived relaxation of the striated periurethral sphincter musculature at the commencement of the act of micturition. The periurethral striated sphincter musculature is under continuous tonic activation, thus resembling the external anal sphincter muscle and the pubo-rectalis muscle. The abductor muscle of the larynx, the cricopharyngeus muscle, the stapedius, and the striated sphincter muscle of the diaphragm at the cardia are similarly under tonic continuous low-level activation. In order to function effectively, the bladder detrusor, and the sphincter musculature and its central motor connections require afferent input and this is achieved through both the autonomic and somatic nervous systems.

Spinal Origin of Innervation of Bladder and Urethral Sphincter

Neuronal nuclei innervating the detrusor muscle of the bladder and the periurethral striated musculature are located in the grey matter of the conus medullaris.

Detrusor motor neurons are found in the intermediolateral cell column in the lumbothoracic outflow of the parasympathetic nervous system. The somatic motor neurons innervating the periurethral striated musculature are contained in a localised nucleus, the Onuf nucleus, that is located in the S2, S3 and S4 segments of the anterior horn [1]. It is probable that the parasympathetic motor neurons innervating the detrusor muscle arise in the intermediolateral cell column at a homologous segmental level to the somatic neurons located in the Onuf nucleus that innervate the sphincter muscle. However, there is no current evidence of functional connection between these two motor neuronal systems at the spinal level [2].

Sympathetic neurons arising in the low thoracic component of the intermediolateral cell column innervate the proximal urethra, and the urinary detrusor muscles via synapses in the pelvic ganglia. These nerve fibres reach their target organs via the inferior mesenteric ganglion and the hypogastric nerve, and also provide innervation to the lower part of the rectum and the internal anal sphincter muscle. The kidney is similarly innervated by components of this sympathetic innervation, as are the external genitalia. The parasympathetic innervation of the detrusor muscle of the bladder is excitatory to the cholinergic muscarinic receptors in the detrusor musculature, and components of this innervation are probably inhibitory to the smooth muscle of the internal urinary sphincter at the bladder neck. As in other autonomic modulatory systems, for example in the gut, the extrinsic innervation of the bladder is not coupled to the bladder musculature by direct synaptic connections, but excites muscle cells by junctions consisting of close appositions between axonal varicosities containing synaptic vesicles, and adjacent muscle cells. The muscle cells are themselves connected by gap junctions and other close appositions of the membranes of adjacent muscle cells so that there is electrical coupling between these muscle fibres, accounting for the co-ordinated contraction of the whole detrusor musculature. There is controversy as to whether or not the detrusor muscle of the bladder contains an intrinsic nervous system, with ganglion cells, resembling that of the myenteric plexus in the gut. Afferent fibres arising in the mucosa and surface layers of the bladder travel with the parasympathetic innervation back to the spinal cord.

The origin and connections of thin unmyelinated axons within the bladder wall are uncertain, but it is believed that these fibres are essentially nociceptive in function, and are actuated only when the bladder is irritated, for example by infection. Similarly, unmyelinated afferents enter the spinal cord at the lower thoracic level from the bladder with the sympathetic nervous system. Myelinated afferents, believed to represent stretch receptor input, arising in the trigone, are also recognised. Lesions of the cauda equina abolish pain resulting from over-distension of the bladder, but section of the hypogastric nerve does not have this effect. Similar unmyelinated sensory receptors are found in the urethral smooth muscle and in the epithelium of the upper urethra. The urethra, in addition, is innervated by somatic sensory receptors that receive axons from the perineal branches of the pudendal nerves [3].

Pelvic Floor

The innervation of the pelvic floor musculature is important in the assessment and understanding of pelvic floor disorder, especially incontinence [4,5]. The pelvic floor musculature consists of two embryological components. The sphincter cloacae components of the pelvic floor muscles receive their innervation from their perineal aspect, that is from the pudendal nerves, and the pelvicaudal component receives its innervation from motor branches derived from the pelvic plexus [6]. This concept has proved particularly important in studies of the anorectal sphincter since there is a clear differentiation between the innervation of the external anal sphincter, from the inferior rectal branches of the pudendal nerves, and the innervation of the puborectalis muscle, from direct pelvic branches of the sacral plexus. Controversy in the anatomical literature on this point [6–9] has been resolved by electrophysiological studies in which recordings were made with EMG needle electrodes from the puborectalis and external anal sphincter muscles during post-anal repair. In these experiments the puborectalis muscle was found to be innervated not by the pudendal nerves but by branches of the pelvic nerves in 19 of the 20 subjects studied [10]. In addition, histopathological investigations of the puborectalis and external anal sphincter muscles in normal subjects, and in patients with idiopathic neurogenic anorectal incontinence, have suggested that these muscles differ in their composition of Type 1 and Type 2 fibres, in their fibre size distribution, and also in their susceptibility to denervation [11,12]. Further, Schroder and Reske-Nielsen [13] have noted the differing resistance of these muscles to denervation in motor neuron disease.

Urethral Sphincter

The anatomy of the innervation of the striated sphincter musculature of the urethra is similarly controversial. Gosling [14] showed that the periurethral striated sphincter muscles throughout the lower third of the urethra, consist largely of Type 1 muscle fibres which, like the muscle fibres of the external anal sphincter and puborectalis muscle, are smaller than those found in other human striated muscles. This muscle is innervated by perineal branches of the pudendal nerves, thus being phylogenetically related to the external anal sphincter muscle, and representing a muscle derived from the sphincter cloacae. Gosling also demonstrated striated muscle fibres in the wall of the middle third of the urethra, the intramural component of this muscle [14,15]. These intramural fibres are also largely Type 1 muscle fibres but the source of their innervation has been uncertain. Gosling suggested that this innervation arose, like that of the puborectalis muscle, from somatic efferents derived from the lumbosacral plexus S2–4 roots accompanying autonomic fibres in the pelvic plexus. The striated ischiocavernosus and bulbocavernosus muscles appear to have a similar pattern of innervation.

Electrophysiological Studies

Electrophysiological observations of the motor latencies of the evoked action potential response in the periurethral striated musculature following pudendal or transcutaneous lumbar stimulation are pertinent to this problem of the innervation of these muscles [16]. The latencies of the compound muscle action potential responses in the external anal sphincter and periurethral striated sphincter muscles, both innervated by the pudendal nerves, differ by about 0.5 ms, a difference consistent with the additional length of the perineal branch of the pudendal nerve innervating the latter muscles (approximately 2.5 cm at a nerve conduction velocity of 50 ms^{-1}. Spinal stimulation at the level of the L1 vertebral spine produces recordable muscle action potentials in the puborectalis, external anal sphincter and urethral striated sphincter muscles. The difference in latency between the compound muscle action potentials evoked in the external anal sphincter and in the urethral striated sphincter muscles after spinal stimulation at L1 is about 0.6 ms. The compound muscle action potential recorded in the puborectalis muscle, after this stimulus, was evoked 0.7 ms earlier than that in the external anal sphincter muscle, suggesting that the innervation of the puborectalis from the point of stimulation at L1 was about 3.5 cm shorter than that to the external anal sphincter (assuming a conduction velocity of 50 ms^{-1}).

In patients with faecal incontinence the pudendal nerve terminal motor latency is increased, and, similarly, in patients with genuine stress urinary incontinence the perineal nerve terminal motor latency is increased – findings suggestive of damage to this innervation. Spinal stimulation at the L1 level in patients with double incontinence shows that the latency of the evoked compound muscle action potentials in the striated urethral sphincter musculature is increased but in 40% of the patients studied it was normal, despite the finding that the perineal nerve terminal motor latency in these patients was greatly increased. This observation suggests that there must be a dual innervation to this urethral sphincter complex and that in these patients only the perineal component, innervated by the perineal branch of the pudendal nerve, was abnormal. Thus, the latency from L1 to the urethral striated sphincter muscle complex was greater than that from transrectal stimulation of the pudendal nerve, despite the much shorter length of the latter nerve. Since the human urinary sphincter muscle complex is composed of two parts, the periurethral and the intramural striated sphincter muscles, these data can be interpreted as supporting the suggestion that these two components have separate innervations. Thus the innervation of the periurethral component is derived from the perineal branch of the pudendal nerves and that of the intramural component is probably derived from supralevator branches of the pelvic nerves, consisting of somatic efferent nerve fibres derived from the S2, S3 and S4 ventral roots. This double innervation of the urethral sphincter complex in the human is thus analogous to the double innervation of the external anal sphincter and puborectalis muscles respectively.

Nonetheless, our physiological observations could not exclude the possibility that the puborectalis and the puboanal sling form a composite muscle with components representing both pelvicaudal and sphincter cloacae derivations. The motor neurons that give rise to the innervation of the urethral and anal sphincter muscles also innervate the ischiocavernosus and bulbocavernosus muscles. They also derive from the Onuf nucleus in the sacral spinal cord. Both the periurethral striated muscle complex and the external anal sphincter muscle contain muscle spindles, representing somatic afferent innervation important in the modulation of ongoing contraction of these muscles in the maintenance of continence.

Conclusion

These observations of the dual nature of the nerve supply of the intramural and periurethral components of the urinary striated sphincter muscle complex are relevant not only to understanding continence and incontinence, but in planning surgical procedures. Clearly, it is important to conserve the supralevator component of the innervation of the urethral sphincter complex in operations in this region.

References

1. Onuf B. On the arrangement and function of the cell groups in the sacral region of the spinal cord. Arch Neurol Psychopathol 1900; 3:387–411.
2. Schroder HD. Organisation of the motoneurons innervating the pelvic muscles of the male rat. J Comp Neurol 1980; 192:567–78.
3. Gosling JA, Dixon JS, Lendon RG. Autonomic innervation of human male and female bladder neck and proximal urethra. J. Urol 1977; 118:302–5.
4. Snooks SJ, Barnes PRH, Swash M. Damage to the innervation of the voluntary anal and peri-urethral striated sphincter musculature in incontinence; an electrophysiological study. J Neurol Neurosurg Psychiat 1984; 47:1269–73.
5. Swash M. New concepts in incontinence. Br Med J 1985; 290:4–5.
6. Wendell-Smith CP. Studies on the morphology of the pelvic floor. London: University of London, 1967 PhD thesis, pp 305.
7. Lawson JON. Pelvic anatomy 1, pelvic floor muscles. Ann R Coll Surg Eng 1974; 54:244–52.
8. Lawson JON. Pelvic anatomy 2, anal canal and associated sphincters. Ann R Coll Surg Eng 1974; 54:288–300.
9. Stelzner F. Uber die Anatomie des Analen sphincterorgans wie sie der Chirurgsieht. J Anat Entwicklingsgesicht 1960; 121:525–35.
10. Percy JP, Neill ME, Swash M, Parks AG. Electrophysiological study of motor nerve supply of pelvic floor. Lancet 1981; 1:16–17
11. Parks AG, Swash M, Urich H. Sphincter denervation in anorectal incontinence and rectal prolapse. Gut 1977; 18:656–65.
12. Beersiek F, Parks AG, Swash M. Pathogenesis of anorectal incontinence; a histometric study of the anal sphincter musculature. J Neurol Sci 1979;42:111–27.
13. Schroder HD, Reske-Nielsen EC. Fibre types in the striated urethral and anal sphincters. Acta Neuropathol (Berl) 1984; 60:278–82.
14. Gosling J. The structure of the bladder and urethra in relation to function. Urol Clin North Am 1979; 6:31–8.
15. Critchley HOD, Dixon JF, Gosling JA. Comparative study of the periurethral and perianal parts of the human levator ani muscle. Urol Int 1980; 35:226–32.
16. Snooks SJ, Swash M. The innervation of the muscles of continence. Ann R Coll Surg Eng 1986; 68:45–9.

Discussion

Stanton: Dr DeLancey certainly puts forward the argument for the use of a sling procedure as a supporting mechanism. One thing I am in some doubt about. He showed a slide of the pressures, which argued in terms of the place at which they are set. I suspect that this is a function of the different operations that have been done. Certainly his peak in pressure is much lower down the urethra than Dr Hilton's peak.

DeLancey: What stimulated my looking into that was the observation with the vulvectomy patients. That was more of an indirect observation than simply trying to understand why, when the distal urethra was excised without change in support or change in resting pressure, they became incontinent.

When we have done pressures they have not always been much higher in the distal urethra than they were in the proximal urethra, but on the other hand they were not lower. If we think of the paradigm with the proximal urethra being intra-abdominal, then we would expect that the pressures in the proximal urethra would be much higher than the pressures in the distal urethra. The point that struck me was that they were not lower as one moved down the urethra until one got to the very distal urethra.

I have looked at a number of different graphs from different people's data and they do seem to vary somewhat. It seems that in that distal portion of the urethra there are still significant increases in intraurethral pressure.

Stanton: Do the anatomical studies confirm there are different mechanisms of achieving continence, and different ways in which surgery operates?

DeLancey: I am hesitant about speculation based on anatomy. It is frustrating because I can tell with great certainty what the structures are, but I am not sure that I can speculate about how they work. I can watch people move their vesical neck: that can be seen fluoroscopically or with the urethroscope or simply by putting a speculum in the vagina. We can also record people's ability to increase intraurethral pressure. What that means in terms of the overall continence mechanism, however, I do not have a good explanation for in terms of what happens surgically.

One thing I am curious about is that there are operations that seek to repair the normal connections of the periurethral tissues to the pelvic side wall, and those seem to be effective. Another is the relationship between continence and voiding, which is something that we all struggle with in our surgical procedures. We are able to make people dry but we are not necessarily able to return normal urinary control to them. The usefulness of looking at structure may be to say what is it in an individual that differs from the normal, and can we restore them to normal? And if we can restore them to normal, does that restore both continence and voiding?

Hudson: Can I gently take issue with the comments about continence after vulvectomy? Dr DeLancey reported a relatively small number. I cannot give facts and figures but it certainly runs counter to my own impression of removal of the distal centimetre, which means taking the vulvectomy operation flush with the pubic bone and leaving the entire subpubic urethra and the intra-abdominal urethra. I would have said that it made no difference to control.

DeLancey: That was what we thought when we started.

Hudson: I should like to see rather more cases.

DeLancey: We are not suggesting that 100% will develop incontinence.

Hudson: Your figures were four out of four.

DeLancey: I am sure if we had looked at 50 we would have had a number who were continent afterwards.

We also realised that there are differences in how surgeons excise the urethra. The surgeon who does the vulvectomies in our institution pulls the vulvectomy specimen towards him as he is coming across the urethra, which tends to pull the more distal part of the urethra out from under the pubic bone a little more. He also uses an electrosurgical unit so that there probably is some damage. He said that he removes 1 cm of the urethra, but when we measured the length actually excised it was 1.3 or 1.4 cm.

Hudson: Probably the answer is in the use of the filleting technique because anything can be filleted out if it is pulled like that. With that description, I should have thought most of the subpubic urethra has been severely damaged if not removed, as opposed to deliberately cutting flush with what from below appears as the perineal membrane.

DeLancey: The curious thing was that previous descriptions had suggested that the distal urethra was useless and that patients should not become incontinent. Of the people looked at, the ones in whom that distal portion was removed did develop incontinence but did not have a change in urethral support, although that is somewhat difficult to measure depending on how hard people are straining. And their resting pressures did not change. It did not seem to be simply denervation of the urethra.

Versi: It depends on whether these patients have an incompetent bladder neck preoperatively. We showed that if these women do have an incompetent bladder neck, then they use their distal sphincter more by augmenting the transmission pressure ratios. Were the four patients known to have an incompetent bladder neck before?

DeLancey: Pressure profilometry showed that their urethras functioned poorly before the operation in that they did not have perfect pressure transmission in the proximal urethra, but we did not fluoroscope them so we do not have direct evidence.

Cardozo: Relating to vulvectomy, it is not important whether or not the end of the urethra is cut, they still become incontinent.

Plevnik: It may not be wise to draw any conclusions from the pressure measurements in the urethra. We have pointed out on several occasions that they are largely artefactual, the artefacts being mainly due to the stiffness of the catheter and its weight.

Sutherst: I wanted to comment on Mr Plevnik's work on conductance and our own studies on fluid bridge testing which show that in the vast majority of patients continence is maintained at the bladder neck.

Plevnik: That is correct.

Sutherst: And the same goes for X-ray studies as well. This particular small group presumably had an incompetent bladder neck.

Stanton: But there is a secondary mechanism lower down. If the secondary mechanism should be damaged, and the primary mechanism in some patients is already damaged, then without studies before operating one cannot be sure what their continence state will then be.

Cardozo: Can I ask for a clarification on what was said about the pubovesical and the pubourethral ligaments?

DeLancey: The confusion that has existed in the past is because the terms pubourethral ligament and pubovesical ligament have been used interchangeably. There is a group of detrusor muscle fibres that leave the detrusor at the vesical neck and insert into the pubic bone in the arcus tendineus. The anatomical term for that is the pubovesical muscle, and when that muscle and its surrounding connective tissue are considered it is called the pubovesical ligament, much as the ligamentum teres is the smooth muscle in the connective tissue of the round ligament. There is a separate issue which is the supportive tissues of the urethra. There is no supportive ligament that goes from the pubic bone to the urethra. I have tried not to use the term pubourethral ligament because that implies that the urethra is firmly fixed by a ligamentous band, which is not anatomically correct.

Pubovesical ligament is a proper anatomical term and refers to the smooth muscle tissue that goes out to the arcus tendineus and to the pubic bone. Pubourethral ligament is a term that we probably should not use because it does not correspond to anything useful.

Cardozo: So when we do retropubic urethropexy we are looking at pubovesical smooth muscle?

DeLancey: Yes.

Swash: In terms of locomotion, ligaments act as an energy store rather than as a structural scaffold. They store the energy of contraction in their elastic tissue – they consist largely of elastic tissue – and then release it. That is how a bird like the ostrich runs so fast; the muscle is all up in the body and the legs have long ligaments in them. The ligaments in the legs are acting simply as elastic energy stores and propelling the animal forward when they are released.

It would make complete sense if the ligaments that are under discussion did have muscle attached to them because they would be able to act as a lively elastic energy-dependent process that would help to restore the anatomy of the system when it has been released.

DeLancey: One of the things that the biomechanicians talked about when we were discussing ligaments was that ligaments are not well suited to maintaining tension over the course of time.

Sutherst: I was comforted by Dr Swash's explanation of why some people with prolapse have stress incontinence and some do not. We all come across it every day and it is hard to explain.

About the innervation of the urethra in someone who has prolapse: is that sufficient to cope with sudden stress?

Swash: It might be. Mr Warrell has studied prolapse in patients with incontinence. I have not done that myself.

Warrell: One of the things I found difficult is the clear distinction of the extrinsic periurethral striated muscle and the so-called intrinsic striated muscle in the sphincter. We all pay lip service to this, but histologically I wonder how good the evidence is for intrinsic striated muscle in the urethral tube.

Stanton: Is this what we would call the rhabdosphincter?

Warrell: To keep the words as simple as possible, there is a band of striated muscle around the thickness of the urethra, the majority of the thickness of the urethra being smooth muscle and elastic tissue and blood vessels. This is what most people call the external sphincter or the striated muscle component of the urethra. What perplexes me is where the other striated muscle is that Dr Swash suggests is supplied by the perineal branch.

Swash: No one need be too concerned about trying to make a distinct anatomical statement about differences between them in spatial terms. All one has to do is to recognise that there does seem to be a double innervation to muscle fibres in that region and that some of those muscle fibres clearly have a different destination. Some are clearly circumferential and some have a different anatomical position. I do not see that one need get too excited about having a separate muscle with a separate fascial band dividing them up.

The same argument has occurred in proctology. All the proctologists got very excited about dissecting and finding the difference between puborectalis and the external anal sphincter, and it actually does not matter. What we are saying is that there is a bit of tissue which is innervated by one nerve and another innervated by another nerve, and they probably have slightly different functions. They are in very close anatomical contiguity and have slightly different functions. That is how I would put it.

Others may have slightly different information about the anatomy, but when the anatomy is so complicated that we have to cut sections in different planes

to be precisely sure what we are looking at, the argument becomes very circumferential.

DeLancey: Clearly there are two different muscles, which can be described in
this way.

When one puts a finger in the vagina on vaginal examination and one feels
the lateral vaginal wall, one can feel the medial border of the levator ani. That
muscle is attached to the connective tissue around the urethra but does not attach
directly to the urethra, and that is one muscle that could influence urethral function
because of its position. The second is a muscle that is intrinsic to the urethral
wall for most of its part: it is circular in its upper portion but in its lower portion
it forms a strap over the top of the urethra.

One muscle is relatively large and bulky and has to do with lots of other things,
such as anorectal angulation. The muscle that is intrinsic to the urethra itself
is primarily slow-twitch muscle and may have autonomic innervation. But there
are those two separate parts to it that are easy to separate anatomically once
we start to look at serial sections.

Swash: But we are not saying that there is a fascial sheath that separates these
two bands of muscle, because the distinction between them fades at the edges.

Warrell: There is clearly attachment between the pelvic floor and the periurethral
fascia. It seems to be accepted that there are two lots of striated muscle in the
urethra, but I do not think this is so. I think there is one lot of striated muscle.
It may have a twin nerve supply but to talk about intramural urethral striated
muscle and striated muscle going mostly round the outside of the urethra is wrong.
Nevertheless, it is in the literature, and what has been said suggests that there
are two lots of striated muscle in the urethral tube. I do not think that is true.

Hudson: Does Mr Warrell recognise a compressor urethra?

Warrell: I do not know what the term means. I agree entirely with what Dr
DeLancey said about striated muscle in the urethra. There is circumferential
striated muscle maximal about mid-urethra and nearer the outside it becomes
more hoop-like rather than striated. Would one call that the compressor urethra?
One could, I suppose.

Hudson: The point was made that the compressor urethra, instead of a circular
or an elliptical form, has an insertion to the subpubic arch. In fact it has a flattening
effect so that some of the sphincter is splayed out and is not sphincteric. In much
the same way, in the anorectal region, the puborectalis comes from bone to bone
round the anorectal ring, and below it are the sphincter muscles of the anal canal.
It is suggested that there is a strap, as it were, across the front of the urethra
which is inserted to the subpubic angle slightly posteriorly, so that it is in a
position to pull the urethra against the vagina, and that this is continuous with
the voluntary circular muscle.

DeLancey: That is correct. They are both continuous and they are just two different aspects of the same musculature.

Hudson: Then the compressor urethra would be the female equivalent presumably of the deep transverse perineal muscle in the male?

DeLancey: Yes. Exactly analogous.

Peattie: I liked Dr Swash's concept of the kinking of the urethra, but at what level does that happen and what causes the kink?

Swash: I was trying to draw an analogy between the bladder neck angulation and the angulation of the anorectum caused by the puborectalis. There is this mechanism at the bladder neck in which one can visualise there being an angulation which might act as a little kink in the urethra. The question is what happens in the rest of the urethra and how much of the continence function relates to the rest of the length of the urethra in relation to what is happening at the bladder neck? I am aware of the difficulty that one experiences in clinical practice in understanding the relationship between those two factors.

Stanton: Dr DeLancey has shown that in his diagrams.

There can be an alternative diagram where the higher pubovesical muscle/ligament is kept firm: that leans against the urethra and underneath that, almost in an opposite direction, the endopelvic fascia tightens in relationship to the tightening of the pelvic floor. That can produce a kink, but it is something to be discussed on a later occasion.

Chapter 3

Neurotransmitters and Receptor Functions in the Human Lower Urinary Tract

K.-E. Andersson

Signal transmission between nerves, and between a nerve and an effector organ, occurs by means of chemical substances, "neurotransmitters", secreted from the presynaptic or prejunctional neurons. According to common textbooks of physiology (e.g. [1]) more than 30 different chemical substances have been either proved or postulated to be synaptic transmitters.

In the lower urinary tract, functional roles for the "classical" transmitters acetylcholine and noradrenaline have been established, but the functions of putative transmitters released from non-adrenergic, non-cholinergic (NANC) nerves are still a matter of controversy. In the evaluation of putative NANC transmitters Daniel [2] has listed the following criteria:

Present in NANC nerve
Present in synaptic vesicle of NANC nerve
Released on nerve stimulation
Mimics action of real transmitter
Mimics postsynaptic electrical actions of real transmitter
Antagonised by receptor antagonists to real transmitter
Potentiated by inhibitors of degradation

The following additional criteria are used in the identification of co-transmitters:

Presence of two transmitters in same nerve endings
Both released from same nerve ending on nerve stimulation
Both act on postsynaptic sites and mimic nerve response

The Micturition Reflex

It is generally agreed that in both animals and man micturition is initiated and maintained through the activation of a spinobulbospinal pathway passing through the micturition centre in the rostral brain stem [3,4]. The pontine micturition centre appears to function as a general integration centre since it regulates spinal storage reflexes and also receives modulatory inputs from other areas in the brain. In its simplest form, where involuntary (reflex) micturition is produced through afferent fibres synapsing directly with the pontine micturition neurons, a four neuron pathway should be considered involving dorsal root ganglia, pontine micturition centre, sacral parasympathetic nucleus and pelvic bladder ganglia [4]. The afferent information to initiate reflex micturition is believed to be generated within the bladder wall through activation of mechanoreceptors coupled in series with the muscle cells. Distension-induced myogenic activity excites mechanoreceptors and generates impulses in afferent fibres (Fig. 3.1).

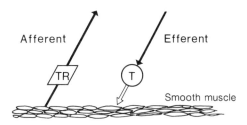

Fig. 3.1.   Afferent and efferent nerves in bladder smooth muscle. T, transmitter; TR, tension receptor.

In the efferent branch of the micturition reflex, descending axons from pontine micturition centre neurons synapse with dendrites of sacral parasympathetic nucleus neurons at sacral cord level. Preganglionic nerve terminals of sacral parasympathetic neurons reach the pelvic ganglia through the pelvic nerves. In the pelvic ganglia there seems to be a gating mechanism which filters out low frequency preganglionic activity during the collection of urine, but amplifies neurotransmission when intravesical pressure approaches a critical level [5]. During the filling phase, sympathetic and somatic inputs to the urethra, which are generated by spinal reflex mechanisms, are active.

The different parts of the micturition reflex arc involve different types of transmitter. In this chapter, the discussion will be limited to neurotransmitters directly involved in regulation of the contractile activity of bladder and urethral smooth muscle (Fig. 3.2).

Acetylcholine (Ach) and Muscarinic Receptor Functions

The human detrusor, and also the trigone and urethra, receive a rich cholinergic innervation [6,7] and it is generally agreed that muscarinic receptors play a crucial role in bladder emptying.

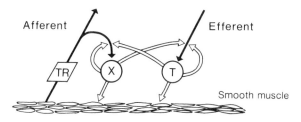

Fig. 3.2. Afferent and efferent nerves in bladder smooth muscle. Possible pre- and postjunctional sites of action of released transmitters are indicated. TR, tension receptor; T, transmitter; X, neuropeptide.

Normal Bladder

In most animal species, detrusor contraction is mediated by both cholinergic and NANC mechanisms [8,9]. In contrast, contraction of the normal human detrusor seems to be mediated almost exclusively through muscarinic receptor stimulation by released acetylcholine [10–13]; for discussion, see [14].

Characteristics of the Postjunctional Muscarinic Receptors

Several investigators using $[^3H]$-QNB binding have found a density of muscarinic receptors in homogenates of the human urinary bladder varying between approximately 60 and 230 fmol mg protein^{-1} [15–18]. Muscarinic receptor antagonists were bound to a virtually uniform population of sites [17], suggesting that it is not possible to obtain a selective effect on the human bladder with presently available antimuscarinic agents.

Zappia et al. [19] investigated the effects of pirenzepine on contractions induced by acetylcholine or bethanechol and by electrical stimulation in isolated strips of human urinary bladder. Pirenzepine was found to behave like atropine, but its potency was 100–300 times lower. It was concluded that according to the M_1/M_2 classification the muscarinic receptors of the human bladder were of M_2-type. This conclusion is supported by receptor-binding experiments [18,20,21]. The findings in human bladder are in line with the results of other investigators studying muscarinic receptor subtypes e.g. in rat urinary bladder [22,23]. Monferini et al. [24] classified by means of AF-DX 116 the muscarinic receptors of the rat bladder (M_2) into cardiac and glandular subtypes and identified a small proportion of glandular muscarinic receptors which could represent the functional receptor responsible for muscarinic agonist-induced contraction. They proposed to call this receptor subtype M_3.

Little is known about the coupling between the muscarinic receptors of the human bladder and intracellular messenger systems. Ruggieri et al. [20] found that carbachol inhibited adenylate cyclase in both rabbit and human urinary bladder. Andersson et al. [25] compared the contractile effects of carbachol and acetylcholine and their abilities to stimulate production of inositol phosphates in human detrusor muscle. Carbachol and acetylcholine (combined with physostigmine) produced almost identical concentration–response curves for contraction, and caused a concentration-dependent increase in the accumulation of inositol phosphates. However, acetylcholine (combined with physostigmine) was significantly less effective than carbachol, suggesting that the importance of inositol phosphates in contraction activation differed between the two agonists.

Prejunctional Muscarinic Receptors

The release of noradrenaline and acetylcholine in the human bladder and urethra can be influenced by prejunctional muscarinic receptors [26–28]. The release of [^{3}H]-noradrenaline from adrenergic nerve terminals could be decreased and increased by carbachol and scopolamine, respectively, in both bladder and urethral tissue, the release being concentration dependent. Muscarinic receptors inhibiting acetylcholine release have been demonstrated on the cholinergic axon terminals in human urethral smooth muscle [28] and in the rat urinary bladder [29].

The importance of prejunctional muscarinic receptors for bladder function can only be speculated upon. Immediately before bladder contraction starts during voiding, the intraurethral pressure falls [30,31]. It cannot be excluded that this fall in intraurethral pressure is caused by stimulation of prejunctional muscarinic receptors on noradrenergic nerves, diminishing noradrenaline release and thereby tone in the proximal urethra [27]. Such an effect would facilitate micturition. There may be a mutual influence of adrenergic and cholinergic nerves at different levels. Thus, de Groat and Saum [5] demonstrated inhibition of the cholinergic influence on the bladder by adrenergic nerves at the ganglionic level. Such an inhibition was also suggested to exist at the axon terminal level [27].

Bladder Dysfunction

Electrically induced contractions, resistant to atropine, have been reported to occur in morphologically and/or functionally changed bladders [10,11,32]. However, Sibley [11] has shown that the atropine-resistant response in hypertrophic bladder muscle was resistant also to tetrodotoxin (TTX), suggesting that this response was not nerve-mediated, but dependent on direct muscle stimulation. Comparison between isolated detrusor muscle from normal bladders, and bladders with different types of hyperactivity (idiopathic instability and hyperreflexia) revealed no significant differences in the degree of inhibition of electrically induced contractions by TTX and atropine [33]. The concentration–response curves for contractions induced by acetylcholine were similar. These data suggest that in both normal and hyperactive detrusor muscle acetylcholine may be the only transmitter involved with contraction.

In bladder tissue from patients with bladder hyperactivity, but without overt neurological disease, there was a significant reduction in the density of muscarinic receptors [34]. In contrast, the density of alpha-adrenoceptors was significantly increased. Whether these changes in receptor densities are a cause of the bladder hyperactivity or a consequence of it, remains to be established.

Parasympathetic denervation or decentralisation leads to an impaired ability of the bladder to empty. An increased responsiveness to muscarinic receptor stimulation can often be demonstrated, and this has been the basis for the use of bethanechol or carbachol as a test to diagnose neurogenic bladder disorders

[35,36]. It is not known if the increased response to cholinergic agents is due primarily to changes in muscarinic receptor functions secondary to the denervation/decentralisation, or can be attributed to changes in morphology, e.g. smooth muscle hypertrophy. Nilvebrant et al. [37] found no changes in the muscarinic receptor density in the denervated rat bladder that could explain supersensitivity and suggested that the regulation of the receptor levels is influenced by the functional state of the bladder. In support of this, Mattiasson et al. [38] were unable to demonstrate any supersensitivity to muscarinic receptor stimulation in decentralised cats provided that the urine was diverted and the bladder did not hypertrophy.

Urethra

The human urethra receives a cholinergic innervation which seems to be less dense than that of the bladder [7]. Isolated urethral muscle preparations show a weak contraction in response to muscarinic receptor stimulation [39,40], suggesting the occurrence of postjunctional muscarinic receptors. Prejunctional muscarinic receptors have been demonstrated on both adrenergic and cholinergic nerve terminals, which on stimulation inhibit the release of transmitter [26–28]. However, the functional role of the cholinergic innervation in the human urethra remains to be established (see above).

Noradrenaline (NA) and Adrenoceptor Functions

Beta-adrenoceptors

There seems to be agreement that the adrenergic innervation of the human detrusor muscle is sparse and non-uniform [8,41,42]. Release of noradrenaline from sympathetic nerve terminals in human detrusor has been demonstrated [27]. In normal detrusor muscle the amine produces relaxation, and functional studies as well as receptor binding studies suggest that in the detrusor beta-adrenoceptors dominate over alpha-adrenoceptors [43,44]. Several investigators have reported that the beta-adrenoceptors of human detrusor muscle have functional characteristics typical of neither beta$_1$- nor beta$_2$-receptors [45,46]. However, receptor binding studies suggest that the beta-adrenoceptors of the human detrusor are primarily, if not exclusively, of beta$_2$-subtype [21]. Unstable human detrusor muscle was reported to show a similar degree of inhibition in response to isoprenaline as normal detrusor. However, the inhibitory effect of isoprenaline on the response to electrical stimulation was less in unstable muscle [47]. Receptor binding studies revealed no difference in the density of beta-adrenoceptors between normal and "hyper-reflexic" bladders [34]. The importance of beta-adrenoceptors for normal detrusor function remains to be settled.

The adrenergic innervation of the human trigone and urethra is more dense than that of the detrusor [8]. Even if noradrenaline has a contractile effect on trigone, bladder base, as well as urethral smooth muscle [39,48,49], relaxation-mediating beta-adrenoceptors can be demonstrated both in vitro [39] and in vivo [50,51]. Their functional role remains unclear.

Alpha-adrenoceptors

In the normal human detrusor, drugs stimulating alpha-adrenoceptors have hardly any contractile effects [41,52,53], but both trigonal and urethral smooth muscle respond to noradrenaline with contraction [39,48,49]. Functional studies and receptor binding studies have shown that the predominating postjunctional alpha-receptor subtype is alpha$_1$ [21,49]. Levin et al. [21] found in receptor binding studies that the distribution of alpha receptor subtypes in the human bladder base was approximately 80% alpha$_1$ and 20% alpha$_2$.

In both detrusor and urethral smooth muscle Mattiasson et al. [26,27] found evidence for the occurrence of alpha$_2$-adrenoceptors on adrenergic nerve terminals, which on stimulation inhibited release of noradrenaline.

There is evidence that the alpha-adrenoceptor function in the detrusor can change, e.g. after bladder outlet obstruction and parasympathetic decentralisation. It may also be different in overactive bladders. Perlberg and Caine [54] showed that in bladders from 11 of 47 patients with bladder outlet obstruction, the response to noradrenaline was changed from relaxation to contraction. In bladder strips from six of 11 patients with bladder instability, they found contraction in response to noradrenaline, whereas in preparations from patients with normal cystometrograms noradrenaline caused contraction in only one out of 16. They suggested that this could be of importance for bladder hyperactivity. In bladders from patients with hyperreflexia, Restorick and Mundy [34] found that there was an almost fourfold increase in the density of alpha-adrenoceptors compared to the density in normal bladders. However, they concluded that whether or not this explains the detrusor overactivity remains an open question. More information is needed to establish a role for noradrenaline and alpha-adrenoceptors in bladder instability.

Non-adrenergic, Non-cholinergic (NANC)-Mediated Transmission

In both the bladder and the urethra ultrastructural studies have demonstrated a population of nerves which differ from the classical types of autonomic nerves. Burnstock et al. [55] demonstrated presumably purinergic nerves in the guinea-pig urinary bladder and several studies in animals and man have demonstrated the occurrence of peptide-containing neurons. There is evidence for the occurrence of NANC transmission in the human lower urinary tract, but so far no NANC-transmitter, excitatory or inhibitory, has been definitively established.

ATP

In isolated human bladder muscle, Husted et al. [56] found that ATP had a concentration-dependent contractile effect, and that ATP influenced the responses to transmural nerve stimulation, probably by both prejunctional and postjunctional effects. Evidence was presented that ATP may release prostaglandins, and that the sensitivity to ATP was higher in hypertrophied than in normal bladder.

However, available information does not support the view that ATP has a transmitter function in the normal human bladder.

Prostanoids

Several investigators have shown that prostaglandins PGF_{2a}, PGE_1, and PGE_2 contract isolated human bladder muscle. On the other hand, PGE_1 and PGE_2 relax contracted human urethral smooth muscle [57,58]. Biopsies of human urinary bladder mucosa were shown to release prostanoids: prostacyclin, PGE_2, PGF_{2a} and thromboxane A_2 [59]. It has been stressed that the response of bladder smooth muscle to prostanoids is slow, and that it is unlikely that these agents are involved in the evacuation of the bladder by exerting direct effects on the bladder smooth muscle. More probably they contribute to tone and spontaneous activity [58].

Maggi et al. [60] produced evidence for the involvement of arachidonic acid metabolites in spontaneous as well as drug-induced contractions of rat urinary bladder, and suggested that some of these were involved in the physiological regulation of the micturition reflex in the rat. The release of prostanoids from rat bladder mucosa was similar to that from human bladder [61]. Even if a transmitter function of prostanoids seems unlikely, it is possible that prostanoids may sensitise sensory nerves and increase the afferent input produced by a given degree of bladder filling.

Peptides

Several peptides, including substance P, vasoactive intestinal polypeptide (VIP), cholecystokinin-gene related peptide (CGRP), somatostatin, enkephalins, neuropeptide Y (NPY), and galanin, have been demonstrated in the human lower urinary tract [4]. According to the criteria required to identify a putative neurotransmitter (see above) few, if any, of these neuropeptides have an established role at any site along the micturition reflex pathway. However, as pointed out by Maggi and Meli [4], there is little doubt that many neuropeptides, including those detected in the bladder and urethral wall and pelvic or bladder ganglia, play some functional role as neurotransmitters and/or neuromodulators. Maggi and Meli [4] reviewed the role of neuropeptides in the regulation of the micturition reflex as studied by means of capsaicin, which is considered to release peptides from sensory afferent nerves. They suggested that peptides released from such nerves by appropriate stimuli have an "efferent" function on the bladder, and may produce various effects including micturition reflex activation, smooth muscle contraction, potentiation of efferent neurotransmission and induction of changes in vascular tone and permeability. An indication that capsaicin-sensitive structures may be present in the human urinary bladder was presented by Maggi et al. [62]. They instilled capsaicin intravesically in nine patients with hypersensitivity disorders of the lower urinary tract. They found that in six of these patients capsaicin produced a concentration-related reduction of the first desire to void, of bladder capacity and of pressure threshold for micturition. Capsaicin produced a burning sensation over the suprapubic area on instillation, but no other side effects. All six responders experienced a relief of their symptoms which disappeared or showed marked improvement for a few days after capsaicin application.

Three distinct functional roles have been proposed for endogenous VIPergic systems in modulating micturition. Thus, VIP may serve: (a) as a sensory neurotransmitter relaying information from pelvic viscera to CNS; (b) as a neuromodulator of ganglionic transmission in pelvic/bladder ganglia and (c) as a neurotransmitter released from postganglionic nerves in the bladder wall [4].

According to Maggi and Meli [4], no physiological or pharmacological evidence is available indicating that VIP plays a role as a sensory neurotransmitter in the micturition reflex pathway. Nor has its role in neurotransmission in bladder/pelvic ganglia been clarified.

VIP inhibits spontaneous contractile activity in isolated human bladder muscle [63–66], but seems to have little effect on contractions induced by muscarinic receptor stimulation or by electrical stimulation of nerves [66]. Maggi and Meli [4] have suggested that the low-amplitude myogenic contractile activity is of primary importance for the genesis of reflex bladder contraction. If this is correct, the direct effects of VIP on bladder smooth muscle, and the findings that VIP levels were markedly reduced in patients suffering from idiopathic detrusor instability [67] or detrusor hyperreflexia [68], suggest that the peptide (or lack of it) may play a role in some forms of bladder overactivity.

Substance P and other neurokinins contract human bladder muscle [69–71]. Kalbfleisch and Daniel [69] found a contractile component of the response to electrical stimulation that was resistant to atropine, and found that a substance P antagonist did not reduce this response. They concluded that substance P was unlikely to be the mediator of the response. Maggi et al. [71] found that the contractile response of the human bladder to neurokinins involved neurokinin (NK)-2 receptors. They also pointed out that the substance P antagonist used by Kalbfleisch and Daniel [69] behaves like a NK-1 tachykinin antagonist, while it has almost no antagonistic activity at NK-2 receptor sites, and concluded that further studies are needed to establish the possible pathophysiological relevance of the contractile response mediated by NK-2 receptors in human detrusor muscle.

It is possible that peptides released from sensory nerves may serve as modulators of neurotransmission in the lower urinary tract. Thus Maggi et al. [72] showed that galanin potently inhibited atropine-sensitive contractions in human detrusor muscle, probably by inhibiting the release of acetylcholine from cholinergic nerves.

In isolated smooth muscle from human trigone and urethra a relaxant response to electrical stimulation has been shown, particularly when tension was increased e.g. by noradrenaline or vasopressin [73–75]. These relaxant responses could be blocked by tetrodotoxin, and were suggested to be produced by a NANC transmitter released from nerves. The nature of this putative transmitter and the functional role of its effect are not known.

Conclusion

There is increasing evidence that in the normal human detrusor (and probably also in the "overactive" detrusor) contraction is initiated by acetylcholine released from nerves stimulating muscarinic receptors on bladder smooth muscle. In the urethra nerve-released noradrenaline contributes to intraurethral pressure by stimulating alpha-receptors on urethral smooth muscle. The definite roles of other transmitters and modulators, established or putative, in the regulation of micturition, remain to be established.

References

1. Guyton AC. Textbook of medical physiology, 7th ed. Philadelphia: WB Saunders, 1986; 552.
2. Daniel EE. Nonadrenergic, noncholinergic (NANC) neuronal inhibitory interactions with smooth muscle. In: Grover AK, Daniel EE, eds. Calcium and contractility. Clifton, NJ: The Humana Press, 1985; 385–425.
3. de Groat WC, Booth AM. Physiology of the urinary bladder and urethra. Ann Int Med 1980; 92:312–15.
4. Maggi CA, Meli A. The role of neuropeptides in the regulation of the micturition reflex. J Auton Pharmacol 1986; 6:133–62.
5. de Groat WC, Saum WR. Sympathetic inhibition of the urinary bladder and of pelvic ganglionic transmission in the cat. J Physiol (Lond) 1972; 220:297–314.
6. Mobley TL, El-Badawi A, McDonald D, Schenk E. Innervation of the human urinary bladder. Surg Forum 1966; 17:505–6.
7. Ek A, Alm P, Andersson K-E, Persson CGA. Adrenergic and cholinergic nerves of the human urethra and urinary bladder. A histochemical study. Acta Physiol Scand 1977; 99:345–52.
8. Ambache H, Zar MA. Non-cholinergic transmission by postganglionic motor neurones in the mammalian bladder. J Physiol (Lond) 1970; 210:761–83.
9. Taira N. The autonomic pharmacology of the bladder. Ann Rev Pharmacol Toxicol 1970; 12:197–208.
10. Sjögren C, Andersson K-E, Husted S, Mattiasson A, Møller-Madsen B. Atropine resistance of the transmurally stimulated isolated human bladder. J Urol 1982; 128:1368–71.
11. Sibley GNA. A comparison of spontaneous and nerve-mediated activity in bladder muscle from man, pig and rabbit. J Physiol (Lond) 1984; 354:431–43.
12. Kinder RB, Mundy AR. Atropine blockade of nerve-mediated stimulation of the human detrusor. Br J Urol 1985; 57:418–21.
13. Craggs MD, Rushton DN, Stephenson JD. A putative non-cholinergic mechanism in urinary bladders of new but not old world primates. J Urol 1986; 136:1348–50.
14. Andersson K-E. Clinical relevance of some findings in neuro-anatomy and neurophysiology of the lower urinary tract. Clin Sci 1986; 70 Suppl 14:21–32.
15. Levin RM, Staskin DR, Wein AJ. The muscarinic cholinergic binding kinetics of the human urinary bladder. Neurourol Urodyn 1982; 1:221–5.
16. Anderson GF, Skender JG, Navarro SP. Quantitation and stability of cholinergic receptors in human bladder tissue from post surgical and postmortem sources. J Urol 1985; 133:897–9.
17. Nilvebrandt L, Andersson K-E, Mattiasson A. Characterization of the muscarinic cholinoceptors in the human detrusor. J Urol 1985; 134:418–23.
18. Batra S, Björklund A, Hedlund H, Andersson K-E. Identification and characterization of muscarinic cholinergic receptors in the human urinary bladder and parotid gland. J Auton Nerv Syst 1987; 20:129–35.
19. Zappia L, Cartella A, Potenzoni D, Bertaccini G. Action of pirenzepine on the human urinary bladder in vitro. J Urol 1986; 136:739–42.
20. Ruggieri MR, Bode DC, Levin RM, Wein AJ. Muscarinic receptor subtypes in human and rabbit bladder. Neurourol Urodyn 1987; 6:119–28.
21. Levin RM, Ruggieri MR, Wein AJ. Identification of receptor subtypes in the rabbit and human urinary bladder by selective radio-ligand binding. J Urol 1988; 139:844–8.
22. Adami M, Bertaccini G, Coruzzi G, Poli E. Characterization of cholinoreceptors in the rat urinary bladder by the use of agonists and antagonists of the cholinergic system. J Auton Pharmacol 1985; 5:197–205.
23. van Charldorp KJ, de Jonge A, Thoolen MJ, van Zwieten PA. Subclassification of muscarinic receptors in the heart, urinary bladder and sympathetic ganglia in the pithed rat. Selectivity of some classical agonists. Naunyn Schmiedebergs Arch Pharmacol 1985; 331:301–6.
24. Monferini E, Giraldo E, Ladinsky H. Characterization of the muscarinic receptor subtypes in the rat urinary bladder. Eur J Pharmacol 1988; 147:453–8.

25. Andersson K-E, Fovaeus M, Hedlund H, Holmquist F, Sundler F. Muscarinic receptor stimulation of phosphoinositide hydrolysis in the human urinary bladder. J Urol 1989; 141:324A (abstract 619).

26. Mattiasson A, Andersson K-E, Sjögren C. Adrenoceptors and cholinoceptors controlling noradrenaline release from adrenergic nerves in the urethra of rabbit and man. J Urol 1984; 131:1190–5.

27. Mattiasson A, Andersson K-E, Elbadawi A, Morgan E, Sjögren C. Interaction between adrenergic and cholinergic nerve terminals in the urinary bladder of rabbit, cat and man. J Urol 1987; 137:1017–19.

28. Mattiasson A, Andersson K-E, Sjögren C. Inhibitory α-adrenoceptors on cholinergic axon terminals in the urethra of rabbit and man. Neurourol Urodyn 1988; 6:449–56.

29. d'Agostino G, Kilbinger H, Chiari MC, Grana E. Presynaptic inhibitory muscarinic receptors modulating ^{3}H-acetylcholine release in the rat urinary bladder. J Pharmacol Exp Ther 1986; 239:522–8.

30. Tanagho EA, Miller ER. Initiation of voiding. Br J Urol 1970; 42:175–83.

31. Rud T, Ulmsten U, Andersson K-E. Initiation of voiding in healthy women and those with stress incontinence. Acta Obstet Gynecol Scand 1978; 57:457–62.

32. Nergårdh A, Kinn A-C. Neurotransmission in activation of the contractile response in the human urinary bladder. Scand J Urol Nephrol 1983; 17:153–7.

33. Kinder RB, Restorick JM, Mundy AR. A comparative study of detrusor muscle from normal, idiopathic unstable and hyperreflexic bladder. In: Proceedings of the 15th Annual Meeting of the International Continence Society. London, 1985,170–1.

34. Restorick JM, Mundy AR. The density of cholinergic and alpha and beta adrenergic receptors in the normal and hyper-reflexic human detrusor. Br J Urol 1989; 63:32–5.

35. Lapides J, Friend CR, Ajemian EP, Reus WF. A new method for diagnosing the neurogenic bladder. Univ Michigan Med Bull 1962; 28:166–40.

36. Glahn BE. Neurogenic bladder diagnosed pharmacologically on the basis of denervation supersensitivity. Scand J Urol Nephrol 1970; 4:13–24.

37. Nilvebrant L, Ekström J, Malmberg L. Muscarinic receptor density in the rat urinary bladder after denervation, hypertrophy and urinary diversion. Acta Pharmacol Toxicol 1986; 59:306–14.

38. Mattiasson A, Andersson K-E, Sjögren C, Sundin T, Uvelius B. Supersensitivity to carbachol in the parasympathetically decentralized feline urinary bladder. J Urol 1984; 131:562–5.

39. Ek A, Alm P, Andersson K-E, Persson CGA. Adrenoceptor and cholinoceptor mediated responses of the isolated human urethra. Scand J Urol Nephrol 1977; 11:97–102.

40. Andersson K-E, Persson CGA, Alm P, Kullander S, Ulmsten U. Effects of acetylcholine, noradrenaline, and prostaglandins on the isolated perfused human fetal urethra. Acta Physiol Scand 1978; 104:394–401.

41. Sundin T, Dahlström A, Norlén L, Svedmyr N. The sympathetic innervation and adrenoceptor function of the human lower urinary tract in the normal state and after parasympathetic denervation. Invest Urol 1977; 14:322–8.

42. Benson GS, McConnell JA, Wood JG. Adrenergic innervation of the human bladder body. J Urol 1979; 122:189–91.

43. Wein AJ, Levin RM. Comparison of adrenergic receptor density in urinary bladder in man dog and rabbit. Surg Forum 1979; 30:576–8.

44. Amark P, Nergårdh A, Kinn AC. The effect of noradrenaline on the contractile response of the urinary bladder. Scand J Urol Nephrol 1986; 20:203–7.

45. Nergårdh A, Boréus LO. Autonomic receptor function in the lower urinary tract of man and cat. Scand J Urol Nephrol 1972; 6:32–6.

46. Larsen JJ. α- and β-adrenoceptors in the detrusor muscle and bladder base of the pig and β-adrenoceptors in the detrusor of man. Br J Pharmacol 1979; 65:215–22.

47. Eaton AC, Bates CP. An in vitro physiological study of normal and unstable human detrusor muscle. Br J Urol 1982; 54:653–7.

48. Benson GS, Wein AJ, Raezer DM, Corriere JJN. Adrenergic and cholinergic stimulation and blockade of the human bladder base. J Urol 1976; 116:174–5.

49. Kunisawa Y, Kawabe K, Nijima T, Honda K, Takenaka T. A pharmacological study of alpha adrenergic receptor subtypes in smooth muscle of human urinary bladder base and prostatic urethra. J Urol 1985; 134:396–8.

50. Rao MS, Bapna BC, Sharma PL, Chary KSN, Vaidyanathan S. Clinical import of beta-adrenergic activity in the proximal urethra. J Urol 1980; 124:254–5.

51. Vaidyanathan S, Rao MS, Bapna BC, Chary KSN, Palaniswamy R. Beta-adrenergic activity in human proximal urethra: a study with terbutaline. J Urol 1980; 124:869–71.

52. Nergårdh A, Boréus LO, Naglo AS. Characterization of the adrenergic beta-receptor in the urinary bladder of man and cat. Acta Pharmacol Toxicol 1977; 40:14–21.
53. Awad AA, Bruce G, Carrocampi JW, Lin M, Marks GS. Distribution of α- β-adrenoceptors in human urinary bladder. Br J Pharmacol 1974; 50:525–9.
54. Perlberg S, Caine M. Adrenergic response of bladder muscle in prostatic obstruction. Urology 1982; 20:524–37.
55. Burnstock G, Cocks T, Crowe R, Kasakov L. Purinergic innervation of the guinea-pig urinary bladder. Br J Pharmacol 1978; 63:125–38.
56. Husted S, Sjögren C, Andersson K-E. Direct effects of adenosine and adenine nucleotides on isolated human urinary bladder and their influence on electrically induced contractions. J Urol 1983; 130:392–8.
57. Andersson K-E, Forman A. Effects of prostaglandins on the smooth muscle of the urinary tract. Acta Pharmacol Toxicol 1978; 43 (Suppl II): 90–5.
58. Andersson K-E, Sjögren C. Aspect on the physiology and pharmacology of the bladder and urethra. Progr Neurobiol 1982; 19:71–81.
59. Jeremy JY, Tsang V, Mikhailidis DP, Rogers H, Morgan RJ, Dandona P. Eicosanoid synthesis by human urinary bladder mucosa: pathological implications. Br J Urol 1987; 59:36–9.
60. Maggi CA, Evangelista S, Grimaldi G, Santicioli P, Gioletti A, Meli A. Evidence for the involvement of arachidonic acid metabolites in spontaneous and drug-induced contractions of rat urinary bladder. J Pharmacol Exp Ther 1984; 230:500–13.
61. Jeremy JY, Mikhailidis DP, Dandona P. The rat urinary bladder produces prostacyclin as well as other prostaglandins. Prostaglandins, Leukotriencs Med 1984; 16:235–48.
62. Maggi CA, Barbanti G, Santicioli P et al. Cystometric evidence that capsaicin-sensitive nerves modulate the afferent branch of micturition reflex in humans. J Urol 1989; 142:150–4.
63. Larsen JJ, Ottesen B, Fahrenkrug J, Fahrenkrug L. Vasoactive intestinal polypeptide (VIP) in the male genitourinary tract. Concentration and motor effect. Invest Urol 1981; 19:211–13.
64. Klarskov P, Gerstenberg T, Hald T. Vasoactive intestinal polypeptide influence on lower urinary tract smooth muscle from human and pig. J Urol 1984; 131:1000–4.
65. Kinder RB, Mundy AR. Inhibition of spontaneous contractile activity in isolated human detrusor muscle strips by vasoactive intestinal polypeptide. Br J Urol 1985; 57:20–3.
66. Sjögren C, Andersson K-E, Mattiasson A. Effects of vasoactive intestinal polypeptide on isolated urethral and urinary bladder smooth muscle from rabbit and man. J Urol 1985; 133:136–40.
67. Gu J, Restorick JM, Blank MA et al. Vasoactive intestinal polypeptide in the normal and unstable bladder. Br J Urol 1983; 55:645–7.
68. Kinder RB, Restorick JM, Mundy AR. Vasoactive intestinal polypeptide in the hyperreflexic neuropathic bladder. Br J Urol; 57:289–91.
69. Kalbfleisch RE, Daniel EE. The role of substance P in the human urinary bladder. Arch Int Pharmacodyn Ther 1987; 285:238–48.
70. Dion S, Corcos J, Carmel M, Drapeau G, Regoli D. Substance P and neurokinins as stimulants of the human isolated urinary bladder. Neuropeptides 1988; 11:83–7.
71. Maggi CA, Santicioli P, Patacchini R et al. Contractile response of the human isolated urinary bladder to neurokinins: involvement of NK-2 receptors. Eur J Pharmacol 1988; 145:335–40.
72. Maggi CA, Santicioli P, Patacchini R et al. Galanin: a potent modulator of excitatory neurotransmission in the human urinary bladder. Eur J Pharmacol 1987; 143:135–7.
73. Andersson K-E, Mattiasson A, Sjögren C. Electrically induced relaxation of the noradrenaline contracted isolated urethra from rabbit and man. J Urol 1983; 129:210–13.
74. Klarskov P, Gerstenberg TC, Ramirez D, Hald T. Non-cholinergic, non-adrenergic nerve mediated relaxation of trigone, bladder neck and urethral smooth muscle in vitro. J Urol 1983; 129:848–50.
75. Speakman MJ, Walmsley D, Brading AF. An in vitro pharmacological study of the human trigone – a site of non-adrenergic, non-cholinergic neurotransmission. Br J Urol 1988; 61:304–9.

Chapter 4

Continence Mechanism

S. Kulseng-Hanssen and B. Klevmark

For a woman to be continent, the urethra must seal properly, the urethral pressure must be higher than the bladder pressure and the bladder must be under control.

Urethral aspects of continence may be divided into passive and active continence. Passive continence is maintained by tension in the urethral wall generated by the urethral smooth and striated muscle. Active continence implies that striated muscle in the urethral wall and the periurethral striated muscle contract by will or reflexly. This chapter is in two parts: urethral closure mechanism and bladder control.

Urethral Closure Mechanism

The term "urethral sphincter" will be used for the urethral muscle itself, comprising both the smooth and striated components, and "periurethral striated sphincter" for the levator ani muscles.

In the male a bladder neck genital sphincter is present which prevents retrograde ejaculation. In the female an analogous sphincter is not present. There is little reason to believe that there is a separate closure mechanism at the bladder neck in the female.

The main sphincter activity is found in the middle of the urethra. Here the vascular plexus is most abundant and the smooth and striated muscles are best developed [1].

Urethral pressure in females decreases with age [2] and increases with bladder filling [3]. It is increased in the standing compared to the supine position [4]. The functional urethral length was found to decrease significantly after the menopause [2].

Urethral pressure variations have been found in normal females [5,6] as well as in incontinent patients. The leaking mechanism in incontinent patients with urethral pressure variations has been found to be a urethral pressure decrease followed by detrusor contraction [7]. Incontinence due to isolated urethral pressure decrease is very rare [8].

The Urethral Seal

Continence depends, apart from urethral compression, on the inner urethral wall softness [9]. The inner urethral epithelial surface is richly folded to allow complete apposition of the mucosa. The submucosa is composed of collagen fibres, elastic tissue and a rich network of veins. This spongy tissue fills the urethral folds and contributes to urethral sealing. If the urethral seal is defective, a larger compressive force is necessary to obtain continence. With age both the sealing and the compressive factors are weakened.

Submucosa

The urethral venous plexus was described by Berkow [10], who suggested that the venous sinuses had a function like a "washer" in a tap. Vascular pulsations in the urethral high pressure zone were described by Enhørning [11], who regarded the rich venous network as an auxiliary closure mechanism. This theory was confirmed by Raz et al. [12] and Rud et al. [13], who recorded a one-third reduction of the urethral pressure after clamping the urethral blood supply in female dogs and in women. Arteriovenous shunts were described by Huisman [1]. Theoretically an active pooling or emptying of the urethral venous plexus might induce changes in urethral pressure. However, the presence of these arteriovenous shunts was not confirmed by Gosling et al. [14], and the theory was not supported by Downie and Lautt [15] who showed that stimulation of the hypogastric nerve produced no change in vascular resistance of the perfused urethra, though it did produce urethral constriction. Neither was it supported by Kulseng-Hanssen and Stranden [16] who found the periurethral vascular plexus to be filled and emptied secondary to urethral striated and smooth muscle activity.

Hormonal Factors

Urethral pressure does not change significantly during the menstrual cycle [2]. However, it decreases with age [2] and after the menopause an atrophic mucosa [17] is found. This may cause a reduced sealing effect. With age, muscle power also decreases and the tendency to become incontinent therefore increases. Oestrogen receptors have been demonstrated in the female urethra [18]. Oestrogen treatment with or without alpha stimulating drugs has largely been used to treat postmenopausal stress incontinence. However, large well-controlled studies to document the effect are sparse.

Smooth Muscle

The urethral smooth muscle consists of a thick inner longitudinal layer and a thin outer circular layer. The function of the inner longitudinal layer is uncertain.

Because the outer circular smooth muscle is so thin, it has been doubted that the urethral smooth muscle is of any importance for the urethral closure mechanism. From a morphological point of view it is difficult to explain how the urethral smooth muscle takes part in urethral closure. However, there are reasons to believe that the smooth muscle is important for urethral closure. Donker et al. [19] found a 65% reduction in urethral pressure after intravenous injection of phentolamine. This was confirmed by Nordling [20] and Mattiasson et al. [21], who found respectively 42% and 36% reductions in urethral pressure after phentolamine. However, the phentolamine may have effects on vascular factors, autonomic ganglia and striated muscle as well.

Urethral pressure variations are generated by a continuously changing mixture of urethral smooth and striated muscle activity [8]. Pudendal anaesthesia was given to women with urethral pressure variations by Kulseng-Hanssen [22]. During the anaesthesia urethral pressure variations of up to 38% of the pre-anaesthesia level were still found. The fluctuation found during the anaesthesia is caused by smooth muscle activity.

Patients have been found to be continent after successful pudendal anaesthesia [23,24]. Some were even able to blow up a column of mercury by mouth to 110 mm after pudendal anaesthesia without becoming incontinent [25]. Assuming that pudendal anaesthesia blocks urethral striated muscle activity completely, smooth muscle and the vascular factor are responsible for continence in these situations.

McGuire and Wagner [26] found that complete bilateral rhizotomy, which denervates the periurethral and urethral striated muscle and the bladder, did not make patients incontinent. However, additional spinal anaesthesia, which included sympathetic innervation, made these patients incontinent.

The innervation of the female urethral smooth muscle is controversial. Ek et al. [27] described scanty sympathetic innervation whereas Gosling et al. [28] described a very poor supply of sympathetic nerves. Nordling [29] found that circulating noradrenaline was not important for urethral pressure regulation and that urethral pressure was controlled by neural activity. According to Mattiasson et al. [30,31] smooth urethral muscle activity is due to continuous stimulation by adrenergic fibres with release of noradrenaline from the nerve endings.

Urethral smooth muscle tonus may be inhibited by parasympathetic stimulation [32]. In isolated human urethra, stimulation of muscarinic receptors caused a significant decrease of electrically induced [^{3}H]noradrenaline release [33]. If such an effect is present in vivo, it may explain the inhibitory parasympathetic effect on the noradrenaline-dependent urethral tone.

Both non-adrenergic, non-cholinergic nerve-mediated contraction and relaxation have been described in the human urethra [30].

Striated Urethral Muscle

According to DeLancey [34], the proximal part of the striated urethral muscle fibres surround the smooth muscle coat circularly. They are incomplete in the ventral aspect of the urethral wall and are found along 18% to 64% of the urethral length. The distal part of the striated urethral muscle lies in the urogenital diaphragm and is found along 54% to 76% of the urethral length. Some fibres encircle both urethra and vagina whereas others pass out laterally and insert into the urogenital diaphragm near the pubic rami. During a "hold urine" manoeuvre two urethral pressure peaks are seen between 15% and 85% along the urethral length [35]. The largest distal peak corresponds to the area with the strongest urethral striated muscle and the most proximal peak is seen in the area influenced by the attachment to the vagina [34]. Urethra and vagina are attached to the levator ani muscles through the pubourethral ligaments [36]. When the striated pelvic floor contracts, the vagina and proximal urethra are elevated. DeLancey [37] suggests that the proximal part of the urethra during a levator ani contraction will be compressed between the vagina and a precervical arch which runs in front of the urethra between the arcus tendineus on each side of the pelvis. In this way the proximal urethral pressure increase may be explained. It is more likely that the levator ani muscle influences urethral pressure in this way than that it provides an occlusive force on the urethral wall as has been suggested by Gosling et al. [14]. Urethral striated muscle is composed mainly of slow twitch fibres in contrast to the periurethral striated muscles, which contain both slow and fast twitch fibres [38]. The slow twitch fibres in the urethral striated muscle are well suited to exert a resting pressure. During a cough a urethral pressure increase is seen at the level of the urethral sphincter, but not more proximally where a transferred abdominal pressure increase should be expected [35]. This suggests that the urethral striated muscle may cause the urethral pressure increase. That this muscle is a slow twitch muscle does not necessarily mean that it is too slow to cause the urethral pressure increase caused by a cough. Little is known about the physiological characteristics of urethral striated muscle.

Attempts have been made to determine what percentage of urethral pressure is caused by striated muscle. A urethral pressure decrease from zero to 39% has been reported by various authors [13,19,39,40] after striated muscle paralysis with different competitive and depolarising muscle blockers. However, the additional anaesthetic drugs these patients were given may have influenced the urethral pressure through effects on the central nervous system, the ganglia, the vascular system and the urethral smooth muscle.

A 20% to 84% reduction in urethral pressure after pudendal anaesthesia was found in patients with urethral pressure variations. The degree of urethral pressure reduction after pudendal anaesthesia depends on the urethral striated muscle activity level before the anaesthesia. This activity level is probably different in different people and in the same person at different times [41].

Pressure Transmission to the Urethra During Cough

Enhørning [11] found that in continent females during a cough the urethral pressure exceeded the bladder pressure. This was not the case in women with stress incontinence. Collins [42] found that when abdominal pressure increases due to the valsalva manoeuvre both urethral and bladder pressure increase. He introduced the concept that this abdominal pressure transmission aided urethral closure during stress. Heidler et al. [43] found the urethral pressure increase during a cough to be more than 100%, indicating an active mechanism. This was supported by Constantinou and Gowan [44], who during a cough found an increased EMG activity preceding the urethral pressure increase. Thus probably the urethral striated muscle causes this extra pressure increase during a cough. Women with stress incontinence have been found to have a pressure transmission less than 100% [45]. This may be due to mechanical damage to the pubourethral ligaments and/or to neurogenic lesions [46].

Bladder Control

During bladder filling when a desire to void is felt the human being can voluntarily inhibit bladder activity for a reasonable amount of time, and within certain limits can decide the moment for micturition. Complicated neurophysiological mechanisms underlie this simple behaviour.

Bladder Filling

During natural filling at an average low rate, which is $1–2\,\mathrm{ml\,kg^{-1}\,h^{-1}}$, there is no bladder pressure rise. However, at higher physiological filling rates bladder pressure will increase due to activation of viscoelastic bladder wall properties [47,48]. During bladder filling, the muscle bundles in the bladder wall undergo reorganisation and the muscle cells are elongated up to four times their minimum length [49]. During filling, mechanoreceptors in the bladder wall are activated [50] and action potentials run with the parasympathetic nerves (pelvic nerves) to the spinal cord at the level of S2 to S4. The ascending pathways in the spinal cord for bladder proprioception are not definitely mapped, and may vary from one individual to another [51]. Action potentials pass upwards and at a certain bladder wall tension a desire to void is felt. Exactly where in the brain the desire to void is felt is not known. The most important cortical areas involved in micturition in humans are found in the superior frontal gyrus and septal area [51]. Lesions in these areas result in lowering of the volume threshold for micturition, with a risk of incontinence. Bladder activity and urethral sphincter activity are always co-ordinated in these supraspinal lesions.

Normally, a person has a certain volume threshold for micturition, determined by her age and life situation. However, this threshold may vary considerably because of psychogenic factors, resulting sometimes in small volumes and frequency, and at other times in increased volumes and retention.

The first feeling of bladder filling is usually easy to suppress. Later the desire to void becomes stronger and ultimately it will be present all the time. Finally it is no longer possible to suppress the pontine micturition centre, and urethral pressure relaxation and detrusor contraction are initiated. In these circumstances continence can be maintained only by squeezing with the urethral and periurethral striated muscles and thereafter only by direct pressure applied to the perineum such as sitting on the heel.

In healthy women the micturition reflex is co-ordinated in the pontine micturition centre [52,53]. Efferent impulses from this centre run in the reticulospinal tracts and stimulate parasympathetic and somatic motor neurons situated in the intermediolateral cell column and in the anterior horn at level S2–S4. The sympathetic efferents arising at the T10–L2 area synapse in the inferior mesenteric and pelvic ganglia. Some also have their ganglia in the sympathetic chain and run with the pelvic nerves [54].

In patients with complete spinal cord lesions, bladder filling is not felt. Their micturition reflex is organised at a sacral spinal level. In such cases the micturition reflex is usually activated at smaller bladder volumes than normal and continuation of voiding is incomplete. These patients have detrusor sphincter dyssynergia due to loss of the co-ordinating activity of the pontine micturition centre. Supraspinal impulses are necessary for continuation until complete bladder emptying. Consequently, these patients empty the bladder by a series of repeated incomplete emptyings. In healthy humans the sacral micturition centre is of secondary importance in relation to the pontine micturition centre.

The pontine micturition centre is controlled by both stimulatory and inhibitory cerebral areas. Several local systems keep the detrusor motor neurons quiet during bladder filling. There is a recurrent inhibition of preganglionic neurons by inhibitory interneurons in the spinal cord [55]. The intensity of impulses in the postganglionic parasympathetic nerves may be controlled in the ganglia by the following mechanisms:

1. Afferent stimulation from the bladder and urethra does not cause efferent activity in postganglionic fibres before a critical level of stimulation occurs [56].
2. In the parasympathetic ganglia, due to sympathetic stimulation, the small intensely fluorescent (SIF) cells release noradrenaline. This activates presynaptic alpha-adrenergic receptors on the preganglionic parasympathetic terminals. Release of acetylcholine is thereby inhibited [57].

Micturition

When the desire to void is felt and the circumstances are appropriate, the micturition reflex is voluntarily elicited. This requires a short mental concentration. The urethral and periurethral striated muscle activity decreases, the urethral pressure decreases and a detrusor contraction follows seconds later, whereby voiding begins. During voiding the bladder pressure remains relatively constant. Urethral and periurethral striated muscles are reflexly relaxed as long as urine is running in the urethra [58]. Micturition is continuous and the bladder is completely emptied. Then the bladder pressure decreases and the urethral pressure increases over the premicturition level and settles to a normal resting level. Normal micturition is performed without contraction of striated muscle. During micturition the flow can be stopped reflexly or voluntarily. Voiding can also be performed without bladder sensation.

Summary

Continence is partly automatically and partly consciously regulated. It is automatically regulated until the desire to void is felt. From then on, micturition reflex elicitation is consciously inhibited. When that is no longer possible the sequence of urethral relaxation and detrusor contraction automatically takes place. Continence may thereafter be consciously maintained through squeezing with striated muscles and then by external mechanical compression of the urethra.

References

1. Huisman A. Morphologie van de vrouwelijke urethra. Thesis, Groningen, The Netherlands, 1979.
2. Rud T. Urethral pressure profile in continent women from childhood to old age. Acta Obstet Gynecol Scand 1980; 59:331–5.

3. Rud T, Ulmsten U, Andersson KE. Initiation of voiding in healthy women and those with stress incontinence. Acta Obstet Gynecol Scand 1978; 57:457–62.
4. George NJR, Feneley RCL. The importance of postural influences on urethral musculature. Proceedings of the 8th Annual Meeting of the International Continence Society, Manchester, 1978: 117.
5. Sørensen S, Kirkeby HJ, Stødkilde Jørgensen H, Djurhus JC. Continuous recording of urethral activity in healthy female volunteers. Neurourol Urodynam 1986; 5:5–16.
6. Kulseng-Hanssen S, Kristoffersen M. Urethral pressure variations in women with and without neurourological symptoms. Neurourol Urodynam 1987; 6:299–306.
7. Kulseng-Hanssen S, Klevmark B. Ambulatory urethro-cystorectometry. A new technique. Neurourol Urodynam 1988; 7:119–30.
8. Kulseng-Hanssen S. Thesis, Oslo, 1988.
9. Zinner NR, Sterling AM, Ritter RC. Role of inner urethral softness in urinary continence. Urol 1980; 16:115–17.
10. Berkow SG. The corpus spongiosum of the urethra: its possible role in urinary control and stress incontinence in women. Am J Obstet Gynecol 1953; 65:346–51.
11. Enhørning G. Simultaneous recording of intravesical and intraurethral pressure. Acta Chir Scand [Suppl.] 1961; 276:1–6.
12. Raz S, Caine M, Ziegler M. The vascular component in the production of intraurethral pressure. J Urol 1972; 108:93–6.
13. Rud T, Andersson KE, Asmussen M, Hunting A, Ulmsten U. Factors maintaining the intraurethral pressure in women. Invest Urol 1980; 17:343–7.
14. Gosling JA, Dixon JS, Humperson JR. Functional anatomy of the urinary tract. London: Gower, 1983.
15. Downie JW, Lautt WW. Is sympathetic control of the urethra mediated through vasomotor action? Neurourol Urodynam 1986; 5:219–25.
16. Kulseng-Hanssen S, Stranden E. Urethral pressure variations in women with neurourological symptoms. III. Relationship to urethral wall venous plexus. Neurourol Urodynam 1987; 6:87–93.
17. Smith P. Age changes in the female urethra. Br J Urol 1972; 44:667–76.
18. Iosif CS, Batra S, Ek A, Astedt B. Estrogen receptors in the human female lower urinary tract. Am J Obstet Gynecol 1981; 141:817–20.
19. Donker PJ, Ivanovici F, Noach EL. Analysis of urethral pressure profile by means of electromyography and administration of drugs. Br J Urol 1972; 44:180–93.
20. Nordling J. Alpha blockers and urethral pressure in neurological patients. Urol Int 1978; 33:304–9.
21. Mattiasson A, Andersson KE, Sjøgren C. Urethral sensitivity to alpha adrenoceptor stimulation and blockade in patients with parasympathetically decentralized lower urinary tract and in healthy volunteers. Neurourol Urodynam 1984; 3:230–234.
22. Kulseng-Hanssen S. Urethral pressure variations in women with neurourological symptoms. II. Relationship to urethral smooth muscle. Neurourol Urodynam 1987; 6:79–85.
23. Lapides J, Grey HO, Rawling JC. Function of the striated muscles in the control of urination: effect of pudendal block. Surg Forum 1955; 6:611–15.
24. Krahn HP, Morales PA. The effect of pudendal nerve anesthesia on urinary continence after prostatectomy. J Urol 1965; 94:282–5.
25. Brindley GS, Rushton DN, Craggs MD. The pressure exerted by the external sphincter of the urethra when its motor nerve fibers are stimulated electrically. Br J Urol 1974; 46:453–62.
26. McGuire EJ, Wagner FC. The effect of complete sacral rhizotomy on bladder and urethral function. Surg Gyn Obstet 1977; 144:343–6.
27. Ek A, Alm P, Andersson KE, Persson CGA. Adrenergic and cholinergic nerves of the human urethra and urinary bladder. A histochemical study. Acta Physiol Scand 1977; 99:345–52.
28. Gosling JA, Dixon JS, Lendon RJ. The autonomic innervation of the male and female bladder neck and proximal urethra. J Urol 1977; 118:302–5.
29. Nordling J. Influence of the sympathetic nervous system on lower urinary tract in man. Neurourol Urodynam 1983; 2:3–26.
30. Mattiasson A, Andersson KE, Sjøgren C. Adrenergic and non-adrenergic contraction of isolated urethral muscle from rabbit and man. J Urol 1985; 133:298–303.
31. Mattiasson A. Receptor functions/neurotransmitters in the lower urinary tract. In: Thorup Andersen J, ed. Proceedings from Scandinavian Course in Neurourology. Mariehamn, 1987.
32. Torrens MJ. Urethral sphincteric responses to stimulation of the sacral nerves in the human female. Urol Int 1978; 33:22–6.
33. Mattiasson A, Andersson KE, Sjøgren C. Adrenoceptors and cholinoceptors controlling the release

of noradrenaline from the adrenergic nerves in the isolated urethra in rabbit and man. J Urol 1984; 131:1190–5.

34. DeLancey JOL. Correlative study of paraurethral anatomy. Obstet Gynecol 1986; 68:91–7.
35. Constantinou CE, Govan DE. Spatial distribution and timing of transmitted and reflexly generated urethral pressures in healthy women. J Urol 1982; 127:964–9.
36. DeLancey JOL. Pubovesical ligament: a separate structure from the urethral supports ("pubo-urethral ligaments"). Neurourol Urodynam 1989; 8:53–61.
37. Delancey JOL. Anatomy and mechanics of structures around the vesical neck: how vesical neck position might affect its closure. Neurourol Urodynam 1988; 7:161–2.
38. Gosling JA, Dixon JS, Critchley HOD, Thompson SA. A comparative study of the human external sphincter and periurethral levator ani muscles. Br J Urol 1981; 53:35–41.
39. Murray A. Predicting the outcome of surgery for urethral incompetence in women by an intraopera-tive fluid bridge test. A feasibility study. MD Thesis, University of Liverpool, Liverpool, 1986.
40. Doyle PT, Briscoe CE. The effect of drugs and anaesthetic agents on the urinary bladder and sphincter. Br J Urol 1976; 48:329–34.
41. Kulseng-Hanssen S, Stien R, Fønstelien E. Urethral pressure variations in women with neurourolo-gical symptoms. I. Relationship to urethral and pelvic floor striated muscle. Neurourol Urodynam 1987; 6:71–8.
42. Collins CD. Electrical stimulation in the treatment of incontinence. ChM Thesis, University of Sheffield, 1972.
43. Heidler H, Wolk H, Jonas U. Urethral closure mechanism under stress conditions. Eur Urol 1979; 5:110–12.
44. Constantinou CE, Gowan DE. Urodynamic analysis of urethral, vesical and perivesical pressure distribution in the healthy female. Urol Int 1980; 35:53–72.
45. Hilton P, Stanton S. Urethral pressure measurements by microtransducer. The results in symptom-free women and in those with genuine stress incontinence. Br J Obstet Gynaecol 1983; 90:919–33.
46. Snooks SJ, Swash M. Abnormalities of the innervation of the urethral striated sphincter muscula-ture in incontinence. Br J Urol 1984; 56:401–5.
47. Klevmark B. Motility of the urinary bladder in cats during filling at physiological rates. I. Intra-vesical pressure patterns studied by a new method of cystometry. Acta Physiol Scand 1974; 90:565–77.
48. Klevmark B. Motility of the urinary bladder in cats during filling at physiological rates II. Effects of extrinsic bladder denervation on intraluminal tension and intravesical pressure patterns. Acta Physiol Scand 1977; 101:176–84.
49. Uvelius B, Gabella G. Relation between cell length and force production in urinary bladder smooth muscle. Acta Physiol Scand 1980; 110:357–65.
50. Winter DL. Receptor characteristics and conduction velocities in bladder efferents. J Psychiat Res 1971; 8:225–35.
51. Torrens M. Human physiology. In: Torrens M, Morrison JFB, eds. The physiology of the lower urinary tract. London: Springer, 1987; 333–50.
52. Barrington FJF. The nervous mechanism of micturition. Q J Exp Physiol 1914; 8:33.
53. de Groat WC. Nervous control of the urinary bladder in the cat. Brain Res 1975; 87:201–11.
54. Blackman JG, Crowcroft PJ, Devine EE, Holman ME, Yonemura K. Transmission from pregang-lionic fibres in the hypogastric nerve to peripheral ganglia of male guinea-pigs. J Physiol 1969; 201:723–43.
55. de Groat WC, Ryall RW. Recurrent inhibition in sacral parasympathetic pathways to the bladder. J Physiol 1968; 196:579–91.
56. de Groat WC, Booth AN. Inhibition and facilitation in parasympathetic ganglia. Fed Proc 1980; 39:2990–6.
57. de Groat WC, Saum WR. Parasympathetic ganglia: activation of an adrenergic inhibitory mecha-nism by cholinomimetic agents. Science 1972; 175:659–61.
58. Barrington FJF. The component reflexes of micturition in the cat. Parts I and II. Brain 1931; 54:177–88.

Discussion

Van Mastrigt: I was fascinated by the notion that for stimulation with prosta-glandins the time course of contraction is so much slower. We have been studying time courses very intensively, though not of prostaglandins. Is there some mechanism of action to explain why this time course should be so much slower, for instance stimulation with acetylcholine or whatever?

The major factor in this time course is the diffusion of the agent reaching the muscle, and the processes in the muscle are usually much faster than this diffusion factor. But obviously if prostaglandins are given there is an even slower factor that dominates the time course.

Andersson: We have no good explanation for the onset of action of prostaglandins, but it is very characteristic. What we know is that it is not very sensitive to removal of extracellular calcium. The action of prostaglandins and what is seen as oscillations of tension in the smooth muscle, which can be found in any type of smooth muscle, are coupled to the mechanism it initiates. Prostaglandin, through action on its receptors, starts a process that is self-perpetuating, so that changes in tone and spontaneous activity of the muscle will develop slowly. There is no effect mediated through nerves. Primarily the effect of prostaglandin on smooth muscle is to increase tone, possibly by releasing intracellular calcium, and also by changing the membrane potential of cells.

Van Mastrigt: So that it would be more likely to increase the intrinsic instability of the muscle than to stimulate it?

Andersson: Yes.

Kirby: I thought there was some effect of prostaglandins on the sensory innervation of the bladder as well.

There is still a need for an agent that activates an acontractile bladder and I wonder whether we ought to go back and take another look at some of the prostaglandin work in the clinical sense.

Andersson: I think it has been shown that prostaglandins are able to increase the firing rate in sensory afferents and this may very well be the mechanism by which they waken activity in the reflex arc. These atonic bladders do not have any activity maintained through the bladder reflex, but if afferent input could be increased there would then be activity in the reflex arc and there could be increased tone in the bladder and it would also be possible to empty it.

If prostaglandins are instilled through the bladder that would always increase tension in the bladder wall, and any increase in tension in the bladder wall will per se influence activity in the mechanoreceptors. So there are two methods. If tension in the muscle is increased, or the sensitivity to the effects of peptide, for example, released from sensory nerves, there will then be two possibilities for influencing activity in the efferent reflex arc. And that is perfectly possible. We know that reflex micturition can return when it has been absent for several years.

Warrell: In healthy, nulliparous women with normal urinary control the bladder neck is normally closed. In the various continence mechanisms Dr Kulseng-

Hanssen has described, which are largely in the urethra, he did not try to explain this. Is this something intrinsic in the muscle which comprises the bladder and the urethra, or is it due to the periurethral structures such as Dr DeLancey has described?

Also, Dr Kulseng-Hanssen showed in one of his slides that when the striated muscle of the urethra was paralysed by blocking the pudendal nerve, there were still intraurethral pressure variations. He suggested this might be due to a sphincter effect exerted by the smooth muscle. Is he satisfied enough about his EMG? An alternative explanation would be that this is the activity of the striated muscle which is supplied directly from the pelvic nerves. In other words, if one thinks that the striated muscle has two nerve supplies, it might still be feasible to block some of the activity by blocking the pudendal nerve. Was he satisfied that the EMG was completely silent: in other words that the remaining striated muscle with its other nerve supply was not giving some sort of sphincter activity?

Kulseng-Hanssen: The second question first. The EMG activity before the block showed a good correlation between urethral pressure and EMG activity. After the block EMG activity was silent. It is not reasonable that striated muscle should cause these urethral pressure variations. Why should another innervation show striated muscle activity that is not reflected in the EMG? I cannot understand it.

Warrell: I accept what Dr Kulseng-Hanssen is saying. I am trying to highlight a very real problem which is that the various neurophysiological experiments suggest that the pudendal nerve is the dominant nerve in the supply to the striated muscle, and the anatomical experience suggests there may be a twin supply. Dr Kulseng-Hanssen suggests that in fact the striated muscle is heavily dependent on the pudendal nerve for its innervation.

Kulseng-Hanssen: I agree.

Warrell: What keeps the bladder neck closed?

Kulseng-Hanssen: It has been shown that the bladder neck can be open in "normal" patients.

Warrell: I do not think it has been shown to be open in healthy nulliparous women.

Kulseng-Hanssen: Very well: I believe it is closed by the smooth muscle and possibly by DeLancey's mechanism with the action of the levator ani muscle. But if we look at the urethra, why should there be a separate closure mechanism for the most proximal part of the urethra? When I look at the urethra it is a continuous smooth muscle and a continuous striated muscle. Why should anyone say there is a separate mechanism via the bladder? I do not think that there is.

Warrell: I suppose because we cannot measure it. In other words, if we measure the occlusive forces at the bladder neck, they are really very weak compared with the urethra.

Versi: May I answer Mr Warrell's point? We have looked at about 200 women during the climacteric, some of them nulliparous and some of them multiparous, but all of them continent. Of these 50% had an incompetent bladder neck on videography.

Dr Janez has used an electrical conductance test to look at a broader age range of women and they concur with our findings around the climacteric that the bladder neck is incompetent in about 50%. With younger women it is competent, but with older women the figure is up to 78%. So there is evidence to suggest that the bladder neck competence deteriorates with age.

It is said that after the menopause urethral pressures deteriorate. We would agree with that. We find many significant negative correlations between menopausal age and urethral pressures. But the problem again arises as to whether this is due to age or oestrogen deficiency. When we have looked at this problem with partial correlations, namely allowing for age and just looking at the effect of menopausal age, most of these correlations disappear statistically. So it is really an age issue more than a hormonal issue.

Mundy: How was the EMG in the urethral fluctuation study recorded?

Kulseng-Hanssen: I had a concentric needle which I placed at 12 o'clock over the external meatus and at an angle to the midline, and then I cannot pick up anything other than the striated muscle in the urethra.

Mundy: When I stimulate the pelvic nerves electrically at operation, there is a rise of urethral pressure. Then various pharmacological manipulations, such as blocking that effect by neuromuscular blockade, suggest to me that there is an innervation from above, which would go against what Dr Kulseng-Hanssen is saying. It is difficult to get a compatible answer between the two.

If the neurovascular bundles alongside the prostate in males and the equivalent nerves in females are picked up and stimulated electrically, there will be a rise in midurethral pressure which can be blocked by neuromuscular blockade. This would suggest that there is an innervation to what could be described as the intrinsic rhabdosphincter running in from above.

Kulseng-Hanssen: Could that not be smooth muscle?

Mundy: I did this work with Brindley who used various pharmacological methods. I am not sure of the pharmacological details, but he was quite happy that this was an innervation of the intrinsic rhabdosphincter from above.

But Dr Kulseng-Hanssen's evidence seems to be directly contradictory to that, which is confusing.

DeLancey: There is an anatomical point that would explain the divergence of these two observations.

A number of years ago people did some pudendal blocks and mixed Hypaque with the anaesthetic so that it could be seen on a radiograph. The pudendal block actually bathes many of the sacral roots. It does not block just the pudendal nerve. The area of distribution of the pudendal block shown in their radiographic studies goes all the way up to the sacral foramen in some instances, and so a pudendal nerve block might have the ability to block both the pudendal nerve and also the autonomic fibres that come from the nervi erigentes. So it may not be as specific as we think in blocking only the pudendal nerve itself.

Mundy: Is there any relation of that observation to the volume injected? Is there a critical volume above which spread will occur and below which it will not?

DeLancey: They used, as I remember, 10 ml on each side. I do not know that anybody has correlated the volume of injection with how far it goes.

Cardozo: It is not just the volume; it is the medium. People have used different media for injecting local anaesthetic to see if they can get it to go less far.

Mundy: In other words, no direct conclusion can be made from a pudendal block unless there is some other corroborative evidence to show that other nerves have not been involved. How would one do that?

DeLancey: I suppose one could try to inject further down in Alcock's canal; come from the spine just below the crease in the vagina down between Alcock's canal and the perineal membrane and it might be possible to hit it there without as much spread.

Mundy: If a pudendal block involved the nervi erigentes, could one pick up abnormalities of sensory distribution in the lower limbs that would show whether or not such spread had occurred?

DeLancey: There are people who have temporary paralysis of a portion of their leg muscle after a pudendal nerve block so it does influence some of the lower leg motor function, and I would assume the sensory function as well. But that would not always be an effect of the block.

Kirby: I would have made the same point about the spread of local anaesthetic from a pudendal nerve block.
    Another piece of evidence in the male is that if one takes great care to spare the nerves coming down behind and underneath the prostate, which are probably the terminal extensions of the pelvic parasympathetic nerves, and then does an EMG on the urethral sphincter a few months later, the urethral sphincter EMG is normal. But if no effort is made to spare them, or if they are deliberately sacrificed, and a urethral sphincter EMG is done subsequently, there are neuropathic motor potentials. The whole sphincter is not completely denervated but

there are neuropathic motor potentials. That seems to suggest that those nerves carry at least some innervation to the striated muscle of the urethral sphincter.

Mundy: And in the female?

Kirby: I have not done the study in the female, but it could be done.

Mundy: These are radical prostatectomy patients. I have done cystectomy and substitution cystoplasty in both male and female patients, and if those nodes are preserved then the patient will be continent and – if male – potent.

   If the nerves remain undamaged they are continent, and if the nerves are damaged they are incontinent. It is as simple as that.

Kirby: After the pudendal nerve block, I agree that EMG activity seemed to diminish and urethral pressure fell. It did not look to me on that slide as though there was electrical silence. There was still some EMG activity there.

Kulseng-Hanssen: But is it possible to get it quite silent?

Kirby: It is with deep general anaesthesia, and neuromuscular paralysis. We have done it in patients.

Kulseng-Hanssen: I have done it with general anaesthesia too, with a concentric neuromuscular blocker, and one sees some activity there.

Kirby: I agree it is very difficult to block. We have done it on only one or two because there did not seem to be much point in doing it.

   With light general anaesthesia I agree that the activity is still there, but with deep curare it disappears.

Kulseng-Hanssen: It may be that they have not been given enough blocker. It has been shown that when the patient stopped breathing due to a blocker the striated muscle in the pelvic floor was still active.

Kirby: In a sense one could differentiate between the pelvic nerves and the pudendal nerves. Assuming the pudendal nerve block is selective, if one first did a pudendal block and then an epidural block or a caudal block, where the whole of the S234 is not blocked, and saw a further reduction, that would be evidence perhaps that at least some of the innervation is coming down from the pelvic nerves rather than all through the pudendal nerve.

Andersson: A comment on the intrinsic sphincter mechanism at the bladder neck.
   The fact that no muscular structure can be found to explain the sphincter func-

tion does not exclude it. There is marked regional variation in innervation; peptidergic innervation for example is concentrated around the bladder neck. I do not know what it means but it might have some implications for sphincter function.

In both males and females there is a concentration of peptidergic nerves around the ureteric orifices and also at the internal meatus. That says nothing about a change in function, but there are morphological differences between the bladder and the urethra.

DeLancey: The controversy about the internal sphincter in the female has gone on for many years and we shall not solve it today. But there is a recognisable, definable layer at the vesical neck, separate from the detrusor musculature, which is circular around the urethra. So there is a morphological structure, whatever people call it, the trigonal ring or the internal sphincter, which is quite easily seen on serial sections.

I was curious about the urinary trigone in phentolamine blocks and atropine blocks: you commented that each diminished the contractility by roughly half. Was this the full thickness?

Kulseng-Hanssen: No. It is the superficial trigone.

DeLancey: Just the superficial trigone? The musculature that encircles the bladder neck is continuous with trigonal musculature. It is identical in appearance, and I would guess probably behaves the same way.

Kulseng-Hanssen: They separated the superficial trigone from the deep one.

Hilton: If I might change the subject slightly and move over to the question of urethral pressure variations.

As Dr Kulseng-Hanssen's own work has pointed out, my work has confirmed, and Ms Cardozo and Mr Versi have also shown, perfectly normally continent patients show urethral pressure variations of considerable magnitude in perhaps 50% or so of normal continent women. Without getting into the argument as to which aspect of morphology may contribute to those variations, do these variations have any role as far as continence is concerned? Alternatively, do they have a role as far as the development of incontinence is concerned?

Kulseng-Hanssen: I do not know if they have any role. Possibly. It is much more difficult to make a biological system that keeps pressure at the same level.

Versi: I can understand the idea of a servomechanism which would correct to the pressure that was wanted. But clearly there are some people who have an abnormally large variation and therein may lie pathology.

Van Mastrigt: But this is obviously not a servomechanism.

Versi: It is the failure of that mechanism perhaps.

Hilton: But why should it fail in such a large proportion of the normal continent population?

Van Mastrigt: To me it seems more likely that it is not a servomechanism, because there is no input to the system. This is just some kind of intrinsic instability in the muscle.

Stanton: I will sum up.

Despite Dr Delancey's elegant lecture, there still seems to be a measure of controversy about which are the constituent muscles of the intrinsic musculature of the urethra, and I note that one of Dr Kulseng-Hanssen's slides did seem to show these layers fairly distinctly.

In relation to that, my attention has been drawn to an article in the *British Journal of Urology*, October 1989, by Chapple [1] and others, showing that in asymptomatic nulliparous women 20% have an open bladder neck as defined by ultrasound; that is within the normal, continent population.

One of Dr Swash's many contributions to the session was the enforcement of the notion that continence is produced by a kinking rather than a squeezing mechanism. This is perhaps a simplistic view of looking at it, but I suspect this is the way in which many of our operations do work.

The lecture by Professor Andersson emphasised the importance of the inter-dependence of neurotransmitters and how we cannot think just of a simple system of adrenergics or cholinergics any longer. It is a lot more complex in terms of the neurotransmitters and in terms of the relationship of these transmitters and their receptors at bladder level.

Finally, Dr Kulseng-Hanssen's talk on the continence mechanism emphasised not only the importance of the relationship of the detrusor to the urethra being seen as one functional unit (even though we tend to talk of them as two separate items), but also that we are still fairly divided as to what maintains continence. To my mind the mid-urethral zone, the main pressurised area, is the main mechanism, with the bladder neck perhaps the first mechanism to go but by no means the major mechanism.

Reference

1. Chapple CR, Helm CW, Blease S, Milroy EJG, Rickards D, Osborne JL. Asymptomatic bladder neck incompetence in nulliparous females. Br J Urol 1989; 64:357–60.

Section II
Investigation

Chapter 5

Application of Animal and Physical Models to Human Cystometry

R. van Mastrigt

Introduction

The purpose of the urinary system is to store as much urine as possible, and to expel it completely at will. From an evolutionary point of view it may also have been important to expel urine as fast as possible. Under physiological circumstances it would therefore seem sufficient to quantify the capacity of the urinary bladder and the volume of residual urine left after micturition (and perhaps the amount of time necessary to evacuate the bladder) to characterise completely the functioning of the urinary system. These parameters may be called *Physiological Parameters*.

In case of dysfunction of the system more parameters are necessary to accurately and completely describe the degree of dysfunction of the system. For instance in the case of involuntary urine loss in the storage phase the amount of lost urine, or the frequency of losses form such additional parameters. These parameters are *Symptomatic Parameters* that objectively quantify the degree of dysfunction of the system.

Curing dysfunction of the urinary system requires information on the cause of the dysfunction. If this information takes the form of objective quantitative parameters these may be called *Diagnostic Parameters*.

The purpose of urodynamic investigation is to apply procedures that yield parameters on which a diagnosis and treatment can be based. From the above it will be clear that only diagnostic parameters can be used to this end. In many cases urodynamic procedures yield parameters that are not diagnostic parameters, but symptomatic parameters at best. The maximum urinary flow measured in the bladder evacuation phase is an example of such a parameter. It quantifies the (possible) degree of dysfunction of the urinary system, but it does not give an indication of the cause of the dysfunction. A diagnosis cannot be based on it. In order to develop methods to derive diagnostic parameters on which diagnosis can be based it is necessary to understand the functioning and dysfunctioning of the system. Models can be used to this end. In this chapter such models will be described. From the models, propositions for diagnostic parameters and methods to calculate these will be derived. In the limited scope of this chapter only models and parameters applying to the evacuation phase of the micturition cycle will be discussed.

The Urinary System in the Evacuation Phase

In the evacuation phase of the micturition cycle, the urinary bladder functions as a pump that forces urine through the urethra, i.e. the bladder generates pressure, and this pressure causes a flow of urine, at a certain flow rate, through the urethra. It is tempting to think that the flow rate is thus determined by the urethra and pressure is caused by the bladder so that (perhaps maximum) flow rate and detrusor pressure are diagnostic parameters that describe the properties of urethra and bladder. This is not the case. The pressure in the urinary bladder is not a constant pressure, but depends among others on the flow rate again. As with any pump, at increasing flow rate, the pressure that the bladder can generate decreases. A relationship exists between pressure generated by the bladder and the flow rate it produces. This relationship will be described in more detail later, but is an essential property of the urinary bladder called *contractility* which can be quantified in such a way that it forms a diagnostic parameter. The urethra, on the other hand, does not accommodate one flow rate at one given pressure head, but yields a different flow rate for each pressure head applied. That is, the essential property of the urethra is its relation between pressure and flow rate, called the *urethral resistance relation*. Again, this urethral resistance relation can be quantified in such a way that it forms a diagnostic parameter. Fig. 5.1 illustrates in one graph the contractility relation characterising detrusor properties and the urethral resistance relation characterising urethral properties. During micturition both properties or relations interact [1] (shown in Fig. 5.1 by projecting one on top of the other). The intersection of both curves determines the actual flow rate and pressure at which micturition takes place.

If the bladder contractility relation and the urethral resistance relation did not change during the act of micturition, one constant detrusor pressure and one constant flow rate throughout micturition would result. We know this to be untrue. Both relations change dramatically during micturition. First, the bladder contractility changes as a result of the emptying of the bladder, which causes shortening of the bladder wall. But also both the bladder contractility and the urethral resistance change as a result of varying stimulation. The relations shown in Fig. 5.1, therefore, should be understood as the intrinsic properties of bladder and urethra at maximum stimulation of the bladder and maximum relaxation of the urethra. In the following sections the properties of bladder and urethra will be separately described in terms of simple models. As the urinary bladder can be thought of

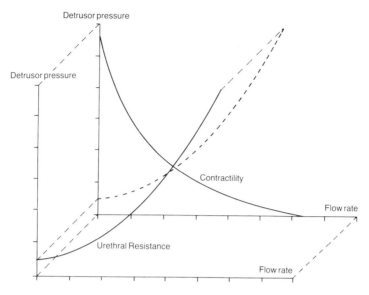

Fig. 5.1. The interaction of the detrusor contractility relation and the urethral resistance relation during micturition. The intersection of both curves determines the detrusor pressure and flow rate at which voiding takes place.

as a hollow spherical organ with a smooth muscular wall, the properties of this wall will be analysed first, before attempting to model the behaviour of the complete bladder.

Modelling the Properties of the Bladder Wall

The bladder wall consists mainly of smooth muscle, and shows both passive and active properties, the latter being those that require energy input from metabolic processes. A widespread and very simple model for striated muscle was published by Hill [2] in 1938. Fig. 5.2 shows a schematic representation of the model, consisting of a contractile element (CE), a series elastic element (SE) and a parallel elastic element (PE). This model has been successfully applied to describe the properties of strips of bladder wall muscle [3,4]. In the model the parallel elastic element describes passive properties of the (bladder wall) muscle. These passive properties do not play an important role in the evacuation phase of the micturition cycle. Furthermore, detailed analysis of these passive properties shows that a much more complicated viscoelastic model consisting of at least four non-linear elastic elements and three non-linear viscous elements is necessary to model these properties adequately [5]. As it was found that passive and active properties are additive [6], a model consisting only of the CE and SE elements can be applied to the active properties of the bladder wall only by subtracting an estimate for the passive force from the actively generated force. The force immediately before stimulation of the muscle can be used to this end.

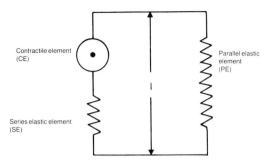

Fig. 5.2. The Hill model for striated muscle.

Properties of the Contractile Element (CE)

The contractile element CE in the model shown in Fig. 5.2 is an element that is thought to shorten upon stimulation. Three variables are of importance in characterising this shortening behaviour: the force opposing the shortening, the length of the muscle, and the rate at which shortening occurs. In the original publication [2] it was concluded on the basis of heat measurements that a hyperbolic relation exists between the rate of shortening and the force exerted by the muscle. Numerous measurements on all muscle types have confirmed that indeed such a relation describes the shortening behaviour of muscle. Fig. 5.3 shows an example of the force–velocity relationship measured on a strip of pig urinary bladder wall [7,8]. The more-detailed models describing muscle contraction on the basis of cross-bridge interaction between actin and myosin filaments developed later [9] can be shown to yield a force–velocity relation which is mathematically differently formulated, but approximates a hyperbola very closely [10]. Such a hyperbolic force–velocity relation is characterised by three parameters: F_0, the intercept with the force axis, or the maximum isometric force the muscle can bear; v_{max}, the intercept with the velocity axis, or the maximum (unloaded) contraction velocity; and aF_0^{-1}, the degree of curvature of the hyperbola. For urinary bladder muscle and many other types of muscle aF_0^{-1} is generally found to be a constant of approximately 0.25 [4,11,12] so that two parameters, F_0 and v_{max} completely characterise the relation between force and shortening velocity of this muscle. Both variables depend severely on the length of the muscle. Fig. 5.4 illustrates the dependence of F_0 on (pig bladder) muscle length, showing a clear optimum "working length" of the muscle, and v_{max} shows a similar length dependence. In striated muscle these length dependencies are explained by varying degrees of overlap of the actin and myosin filaments, which directly influence the number of cross-bridges that can be formed. For smooth muscle a similar mechanism has been proposed, but since a regular filament arrangement is lacking in this type of muscle, there is no basis for such a mechanism. Indeed a length-dependent activation of smooth muscle has been proposed to account for the observed length dependencies [13,14]. Apart from their dependence on length, F_0 and v_{max} also depend on the degree of activation of the muscle. In an inactive muscle, both F_0 and v_{max} are zero, and during the onset of stimulation both parameters somehow increase to a maximum that is maintained for some time

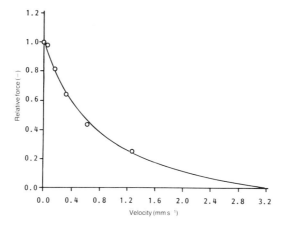

Fig. 5.3. The force–velocity relationship, defining the contractile element (CE) in the model shown in Fig. 5.2. Relationship measured on strips of pig urinary bladder smooth muscle.

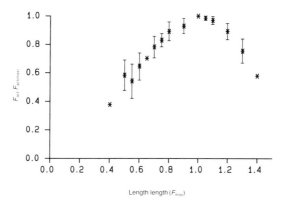

Fig. 5.4. The length dependence of the maximum isometric force F_0, or the intercept of the force–velocity relationship shown in Fig. 5.3 on the force axis as a function of muscle length. Data measured on pig urinary smooth muscle.

depending on stimulus conditions. It is this maximum that is representative for the (myogenic) contractile properties of the muscle. Muscle activation is further discussed on p. 64.

Properties of the Series Elastic Element (SE)

In the model shown in Fig. 5.2, force is developed during an isometric contraction by the shortening of the contractile element which causes stretching of the series elasticity. In this model the series elasticity is symbolised as one discrete elastic element. If this element could be characterised by an unchanging relation between length and force then the shortening of the contractile element could be calculated during isometric contractions and the force–velocity relationship characterising the contractile element CE could be derived from such isometric contractions (for each force the length of the series elasticity could be calculated, so with changing force a changing length would be obtained, which is a velocity). In effect methods have been proposed for estimating smooth muscle contractility from isometric contractions in this way, or involving part of isometric contractions [15–17]. Unfortunately the series elasticity of (smooth) muscle is not discrete, but distributed throughout the muscle. To a large degree it is found in the cross-bridges themselves [18,19]. As a consequence the stiffness of the muscle (or its series elasticity) is roughly proportional to the force developed by the muscle and it is not possible to derive the properties of the contractile element from isometric contractions.

The Activation of Bladder Wall Muscle During Isometric Contractions

As an alternative, it was investigated whether the time course of (isometric) force development is related to contractile properties at all. Phase plots form an attractive approach for the detailed analysis of this time course [20]. Fig. 5.5 shows the isometric force development resulting from electrical field stimulation in a strip of bladder wall muscle. Fig. 5.6 shows a phase plot calculated from these data, i.e. a plot of the rate of change of force as a function of force itself. Such a plot is dominated by a straight line, the slope of which characterises the limiting rate constant of force development, i.e. a characteristic time interval, that represents the slowest process involved in the development of force in this muscle type. It was found that this time constant was fairly constant even under extreme circumstances such as reduction of extracellular calcium as shown in Fig. 5.7, and it was concluded that it was probably related to the process of intracellular calcium release [7] i.e. related to the "activation" of the contractile element CE in Fig. 5.2, and not to its shortening behaviour.

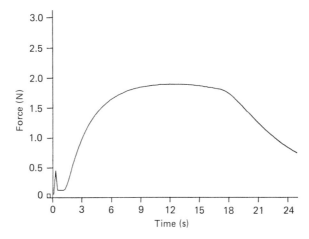

Fig. 5.5. An isometric contraction of an electrically stimulated strip of pig urinary bladder smooth muscle.

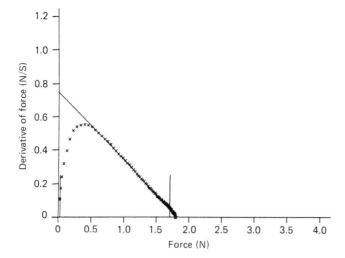

Fig. 5.6. A phase plot of the data shown in Fig. 5.5. The rate of change of force is plotted as a function of force itself. The crosses represent the calculated data, the straight line was fitted to these data. The two short vertical lines indicate the moments of switching on and off the electrical stimulation.

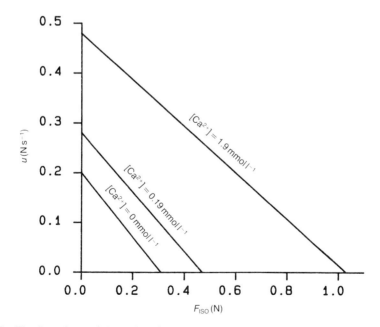

Fig. 5.7. The dependence of the straight line part in phase plots of isometric contractions measured on pig urinary bladder smooth muscle strips on the extracellular calcium level. This straight line characterises the limiting rate constant in muscle activation.

Active Properties of the Complete Urinary Bladder

The urinary bladder can be roughly described as a sphere constructed from smooth muscle tissue. The properties of this tissue were described above in terms of the variables length, contraction velocity and force. In the total bladder the equivalent variables are volume, flow rate and pressure. If shortening of the bladder wall is assumed to be uniform, the relevant muscle length to be taken into account in the case of complete bladder emptying is the circumference of the bladder. On this basis the contraction velocity of the wall can be calculated from flow rate using a simple geometric relationship [21]. Similarly force (being taken as the total force acting around the bladder circumference) can be related to the pressure in the bladder lumen [4]. It follows that from flow rate and pressure, measured during micturition, the contraction velocity and force of the bladder wall can be calculated, or, alternatively, that the force–velocity relationship of the bladder wall muscle is reflected in the "contractility" relation between detrusor pressure and flow rate as shown in Fig. 5.1. Fig. 5.8 shows such a relation measured on a complete urinary bladder. As detrusor pressure and bladder wall force are linearly related, the normalised force (i.e. force at a certain shortening velocity divided by maximum isometric force) plotted on the vertical axis equals a similar normalised pressure.

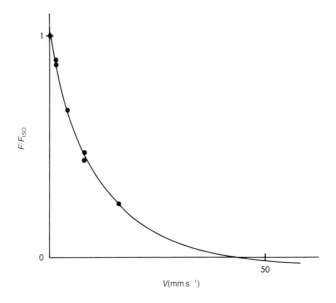

Fig. 5.8.   The force–velocity relationship of bladder wall muscle calculated from measurements of pressure and flow rate made on complete pig urinary bladder in vitro.

Practical Methods for Estimating Contractility

Estimating Contractility from Detrusor Pressure Alone

If the series elasticity of smooth muscle formed a constant, i.e. obeyed one unchanging relation between its length and force, it would be possible to calculate properties of the contractile element from the time course of the development of isometric force or pressure in the urinary bladder. Unfortunately, as described above this is not the case. Alternatively, it was shown by phase plot analysis that isometric force development in vitro is related to activation of the contractile element rather than its shortening. In phase plots made from clinically measured isometric contractions, i.e. the detrusor pressure rise before the onset of micturition, a straight line part is much more difficult to recognise (Fig. 5.9), than in phase plots from isometric contractions measured in vitro (Fig. 5.6). By fitting a straight line with preset slope to such "clinical" phase plots, a parameter (U) was obtained that was normalised by dividing it by the bladder circumference [22]. The normalised parameter Ul^{-1} was extensively evaluated, by including it in a computer program (CLIM) which is used for the storage and analysis of urodynamic data in several academic urodynamic centres [23–25]. It was concluded that the parameter Ul^{-1} derived from phase plots of the isometric detrusor pressure rise before the onset of micturition is biased by the urethral opening pressure to such a degree, that it can be used as a measure for the degree of obstruction. This application will be further discussed below. Here it must be concluded that under clinical circumstances the information in the isometric development of pressure in the urinary bladder before the onset of micturition might be very useful, but not with respect to measuring contractility.

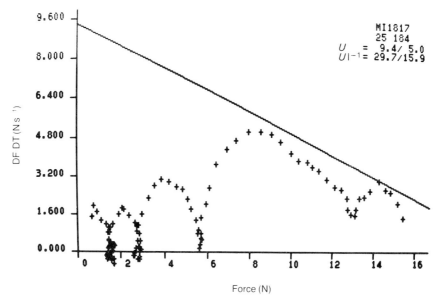

Fig. 5.9. An example of a phase plot of the isometric detrusor pressure rise before the onset of micturition.

Estimating Contractility from Pressure-Flow Studies

Fig. 5.10 shows a plot of detrusor pressure as a function of contraction velocity as calculated from flow rate during micturition. The illustration is certainly not a typical one; in this measurement, a rapid fluctuation in the urethral resistance relationship caused part of the force–velocity relation to be traced out. (See Fig. 5.1, if the urethral resistance relation changes while the contractility relation remains constant, the intersection of both curves will shift along the latter.) In a retrospective study on 2073 micturitions this was the case with 241 measurements or approximately 12% [26]. To these 241 measurements a hyperbolic force–velocity relation with preset curvature aP_0^{-1} could be fitted to yield the parameters P_0 and v_{max} (Fig. 5.11). It was found in this study that P_0 and v_{max} were not correlated, i.e. these parameters form two independent measures of different aspects of contractility.

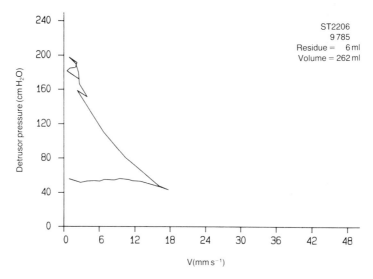

Fig. 5.10. Detrusor pressure as a function of bladder wall contraction velocity as calculated from flow rate during micturition. A non-typical example out of a subpopulation of 12% of pressure flow studies that trace part of the force–velocity relationship of contracting muscle.

In the test population of 241 measurements it was found that an experimental relationship could be established between P_0 and a number of other variables such as the maximum pressure during micturition, the pressure during maximum flow, the maximum wall contraction velocity during micturition, and the bladder volume before micturition. Fig. 5.12 shows a comparison of an estimate for P_0, called P_{est}, calculated from this relationship and the real P_0, showing a very good correlation indeed (Spearman's rank correlation coefficient 0.73). By calculating a hyperbolic relation with $aP_0^{-1} = 0.25$ through P_{est} and the point in the pressure–velocity data with the highest velocity value or the rightmost point in Fig. 5.10, an approximation of the "real" pressure or force–velocity curve can be obtained. The intersection of this approximated curve with the velocity axis forms an estimated maximum contraction velocity called v_{est}. Fig. 5.13 shows

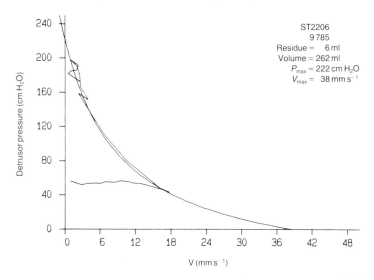

Fig. 5.11. The data in Fig. 5.10 fitted with a hyperbola with preset curvature $aP_0^{-1} = 0.25$.

a scatter plot of v_{est} and the "true" v_{max} for the test population of 241 measurements, indicating a good correlation (Spearman's rank correlation coefficient 0.69). The importance of this method for estimating v_{max} is that the estimation process can be performed on any pressure–flow study, and not just on those 12% that allow fitting of the pressure–velocity relation. The described procedure thus forms a practical method for separately estimating the two parameters, P_0 and v_{max}, that describe the two different aspects of contractility.

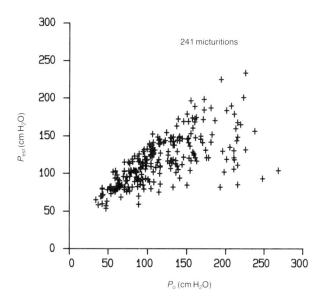

Fig. 5.12. A comparison of the contractility parameter P_0 and P_{est} an estimate for P_0 derived from other variables (see text) for 241 micturition studies as shown in Fig. 5.10.

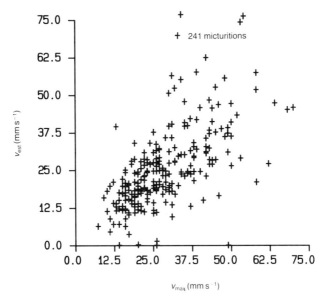

Fig. 5.13. A comparison of the estimated maximum contraction velocity v_{est} and the "true" parameter v_{max} for 241 micturition studies as shown in Fig. 5.10. v_{est} is based on a calculated hyperbolic curve through P_{est} and the maximum contraction velocity in the pressure–velocity data.

As an alternative a method was developed that allows calculation of one combined index of contractility, i.e. one parameter that combines the information in the parameters P_0 and v_{max}. This parameter has the dimension of a power per (bladder wall) surface area and is in fact the maximum of a variable that can be calculated from detrusor pressure and contraction velocity throughout micturition to represent contraction strength. Power itself is not a useful variable to represent contraction strength as it is zero for zero pressure or zero flow rate. As a consequence, the power in a very high isometric contraction is zero, as is the power in a voiding with high flow rate at (almost) zero pressure, which is often seen in normal females. The proposed variable, w, overcomes this problem as it contains additive terms based on Hill's equation that make it non-zero if either flow rate or detrusor pressure is non-zero [21]. Fig. 5.14 shows an example of the calculated variable w as a function of bladder volume during bladder emptying. In the normal case w slowly rises on bladder emptying as a result of the length dependence of P_0 and v_{max}. In case of a failing voiding, w decreases prematurely, as shown in Fig. 5.15, leaving residual urine. The maximum of w during bladder emptying can be taken as a parameter of contractility; w_{max} equals the product of P_0 with v_{max} and a constant.

It is concluded from this section, that bladder function in the evacuation phase is completely characterised by the force or pressure velocity relationship which is determined by the parameters P_0 (isometric pressure) and v_{max} (maximum contraction velocity). A method for estimating these from pressure–flow studies has been described. Also a parameter (w_{max}) can be derived that combines both aspects of contractility into one parameter. It is not possible to derive these parameters from isometric contractions. Examples of practical application of the discussed parameters are given on p. 74.

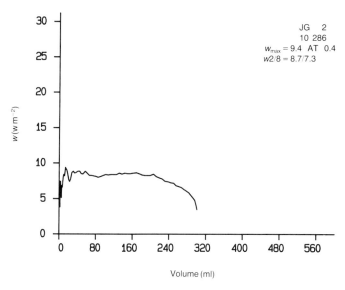

Fig. 5.14. Detrusor contraction strength quantified by the variable w as a function of bladder volume during normal micturition.

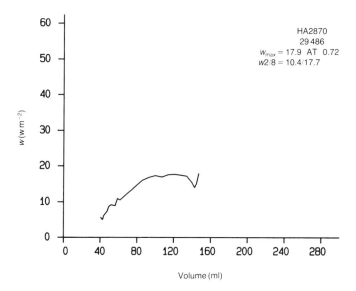

Fig. 5.15. Detrusor contraction strength quantified by the variable w as a function of bladder volume during failing voiding, leaving residual urine.

Practical Methods for Estimating Urethral Resistance

The urethra can be adequately characterised by its relation between flow rate and pressure. Fig. 5.16 shows an example of a plot of flow rate against pressure for a normal, unobstructed voiding. Such a relation results both from passive and active properties of the urethra and surrounding structures and musculature. In contrast to the bladder, where active properties dominate in the evacuation phase, the passive properties of the urethra, being simple elasticity, dominate its voiding behaviour in the ideal case. These properties can be described with a quadratic relation between pressure and flow rate, i.e. a parabolic curve that intercepts the pressure axis at a certain minimum pressure, required for "opening" the urethra [1,27,28]. Active properties of the urethra (partial) contractions of the musculature, yield pressure increases that are added to the passive pressure at a certain flow rate, so that for a quantitative description of urethral properties a quadratic relation should be fitted to the lowest part of the data in the pressure–flow rate plot. Fig. 5.17 shows an example of such fitting. In case of urethral obstruction, the data and fitted quadratic curve shift considerably in the vertical direction, and also the curve is "steeper", as illustrated in Fig. 5.18. The quadratic relation is characterised by two parameters, its intercept on the pressure axis, and its curvature. Experimentally it was established that a group-specific relation exists between these two parameters, i.e. that steeper curves generally also intercept the pressure axis at a higher value. This means that within a group of patients (e.g. adult patients) the urethral resistance can be characterised with one parameter only. This one parameter can simply be calculated from one representative point in the pressure–flow data, for instance the point of maximum flow. Arbitrarily the intercept on the pressure axis was chosen as the one representative parameter (URA) [27].

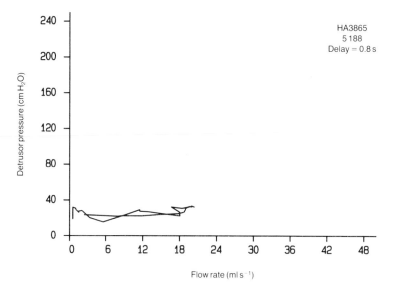

Fig. 5.16. Detrusor pressure as a function of flow rate during voiding of a normal, unobstructed subject.

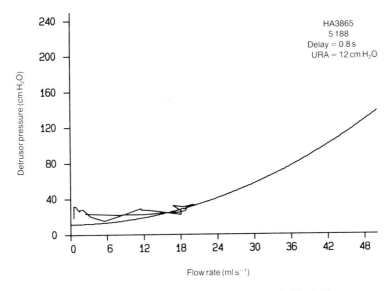

Fig. 5.17. A quadratic curve fitted to the data shown in Fig. 5.16.

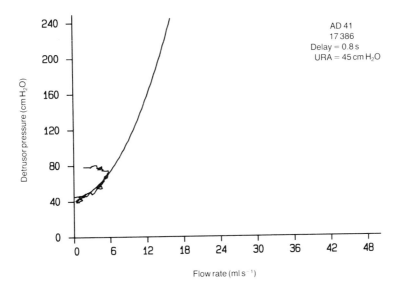

Fig. 5.18. A quadratic curve fitted to a plot of detrusor pressure as a function of flow rate measured during voiding of a patient showing urethral obstruction resulting from benign prostatic hyperplasia.

In a purely practical sense, another parameter can be used for characterising urethral resistance. Earlier it was noted that the parameter Ul^{-1}, derived from phase plots of the isometric pressure rise before the onset of micturition is biased by the urethral opening pressure to such a degree that it can be used as an obstruction parameter. Figure 5.19 shows the frequency distributions of the parameter

Ul^{-1} for groups of obstructed and unobstructed patients of mixed pathology, both male and female. The groups were discriminated on the basis of the pressure–flow relationship [29]. Although the parameter Ul^{-1} is based on pressure data only, both groups can be separated clearly using this parameter, the use of a critical value of 57 would yield both a sensitivity (chance of correctly identifying a diseased subject) and a specificity (chance of correctly identifying a healthy subject) of 92%.

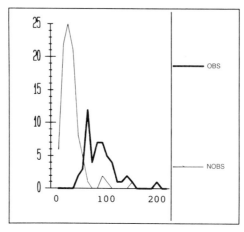

Fig. 5.19.   The frequency distribution of the parameter Ul^{-1} for groups of obstructed (——) and unobstructed (——) adult patients of mixed pathology.

Examples of Application of Contractility and Urethral Resistance Parameters

A computer program (CLIM [23–25]) was developed that allows the interactive storage of detrusor pressure events, such as contractions, and pressure-flow studies in a database, and an interactive graphical analysis immediately following the urodynamic investigation, yielding the described parameters. The program is used in a number of academic centres. The results of two series of measurements will be briefly described and summarised here.

In the first series 22 patients in whom transurethral resection of the prostate was indicated on the basis of conventional diagnosis were evaluated before and after surgical treatment [30,31]. Patients were suprapubically punctured and their bladders were filled three times in succession. Detrusor pressure and flow rate signals during voiding, as well as the isometric detrusor pressure rise just before flow started, were stored as described. In subsequent analysis, the conventional, symptomatic parameters Q_{max} (maximum flow) and $p(Q_{max})$ (detrusor pressure at maximum flow) and the discussed diagnostic parameters Ul^{-1}, URA and w_{max} were evaluated. Both preoperatively and postoperatively patients were divided into obstructed and non-obstructed groups on the basis of randomised inspection of pressure-flow plots. Table 5.1 shows, that for all parameters there was a significant difference between the average values for the unobstructed and obstructed groups. On the basis of an average value for each patient the parameters Ul^{-1} and URA performed best in discriminating both groups. Using a discrimination value of 54 $W m^{-2}$ sensitivity and specificity of Ul^{-1} were 100% and 95% respectively, whereas URA yielded 94% and 100% using a discrimination level of 29 cm H_2O. By combining both parameters the limited set of obstructed and unobstructed patients could be discriminated with 100% sensitivity and 100% specificity, i.e. without any misclassifications. Fig. 5.20 shows a scatterplot of URA and Ul^{-1} with each patient represented by an N (for non-obstructed) or O (for obstructed) and the optimal linear discrimination function separating both groups. This function was constructed interactively using the ISPAHAN [32] program for statistical pattern recognition.

Postoperatively patients were divided into two groups, one with average residual urine exceeding 50 ml, the other with average residual urine less than 50 ml. Preoperatively, patients in the group with significant postoperative residual urine had a significantly lower w_{max} and $p(Q_{max})$ as shown in Table 5.2. w_{max} allows the optimal discrimination of such patients preoperatively: at a discrimination level of 10.85 $W m^{-2}$ a sensitivity of 100% and a specificity of 72% were obtained. From these data it can be concluded that both Ul^{-1} and URA are reliable parameters for detecting obstruction and that w_{max} characterises urinary bladder contractility. If this contractility parameter is low preoperatively then there is a predictable risk of significant residual urine postoperatively.

The second series of measurements was the series of 241 pressure–flow studies selected from 2073 micturitions which was discussed on p. 68 [26]. Using the urethral resistance parameter URA and a discrimination value for this parameter of 28.5 cm H_2O [33] the 241 measurements were split into 66 measurements from obstructed and 175 from unobstructed patients. Differences between parameter values for both groups were tested for significance using the Mann–Whitney U-test. In a first approximation no difference in contractility between measurements from obstructed and non-obstructed patients would be expected. To complicate matters, patients' bladders and thus their contractility may be changed secondary to the obstruction. Table 5.3 shows that there was no significant difference in v_{max} between the two groups, and this lack of difference was faithfully reflected in the estimated parameter v_{est}. P_0 was significantly lower in the unobstructed group, and this was reflected in w_{max} (which combines P_0 and v_{max}). Table 5.3 thus shows that v_{max} (and its estimation v_{est}) and P_0 carry different information which is combined in w_{max}.

The group of 175 measurements from unobstructed patients was further split into 38 micturitions with residual volume larger than or equal to 50 ml, and 137 micturitions with residual volume less than 50 ml. The differences between these groups must surely be due to a difference in contractility, which is reflected in all the parameters shown in Table 5.4.

Conclusions

The behaviour of the urinary system in the evacuation phase is determined by the contractility of the urinary bladder and the urethral resistance. Malfunction of the system can be objectively quantified by physiological parameters such as the amount of residual urine left after voiding, and traditional urodynamic

Table 5.1. Differences in average parameter values between a group of 16 obstructed and 22 unobstructed patients, together with sensitivity and specificity of some of the shown parameters for discriminating both groups, based on an averaged parameter value for each patient

Parameter	NOBS (n = 22)	OBS (n = 16)	Units	Significance U-test	Cut-off point	Sensitivity (%)	Specificity (%)
Residue	92 (142)	199 (110)	ml	0.0018			
Q_{max}	13.6 (5.8)	5.9 (2.6)	$ml\,s^{-1}$	<0.0001	8.5	81	91
$p(Q_{max})$	39 (10)	84 (29)	$cm\,H_2O$	<0.0001	54.5	94	91
w_{max}	10.2 (4.1)	12.1 (4.2)	$W\,m^{-2}$	0.047			
$UI1^{-1}$	33 (14)	84 (24)	$W\,m^{-2}$	<0.0001	54	100	95
URA	18 (6)	53 (21)	$cm\,H_2O$	<0.0001	29	94	100

Values in parentheses are standard deviations.

Table 5.2. Pre- and postoperative differences in average parameter values (standard deviations between parentheses) for ten patients with and six without postoperative residual urine > 50 ml after transurethral resection of the prostate

Parameter	Preoperative measurements			Postoperative measurements			Units
	Postoperative residue <50 (n = 10)	Significance U-test	Postoperative residue >50 (n = 6)	Postoperative residue <50 (n = 10)	Significance U-test	Postoperative residue >50 (n = 6)	
Residue	180 (124)	0.51	231 (83)	14 (20)	0.039	150 (93)	ml
Q_{max}	5.6 (2.2)	0.017	6.4 (3.2)	17.3 (6.5)	0.42	11.6 (2.9)	$ml\,s^{-1}$
$p(Q_{max})$	96 (30)	0.026	64 (12)	37 (10)	0.0056	40 (8)	$cm\,H_2O$
w_{max}	13.7 (4.6)	0.23	9.4 (1.1)	12.9 (4.7)	0.19	7.4 (0.8)	$W\,m^{-2}$
$UI1^{-1}$	91 (26)	0.13	72 (15)	29 (17)	0.17	33 (11)	$W\,m^{-2}$
URA	59 (22)		42 (14)	15 (5)		20 (4)	$cm\,H_2O$

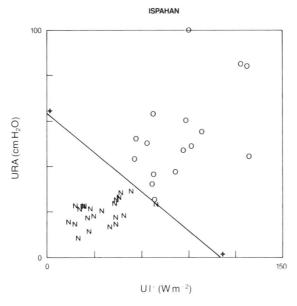

ISPAHAN

URA (cm H$_2$O)

UI$^-$ (W m^{-2})

Fig. 5.20. A scatterplot of the parameters URA and UI^{-1} and a linear discriminant function optimally separating the groups of non-obstructed (N) and obstructed (O) patients.

parameters, or symptomatic parameters, as Q_{max}, the maximum flow rate during voiding, and $p(Q_{max})$ the detrusor pressure measured at this maximum flow rate. A diagnosis cannot be based on these symptomatic parameters as they do not allow a discrimination of properties of the bladder and the urethra. Diagnostic parameters that do allow such discrimination can be derived from detrusor pressure and flow rate measured throughout micturition. P_0 (maximum isometric pressure) and v_{max} (maximum contraction velocity) are the diagnostic parameters characterising the urinary bladder contractility. These two parameters represent different aspects of contractility, that are both clinically relevant. They can only be calculated in about 12% of measured voiding studies. From all studies an approximate value of the parameters can be estimated, however, and the parameter w_{max} that combines the information in P_0 and v_{max} can also be derived. The clinical relevance of the use of these contractility parameters was illustrated in a study on patients subjected to transurethral resection of the prostate. Voiding with a significant amount of residual urine after the operation could be predicted before the operation. The urethral resistance relationship can be characterised by the group-specific parameter URA that can be derived from pressure–flow studies, or the parameter UI^{-1} that can be calculated from phase plots of the isometric detrusor pressure rise before the onset of micturition. Both parameters are highly specific in discriminating obstructed and unobstructed patients. In the same study on transurethral resection patients it was found that approximately 25% of patients subjected to the procedure on the basis of traditional clinical findings was not obstructed. It is concluded that an objective diagnosis in lower urinary tract malfunction should be based on the described diagnostic parameters characterising urinary bladder contractility and urethral resistance.

Table 5.3. Differences between parameters determined in a test population of 241 micturitions from obstructed and unobstructed patients for which P_0 and v_{max} could be determined. The parameter URA was used to separate both groups

Parameter	Obstructed ($n = 66$)	Significance[a]	Unobstructed ($n = 175$)	Units
P_0	143 (39)	<0.0001	108 (49)	cm H_2O
v_{max}	28.9 (13.2)	0.77	28.8 (11.8)	mm s^{-1}
w_{max} 14.5 (3.8)	<0.0001	12.0 (5.3)		W m^{-2}
v_{est}	23.9 (10.7)	0.31	27.5 (15.7)	mm s^{-1}

Standard deviations are in parentheses.
[a] Tested using Mann–Whitney U-test.

Table 5.4. Differences between parameters determined from flow and detrusor pressure during micturition of unobstructed patients, for micturitions ending with or without significant residual urine

Parameter	Residue < 50 ml ($n = 137$)	Significance[a]	Residue > 50 ml ($n = 38$)	Units
P_0	117 (50)	<0.0001	73 (24)	cm H_2O
v_{max}	30.3 (12.3)	0.0012	23.4 (8.0)	mm s^{-1}
w_{max}	13.1 (5.3)	<0.0001	7.9 (2.4)	W m^{-2}
v_{est}	30.8 (16.0)	<0.0001	15.9 (5.4)	mm s^{-1}

Standard deviations are given in parentheses.
[a] Tested using Mann–Whitney U-test.

References

1. Griffiths DJ. Urodynamics: the mechanics and hydrodynamics of the lower urinary tract. Medical Physics Handbooks 4, Bristol: Adam Hilger Ltd, 1980.
2. Hill AV. The heat of shortening and the dynamic constants of muscle. Proc R Soc Lond B 1938; 126:136–95.
3. Griffiths DJ, van Mastrigt R, van Duyl WA, Coolsaet, BLRA. Active properties of the smooth muscle of the urinary bladder. Med Biol Eng Comput 1979; 17:281–90.
4. van Mastrigt R, Griffiths DJ. Contractility of the urinary bladder. Urol Int 1979; 34:410–20.
5. van Mastrigt R, Coolsaet BLRA, van Duyl WA. Passive properties of the urinary bladder in the collection phase. Med Biol Eng Comput 1978; 16:471–82.
6. Coolsaet BLRA, van Duyl WA, van Mastrigt R, van der Zwart A. Visco-elastic properties of the bladder wall. Urol Int 1975; 30:16–26.
7. van Mastrigt R, Koopal JWB, Hak J, van de Wetering J. Modeling the contractility of urinary bladder smooth muscle using isometric contractions. Am J Physiol 1986; 251:R978–R983.
8. van Mastrigt R, Glerum JJ. In vitro comparison of isometric and stop-test contractility parameters for the urinary bladder. Urol Res 1984; 13:11–17.
9. Huxley AF. Muscle structure and theories of contraction. Prog Biophys Chem 1957; 7:255–318.
10. Huxley AF. Review lecture. Muscular contraction. J Physiol 1974; 243:1–43.
11. Hellstrand P. Mechanical and metabolic properties related to contraction in smooth muscle. Acta Physiol Scand Suppl 1979; 464.
12. Murphy RA. Contractile system function in mammalian smooth muscle. Blood Vessels 1976; 13:1–23.
13. Wohlfart B, Noble MIN. The cardiac excitation–contraction cycle. Pharmacol Ther 1982; 16:1–43.

14. Arner A, Hellstrand P. Activation of contraction and ATPase activity in intact and chemically skinned smooth muscle of rat portal vein. Circ Res 1983; 53:695–702.
15. van Mastrigt R. Determination of the contractility of children's bladders from isometric contractions. Urol Int 1983; 38:354–62.
16. van Mastrigt R. The on-line determination of maximal contraction velocity of the urinary bladder from an isometric contraction. Proceedings of the first joint meeting of the International Continence Society and Urodynamic Society, Los Angeles, 1980:175–8.
17. Schafer W. The separate identification of urethral and vesical function during voiding. Proceedings of the first joint meeting of the International Continence Society and Urodynamic Society, Los Angeles, 1980:315.
18. van Mastrigt R, Tauecchio EA. Series elastic properties of strips of smooth muscle from pig urinary bladder. Med Biol Eng Comput 1982; 20:585–94.
19. van Mastrigt R. The length dependence of the series elasticity of pig urinary bladder smooth muscle. J Muscle Res Cell Motil 1988; 9:525–32.
20. van Mastrigt R, Glerum JJ. Electrical stimulation of smooth muscle strips from the urinary bladder of the pig. J Biomed Eng 1985; 7:2–8
21. Griffiths DJ, Constantinou CE, van Mastrigt R. Urinary bladder function and its control in healthy females. Am J Physiol 1986; 251:R225–R230.
22. van Mastrigt R, Griffiths DJ. An evaluation of contractility parameters determined from isometric contractions and micturition studies. Urol Res 1986; 14:45–52.
23. van Mastrigt R. A computer program for on-line measurement, storage, analysis and retrieval of urodynamic data. Comp Prog Biomed 1984; 18:109–17.
24. van Mastrigt R. Computer programs for urodynamics. Neurourol Urodynam 1984; 3:141–2.
25. van Mastrigt R. Urodynamic analysis using an on-line computer. Neurourol Urodynam 1987; 6:206–7.
26. van Mastrigt R. Estimation of the maximum contraction velocity of the urinary bladder from pressure and flow throughout micturition. Urol Res 1989; (in press).
27. Griffiths DJ, van Mastrigt R, Bosch R. Quantification of urethral resistance and bladder function during voiding, with special reference to the effects of prostate size reduction on urethral obstruction due to benign prostatic hyperplasia. Neurourol Urodynam 1989; 8:17–27.
28. Schafer W. Urethral resistance? Urodynamic concepts of physiological and pathological bladder outlet function during voiding. Neurourol Urodynam 1985; 4:161–201.
29. van Mastrigt R, Griffiths DJ. An obstruction parameter based on the isometric pressure rise preceding micturition. Proceedings of the 17th annual meeting of the International Continence Society, Bristol, 1987; 214–15.
30. Rollema HJ, van Mastrigt R. The prognostic value of detrusor contractility in prostatectomy. J Urol 1988; 4–2:274A.
31. Rollema HJ, van Mastrigt R. Detrusor contractility before and after prostatectomy. Neurourol Urodynam 1987; 6:220–1.
32. Gelsema ES. ISPAHAN: an interactive system for pattern analysis. In: Gelsema ES, Kanal LN, eds. Pattern recognition in practice. Amsterdam: North Holland Publishing, 1980; 481–91.
33. van Mastrigt R, Rollema HJ. Urethral resistance and urinary bladder contractility before and after transurethral resection as determined by the computer program CLIM. Neurourol Urodynam 188; 7:226–8.

Chapter 6

Relevance of Urethral Pressure Profilometry To Date

E. Versi

Introduction

Continence is maintained when the intraurethral pressure exceeds intravesical pressure be it at rest or during activity [1]. Therefore measurement of urethral pressures is intuitively logical and so should be a fundamental part of the investigation of the lower urinary tract.

Historical

The pressure within the urethra is not uniform but changes with distance from the bladder neck achieving a peak approximately at the mid-urethral point. The first attempt to measure this maximum urethral pressure (MUP) was published in 1923 by Victor Bonney [2] who used the technique of retrograde sphinctero-metry. This method was replaced by a balloon catheter in 1936 [3] which was then subsequently refined in 1964 and 1969 [4,5].

Karlson [6] introduced the technique of simultaneous measurement of intra-urethral and intravesical pressure (urethrocystometry). Hodkinson [7] and Enhorn-ing [8] used membrane catheters. In 1967 the fluid perfusion method was described by Toews [9] and this was then made popular by Brown and Wickham [10]. The problem with the latter technique is that the response time is too slow to allow accurate assessment of urethral pressures during the cough impulse. To overcome this limitation it was necessary to introduce solid-state transducer technology with placement of the receptors inside the lumen of the urethra [11]. This allows the assessment of the lower urinary tract during stress.

The microtip transducer technique as described by Asmussen and Ulmsten [12,13] is now widely used for simultaneous urethrocystometry and urethral pressure profilometry (UPP). This involves the use of a catheter with two microtransducers mounted six centimetres apart.

Physics

When the lumen of the urethra is filled with fluid (stationary or under steady flow), the pressure in the fluid is in equilibrium with the stress exerted by the urethral walls at right angles [14]. In practice, however, when urethral pressures are determined the urethra is in fact empty and collapsed, and therefore difficulties arise in understanding what is in fact being measured.

Balloons

This technique employs a cylindrical balloon mounted concentrically on a catheter. It is inflated to just above atmospheric pressure and inserted into the urethra. A true hydrostatic pressure is obtained which is close to the ideal of the fluid-filled urethra. As the balloon is pulled through the urethra a pressure profile is obtained. Unfortunately over short axial distances along the urethra there are significant pressure variations and such a balloon technique results in the averaging out of these variations and therefore the profile obtained is distorted.

Infusion Methods

The Brown and Wickham method uses a catheter with one or more side holes which is perfused at a constant rate. As this catheter is withdrawn along the length of the urethra so the force required to allow the fluid to escape varies inversely with the pressure within the urethra at that point. In effect this is a measurement of resistance to flow, but in practice it reflects the urethral pressure provided that the urethra is highly distensible.

The maximum rate of rise in pressure is a function not only of the compliance of the catheter and measuring system, but also of the volume rate of infusion. To minimise the error of measuring the resting UPP, the compliance of the catheter should be kept as small as possible and the speed of withdrawal kept low. In practice the infusion flow rate using an aqueous fluid should be at $1\,\mathrm{ml\,min^{-1}}$ or more, irrespective of withdrawal rate. With gas infusion the rate has to be much higher.

Catheter Tip Transducers

The transducer used in this technique measures not the hydrostatic pressure but the stress component at right angles to its surface. This results in a slight difference in the pressures measured depending upon the orientation, with greatest pressures being measured when the receptor is placed anteriorly and the lowest when the receptor is facing posteriorly. Lateral orientation provides an average measurement. Because the solid-state transducers allow for a rapid rise time in pressure it is possible to use these receptors for measuring the stress profile in that the rapid increases in pressure due to a cough are faithfully recorded by the system.

Technique

Urethral pressures can be measured by positioning the microtransducer at any point along the urethra to measure the pressure at that point. The use of catheters fitted with several receptors allows the simultaneous measurements of pressures at several points along the urethra while also monitoring bladder pressure. For these measurements the catheter remains stationary within the urethra but the readings can be obtained not only at rest but also while the patient is coughing. Unfortunately the cost of the equipment increases in proportion to the number of microtransducers used and so in practice most urodynamic units use catheters with dual sensors mounted (usually) 6 cm apart. These catheters are employed to obtain UPPs at rest and while the patient is coughing (stress). They can also be used to measure changes in pressure at the MUP point.

In 1983 Hilton and Stanton [15] suggested a standard method for the measurement of UPPs which has been adopted by many centres. Recordings are taken in the supine position with the patients having 250 ml of physiological saline in their bladder. The orientation of the transducers is lateral (9 o'clock) and the withdrawal device is adjusted so that it is at the level of the urethra. The following account of the author's technique is only a slight modification [16] of the original technique.

Initially the dual sensor is passed through the urethra such that both transducers are in the bladder. The catheter is then withdrawn at a speed of 2.5 mm s^{-1} and as the proximal transducer passes through the urethra, it records the resting profile (Fig. 6.1). The same procedure is carried out with the patient repeatedly coughing to obtain a stress profile. Fig. 6.2 depicts the recordings from the urethral and bladder transducers with the middle trace being the electronic subtraction. The stress profile (Fig. 6.3) is just the subtraction trace with the dotted line outlining the profile.

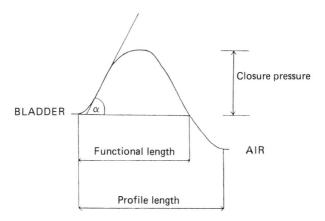

Fig. 6.1. The resting profile. This profile is obtained by pulling the catheter through the urethra so that the proximal sensor passes through the bladder neck and passes out through the external meatus while the distal sensor remains in the bladder throughout. From this profile measures can be made of the maximal urethral pressures, the rate of increase of pressure in the proximal urethra and also the profile lengths (Versi et al., Br J Obstet Gynaecol 1988; 95:147–52).

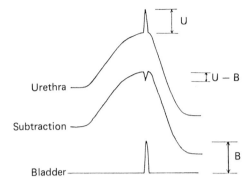

Fig. 6.2. This shows how a stress profile is recorded. The top line shows the pressures at the proximal sensor as it passes through the urethra and the bottom line shows the pressures at the distal sensor which remains in the bladder throughout. The middle trace is the electronic subtraction. A cough spike is shown on the urethral and the bladder trace. Note the notch in the subtraction trace due to the cough impulse being greater in the bladder than in the urethra (Versi et al., Br Med J 1986; 292:166–7).

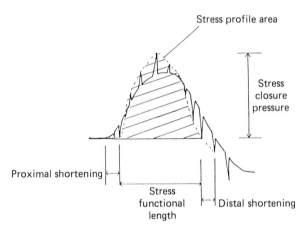

Fig. 6.3. The stress profile. This is the subtraction trace and the dotted line defines the profile. From it can be measured proximal shortening, stress functional urethral length, distal shortening as well as the stress maximum urethral closure pressure and the shaded area under the profile (Versi and Cardozo, Progress in Obstet Gynaecol 1990; Vol 8: in press).

Recordings of resting (Fig. 6.1) and stress (Fig. 6.3) profiles are regarded as satisfactory if two consecutive profiles are the same. Measurements are also taken with the urethral sensor at the point of maximum urethral pressure. For this the patient has to lie perfectly still for 2 to 3 minutes while a pressure trace is obtained. Then the patient is asked to cough once to measure the response to this. Finally the patient is asked to cough six times and the response to this is also recorded (Fig. 6.4).

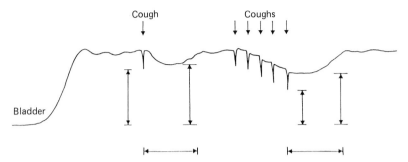

Fig. 6.4. This shows recordings taken as the catheter is pulled out to the maximum urethral pressure point and then stopped. The effects of a single cough and multiple coughs are demonstrated at the point of maximum pressure (Versi et al., Br J Obstet Gynaecol 1988; 95:147–52).

Measurement and Analysis

Variables of resting and stress pressure profiles were measured as depicted in Figs 6.1 and 6.3 respectively. A digitiser software program can be employed to measure the areas under the resting and stress profiles. To estimate the rate of change of pressure in the proximal urethra a regression line can be fitted to the digitised points on the curve, proximal to the peak point. The gradient of this line is then used to reflect the rate of change of pressure in the proximal urethra (see Fig. 6.1).

The response to a single cough and to multiple coughs (Fig. 6.4) is measured on the subtraction trace by noting the instantaneous minimum pressure during the cough, the sustained urethral closure pressure following the cough(s) and the recovery time to the maximum urethral pressure (MUP). The vascular pulsations (seen as small oscillations on the trace at the MUP) and the variations in the MUP can also be measured.

Transmission pressure ratios (TPR) are a measure of the differential transmission of the cough impulse to the urethra and bladder and are calculated as shown in Fig. 6.5. For each patient the TPR of every cough in the stress profile is calculated. The functional urethral length can be divided into four equal lengths and the mean TPR computed for each quartile for each patient. The maximum TPR (TPR-max) can be noted for each patient as can the point on the urethra where it occurs (TPR-mode) as shown in Fig. 6.6.

Reproducibility

Clearly for any technique to be used clinically it has to be shown to be reproducible. As mentioned previously the orientation is important [17,18]. The bladder volume is also important in that urethral pressures increase with increasing bladder volume, so the bladder volume should be standardised. The position of the patient is also important as measurements in the supine position are not the same as those found in the erect position. Finally the cough strength is also important as Schick [19] has shown that the TPR decreases with increasing strength of the cough; so reproducibility would have to ensure comparable coughs in the stress

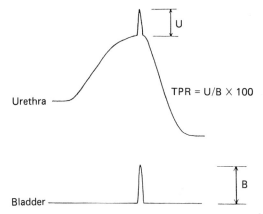

Fig. 6.5. Calculation of the transmission pressure ratio (TPR) (Versi et al., Br J Obstet Gynaecol 1988; 95:147–52).

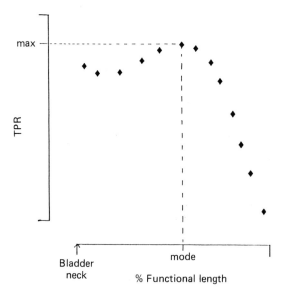

Fig. 6.6. The transmission pressure ratio (TPR) distribution throughout the urethra. Note that for each patient there will be one cough that produces the maximum TPR (TPR-max) and the point where it occurs on the urethra is denoted as TPR-mode (Versi et al., Neurourol Urodynam 1990; in press).

profile. Unless these features are comparable it is difficult to compare studies from different workers and variation in the above may result in difficulties in the accuracy of the UPP technique as a diagnostic tool.

An analysis of variance of the UPP at rest [20] showed that the repeatability of the parameters measured was influenced by the rate of catheter withdrawal, the optimum being $2.5\,\mathrm{mm\,s^{-1}}$. It also showed that profiles recorded by the microtransducer technique showed greater consistency than those recorded by the perfusion method in terms of parameters of urethral length. The fluid perfusion technique had previously been shown to have a significant component of variance due to time, however this was not the case with the microtransducer method. Urethral pressures measured by the latter technique do have a significant time dependence when recorded during the menstrual cycle in women of reproductive age and so comparative studies would also have to control for this variable.

Application

This technique is used for clinical assessment and also for research. The UPP catheter can of course be used merely as a pressure sensor in cystometry but this aspect of its use will not be considered any further. The rest of this chapter will be a critique of its clinical use to date and an attempt will be made to review the data to examine the justification for its use. Other clinical applications resulting from research information will also be mentioned. Finally mention will be made of some of its research use and potential with concluding remarks about the problems associated with the technique.

Clinical Use

The technique has been used for diagnostic purposes as well as for determining the prognosis and to monitor treatment. Its main diagnostic use has been for the assessment of sphincteric incompetence implying a diagnosis of genuine stress incontinence (GSI). Less often it has also been used to detect urethral instability, pressure variations, diverticula and strictures.

Diagnostic

Urethral Diverticula

The classical symptoms of suburethral swelling, post-micturition dribbling, dyspareunia, and the exudation of purulent material on urethral massage are often absent in patients with a urethral diverticulum [21]. While urethral diverticula can be demonstrated by radiological techniques with voiding cystourethrograms, it is also possible to detect them with urethral pressure profilometry. The typical profile picture is that of a loss of urethral pressure which can occur either before, at or after the MUP (Fig. 6.7). Why this loss of pressure should occur during the profile is not certain. It may be due to that portion of the urethral segment becoming inactive, possibly due to denervation and scarring associated with the presence of the diverticulum. Bhatia et al. [21] have, however, recommended UPP studies in the management of urethral diverticula. They suggest that should the diverticulum be found to be proximal to the MUP then the treatment of choice

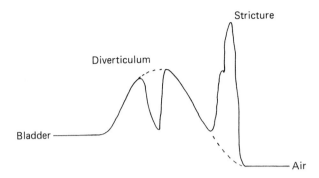

Fig. 6.7. Schematic representation of what a urethral diverticulum and stricture can look like on a resting profile. The "dip" implies the presence of a diverticulum and may be located at any place along the urethra. A stricture is seen as an area of increased pressure.

would be total surgical excision; whereas if it was distal to the MUP then marsupialisation may be a better option.

Urethral Stricture

Urethral strictures may be caused by an infection, but can also be caused iatrogenically following urethral dilatation. In postmenopausal women, due to senile atrophy, there may be distal stenosis of the urethral sphincter. In clinical practice voiding difficulties in females are rarely due to outflow obstruction but UPP studies would be able to demonstrate the presence of a stricture (Fig. 6.7). However, their more important use might be to demonstrate the absence of a stricture and therefore obviate the need for an unnecessary urethral dilatation in cases of female voiding difficulties.

Urethral Instability

When measurements are made of the urethral pressure at the MUP it is not uncommon to note fluctuations in pressure. There is a fluctuation that is synchronous with the heartbeat which is due to a urethral vascular pulse, but also there tend to be fluctuations of the baseline with a lower frequency than the heartbeat. The International Continence Society (ICS) defines urethral instability as a situation where there is total loss of closure pressure and hence incontinence. This is analogous to what occurs during normal micturition and is found in some patients with detrusor instability. Prior to the detrusor contraction there is urethral relaxation. When this urethral relaxation occurs without the ensuing detrusor contraction, the condition is termed urethral instability. It could be argued, however, that this is a form of detrusor instability where the detrusor contraction does not always occur or that the contraction is not perceived (intravesical pressure) as the urethra is open and so an equilibrium does not exist. Urethral instability is well documented [22] but is not very common.

Urethral Pressure Variations

Whilst recording urethral pressures at the MUP in some patients excessive fluctuations in the MUP have been noted. Various authors have defined variations in excess of 10 cm H_2O [23], 15 cm H_2O [24–26], 20 cm H_2O [27] or 25 cm H_2O [28] as indicating an abnormality. Versi and Cardozo [29] demonstrated that on a statistical basis using outlier analysis that the cut-off point should be 25 cm H_2O variation. However, they argued that rather than have an absolute cut-off point it might be more pertinent to examine the ratio of the fluctuations in relation to the resting MUP. By carrying out a similar analysis they found that on a statistical basis any fluctuation of greater than 33% of the resting MUP could be regarded as abnormal (Δ MUP:MUP > 33%). This idea was later supported by Hilton [30]. However, on a subsequent analysis Tapp et al. [31] were unable to detect any difference in symptoms when comparing women with significant variations in the MUP against those who did not have any variations in the MUP. This analysis was carried out for various absolute cut-off points (15, 20, 25 cm H_2O) and also for the ratio of Δ MUP to resting MUP (> 33%) but were unable to find any statistical difference in symptoms between the groups. Their data would suggest therefore that these variations in MUP are not clinically significant.

Genuine Stress Incontinence

The vast majority of urodynamic units utilising the UPP technique use it for the diagnosis of genuine stress incontinence (GSI) because of a highly significant statistical difference in UPP variable between patients with a competent sphincter and those who have GSI. Whilst this is undoubtedly true, there is however an enormous overlap between the two categories. Versi et al. [32] examined 24 UPP variables and employed the Kappa statistic to determine which variable was the more discriminatory. In their analysis they found that the area under the stress profile (Fig. 6.8) is the most discriminatory but the overlap is too great to allow this variable to be used diagnostically for the differentiation of women with GSI from those who have an intact sphincter. Fig. 6.9 shows the data for the MUP from the same study indicating that the overlap for this variable is even greater than that for the area under the stress profile. They therefore went on to conclude that no single variable within a UPP study could be used for the diagnosis of GSI. However, during their analysis they only examined patients in the supine position because the reproducibility data for this condition had been well documented. It may be that if a similar study was repeated with patients in the erect position then this technique may prove to be more promising diagnostically. Richardson [33] examining the stress profile came to a similar conclusion about the usefulness of the test. Bump et al. [34] maintain that TPR analysis of the proximal urethra is diagnostically useful. However, in their study GSI was diagnosed by exclusion and they admitted to a specificity of only 56% which is unacceptably low. Versi et al. [32] showed that the rate of change of pressure in the proximal stress profile was not a useful discriminator.

The results of the discriminant function analysis, whilst producing a better separation than any single UPP variable, still do not allow for an adequate separation of the data (Fig. 6.10). However, a probability function can be computed such that the probability of GSI can be expressed in terms of the discriminant

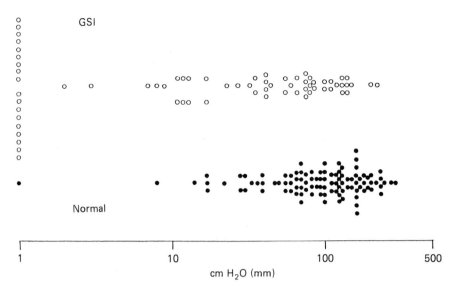

Fig. 6.8. This is the distribution of area under the stress profile in patients with genuine stress incontinence (GSI) and those who are urodynamically normal. Note the logarithmic scale and the excessive overlap (Versi and Cardozo, Prog Obstet Gynaecol, Vol 8: 1990).

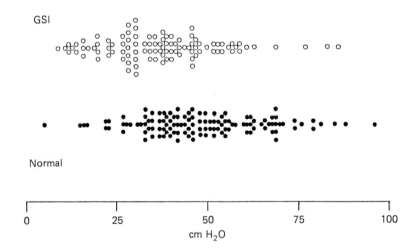

Fig. 6.9. This shows a distribution of the maximum urethral pressure in patients with genuine stress incontinence (GSI) and those who are urodynamically normal. Note that the overlap here is even greater than that in Fig. 6.8 (Versi et al., World J Urol 1986; 4:6–9).

score (Fig. 6.11). In this way the patients with equivocal scores can be determined and so referred for a more definitive test, e.g. videocystourethrography. This would allow the UPP technique to function as a diagnostic test for GSI with the proviso that certain patients will require further investigation. A further development of this technique is the combination of symptoms analysis with UPP analysis. Again utilising discriminant function it is possible to improve on the separation between normal and GSI patients. This analysis reveals correct classification of 93% with a sensitivity of 90% [35]. In a similar manner a probability function can be computed for this (Fig. 6.12). From this figure it can be seen that the slope of the sigmoid curve is steeper than that in Fig. 6.11, implying a better diagnostic separation between normal and GSI patients. In the same way the ambiguous cases can be identified and referred for further analysis with video-cystourethrography. This model can be incorporated into an intelligent system. A package could be developed whereby a microcomputer is used to store the symptoms data from a patient and then to store the UPP information. The system would in fact be very user friendly because it could be programmed to merely output an answer of (a) genuine stress incontinence, (b) intact sphincter, (c) equivocal.

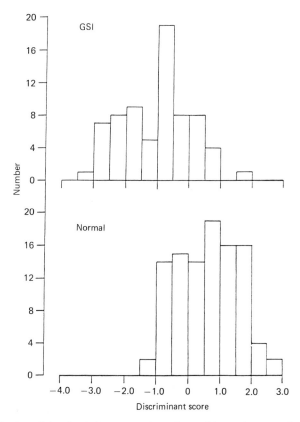

Fig. 6.10. Distribution of the discriminant score in patients with genuine stress incontinence (GSI) and those who are urodynamically normal. Note that even with this technique there is a considerable overlap (Versi, Br J Obstet Gynaecol 1990; in press).

However before such a system could be developed it would have to be tested in the field to determine its robustness.

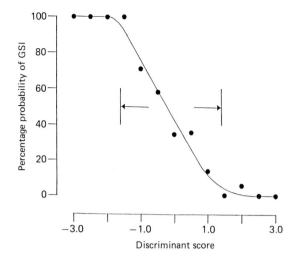

Fig. 6.11. Probability function to define the probability of genuine stress incontinence given the discriminant score from the UPP study. Note that the equivocal range as defined by the bars is wide (Versi, Br J Obstet Gynaecol 1990; in press).

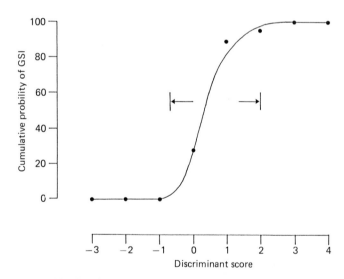

Fig. 6.12. The probability function to define the probability of GSI given the discriminant score from data of the UPP study and symptoms analysis. Note that the sigmoid curve is steeper than that in Fig. 6.11 and that the equivocal range is narrower implying that this function is more diagnostic.

Prognosis

Female continence is maintained by the bladder neck and when this fails the distal sphincter mechanisms act as a back up system. When both fail, GSI ensues. Studies on the prevalence of bladder neck incompetence [36] revealed that it is present in 51% of continent climacteric women and this prevalence appears to increase with age (Janez, personal communication). Versi et al. [37] investigated this phenomenon and found that continence in women with an incompetent bladder neck was achieved by these women because they augmented their distal sphincter mechanisms. On UPP studies this was observed as an increase in the distal TPR and the finding that TPR-mode was located more distally. There may be some clinical consequences of this finding.

Oncological Surgery

In continent women undergoing videocystourethrography it is common to find a closed bladder neck at rest but to note that the bladder neck becomes incompetent on coughing, although the contrast medium does not go past the mid-urethral point [36]. UPP studies carried out on these patients revealed a degree of proximal shortening (Fig. 6.13), but analysis of the stress functional urethral length shows no difference between patients with an incompetent bladder neck and those with a competent bladder neck [13]. The reason for this is that those with an incompetent bladder neck maintain their stress functional length by not having such a reduction in distal shortening. TPR analysis can be used to see how this is achieved. Fig. 6.14 shows that patients with an incompetent bladder neck do not have such a reduction in their TPRs in the distal quartile as do those with a competent bladder neck. In other words continent women with an incompetent bladder neck maintain their stress functional urethral length by augmenting their distal TPRs. When carrying out a stress profile, for every patient there will be one cough that will generate the maximum TPR and the point where it occurs along the urethra has been termed TPR-mode (Fig. 6.6). When comparing the distribution of TPR-mode between patients with a competent bladder neck and those with an incompetent bladder neck (Fig. 6.15) it is found that the latter have a TPR-mode distribution which is shifted distally, again indicating that they use more of their distal urethra.

Shingleton's group [38] showed that continent women with an incompetent bladder neck develop GSI after radical hysterectomy and Versi and Cardozo [39] suggested that this may be due to their inability postoperatively to augment their distal TPRs. Some women become incontinent after radical vulvectomy (Delancey, Chapter 1) and this may be an analogous situation. As pointed out, continent women with an incompetent bladder neck have their TPR-mode located more distally. As this is the most important part of their urethra, its excision during a radical vulvectomy or interference with its function due to surgical insult at radical hysterectomy would result in incontinence. Preoperative UPP studies could therefore identify patients at risk.

Physiotherapy

Whilst it is generally recognised that conservative management of GSI in the form of physiotherapy is a highly desirable treatment modality, efficacy data on the usefulness of this technique are still relatively lacking [40]. The published data to date suggest that physiotherapy success rates vary from 60% to 90% (Shepherd, Chapter 13) but a recent study by Tapp et al. [41] suggested that the success rate was as low as 25% when the assessment was objectively carried out with videocystourethrography. However, an analysis to determine predictor variables

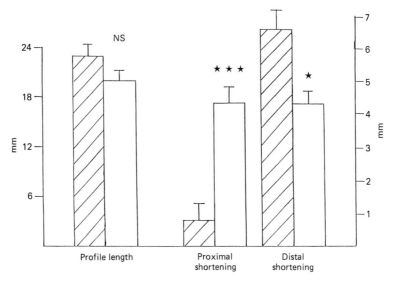

Fig. 6.13. A comparison of the stress profile variables in continent women with a competent bladder neck (shaded) and those with an incompetent bladder neck (not shaded). Note the difference in proximal (∗∗∗: $P < 0.001$) and distal shortening (∗: $P < 0.05$) with no difference in the stress functional length (Versi et al., Neurourol Urodynam 1990; in press).

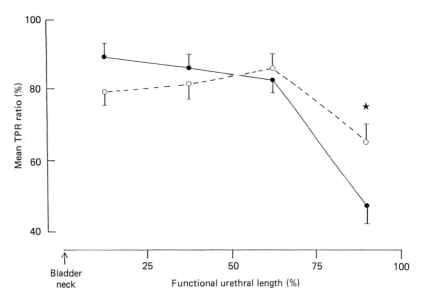

Fig. 6.14. A comparison of the mean TPR values in each quartile of the functional urethral length in women with a competent (●) and an incompetent (○) bladder neck. Note the significant difference ($P < 0.05$) in the distal TPR (Versi et al., Neurourol Urodynam 1990; in press).

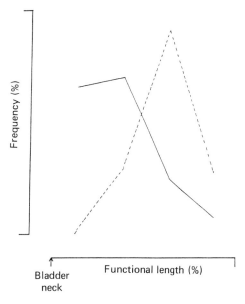

Fig. 6.15. A comparison of the distribution of TPR-mode in continent women with a competent bladder neck (————) with those with an incompetent bladder neck (– – – –). Note that the distribution is shifted distally in those with an incompetent bladder neck.

showed that when the pretreatment stress functional length was greater than 5 mm and the stress MUP greater than 9.4 cm H_2O, the success rate was greatly increased. Clearly if UPP studies could be used for predicting which patients would benefit from physiotherapy, then the treatment would be much more cost effective [40].

Monitoring Treatment

Physiotherapy

Fig. 6.16 shows the distribution of TPR-mode in continent and GSI patients (unpublished observations). There is a significant shift of the median value to the distal urethra (to the right) in the group of women who were continent. This is because some of them have an incompetent bladder neck and so as discussed above, their TPR-mode is shifted distally. Patients with GSI all have an incompetent bladder neck and if the function of physiotherapy is to strengthen the distal sphincter, then any success could be monitored by noting the distal shift of TPR-mode. In this way UPP studies could be used not only to select patients for physiotherapy but also to monitor their progress.

Bladder Neck Surgery

It is recognised now that when bladder surgery is successful, the TPR in the proximal urethra are augmented to well over 100%. Therefore in cases where there is incontinence postoperatively a UPP study could be used to determine whether further bladder neck surgery is indicated on the basis of proximal TPR analysis.

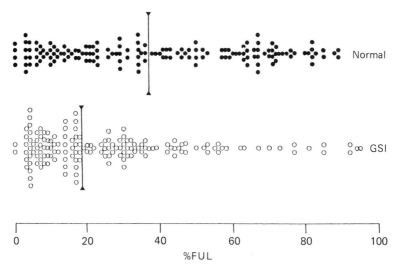

Fig. 6.16. The distribution of TPR-mode in patients who have genuine stress incontinence and those who are urodynamically normal. Note that the median value is distal (shifted to the right) in those patients who are normal.

Hormone Replacement Therapy

It is unlikely that hormone replacement therapy in the long term has any beneficial effect in postmenopausal women with GSI [42], but short-term studies have revealed some benefit [43]. Hilton and Stanton [44] suggested that with hormone replacement therapy in postmenopausal women, the profile of the TPR distribution changes from the typical one seen in GSI towards that seen in symptom-free women. Their study consisted of only ten patients and this preliminary work needs to be extended.

Research

It is not the remit of this chapter to enumerate all the advances that have been made in research with the use of UPP studies. However, mention will be made of just three aspects.

Anatomical Correlates

UPP studies in conjunction with lateral bead chain cystography have resulted in useful information [45] about principles and the mechanisms underlying sphincter incompetence. The bladder neck studies mentioned above have also been important in understanding the genesis of GSI.

Mechanisms of Urethral Closure

Understanding of the sphincteric mechanisms have been aided considerably by the UPP catheter. The work of Raz et al. [46] and Rud et al. [47] has resulted in our understanding that a third of the MUP is due to the vascular component and that a third is due to the muscular input.

Mechanisms of Hormone Action

The distal urethral epithelium is sensitive to oestrogen action [48] and it is said that senile atrophic urethritis can be prevented with hormone replacement therapy. The rich vascular plexuses that serve the urethra also contribute to the closure mechanism [46,47] and these appear to be under hormone control in that after the menopause they tend to decrease but hormone replacement therapy reverses this as witnessed on UPP studies [49]. A significant component of the urethral connective tissue is collagen, and it is known that skin collagen is hormone dependent [50] in that it declines after the menopause and increases with hormone replacement therapy. Versi et al. [51] demonstrated that skin collagen content correlates with many of the variables of UPP.

Problems

For UPP studies to represent urethral pressures and sphincter mechanisms accurately it is essential that the system should be free from artefacts. However, it is difficult to avoid these. The size of the catheter is important and should be as small as possible. It should also be as soft as possible but both of these features are difficult to maintain because the microtransducer does have a size-limiting feature and also increases catheter stiffness, especially if several transducers are mounted on one catheter. Also for accurate measurement, as has been mentioned above, the reproducibility features are crucial.

Conclusion

There is a wealth of data showing that the microtransducer has been an invaluable tool for research into lower urinary tract function. However, its clinical uses are limited and therefore it cannot rank with the first line urodynamic tests such as uroflowmetry and cystometry.

References

1. Barnes AC. The method of evaluating the stress of urinary incontinence. Am J Obstet Gynecol 1940; 40:381–90.
2. Bonney V. On diurnal incontinence of urine in women. J Obstet Gynaecol Br Emp 1923; 30:358–65.
3. Simons I. Studies on bladder function. The Sphincterometer. Urol 1936; 35:96–102.

4. Enhorning G, Miller ER, Hinman F. Urethral closure studies with cine roentgenography and bladder urethral recording. Surg Gynecol Obstet 1964; 118:507–16.
5. Tanagho EA, Meyers FH, Smith DR. Urethral resistance: its components and implications I. Invest Urol 1969; 7:136–49.
6. Karlson S. Experimental studies in the functioning of the female urinary bladder and urethra. Acta Obstet Gynecol Scand 1953; 32:285–397.
7. Hodkinson CP. Direct cystometry. Am J Obstet Gynecol 1960; 79:648–64.
8. Enhorning GE. Simultaneous recording of the intravesical and intraurethral pressure. Acta Chir Scand (Suppl) 1961; 276:1–68.
9. Toews H. Intra-urethral and intra-vesical pressure in normal and stress incontinent women. Obstet Gynecol 1967; 29:613.
10. Brown M, Wickham JEA. The urethral pressure profile. Br J Urol 1969; 41:211–17.
11. Millar HD, Baker LE. Stable ultraminiature catheter tip pressure transducer. Med Biol Eng 1973; 11:86–9.
12. Asmussen M, Ulmsten U. Simultaneous urethrocystometry with a user technique. Scand J Urol Nephrol 1976; 10:7–11.
13. Asmussen M, Miller A. Clinical gynaecological urology. Oxford: Blackwell Scientific Publications, 1983:20–4.
14. Griffiths DJ. Urodynamics: medical physics handbooks 4. Bristol: Adams Hilger, 1980.
15. Hilton P, Stanton SL. Urethral pressure measurements by microtransducer: the results in symptom-free women and those with genuine stress incontinence. Br J Obstet Gynaecol 1983; 90:919–33.
16. Versi E. Discriminant analysis of urethral pressure profilometry data for the diagnosis of genuine stress incontinence. Br J Obstet Gynaecol 1990; (in press).
17. Anderson RS, Shepherd AM, Feneley RCL. Microtransducer urethral profile methodology: variations caused by transducer orientation. J Urol 1983; 130:727–8.
18. Griffiths DJ. The pressure in a collapsed tube, with special reference to urethral pressure. Phys Med Biol 1985; 30:951–63.
19. Schick E. Objective assessment of resistance of female urethra to stress. Urology 1985; 26:518–26.
20. Hilton P. The urethral pressure profile at rest: an analysis of variance. Neurourol Urodynam 1982; 1:303–11.
21. Bhatia MN, McCarthy TA, Ostergard D. Urethral diverticula: urethral closure profile: a preliminary report. Prog Clin Biol Res 1981; 78:239–42.
22. Sand KP, Bowers LW, Ostergard DR. Uninhibited urethral relaxation: an unusual cause of incontinence. Obstet Gynecol 1986; 68:645–8.
23. Plevnic S, Janez J. Urethral pressure variations. Urology 1983; 21:207–9.
24. Ulmsten U, Hendriksson L, Iosif S. The unstable female urethra. Am J Obstet Gynecol 1982; 144:93–7.
25. Herbert DB, Ostergard DR. Vesical instability. Urodynamic parameters by microtip transducer catheters. Obstet Gynecol 1982; 60:331–7.
26. Vereecken RL, Das J. Urethral instability: related to stress and/or urge incontinence? J Urol 1985; 134:698–701.
27. Kulseng-Hanssen S. Prevalence and pattern of unstable urethral pressure in one hundred and seventy four gynecological patients referred for urodynamic investigation. Am J Obstet Gynecol 1983; 146:895–900.
28. Cardozo LD, Versi E. Urethral instability in normal postmenopausal women. Proc Int Cont Soc 1985; 15:115–16.
29. Versi E, Cardozo LD. Urethral instability: diagnosis based on variations of the maximum urethral pressure in normal climacteric women. Neurourol Urodynam 1986; 5:535–41.
30. Hilton P. Unstable urethral pressure: toward a more relevant definition. Neurourol Urodynam 1988; 6:411–18.
31. Tapp A, Cardozo LD, Versi E, Studd JWW. The prevalence of variation of resting urethral pressure in women and its association with lower urinary tract infection. Br J Urol 1988; 61:314–7.
32. Versi E, Cardozo LD, Studd J, Cooper D. Evaluation of urethral pressure profilometry for the diagnosis of genuine stress incontinence. World J Urol 1986; 4:6–9.
33. Richardson DA. Value of the cough profile in the evaluation of patients with stress incontinence. Am J Obstet Gynecol 1986; 155:808–11.
34. Bump RC, Copeland WE, Hart WG, Fantl JA. Dynamic urethral pressure transmission ratio determination in stress incontinent subjects. Am J Obstet Gynecol 1988; 159:749–55.
35. Versi E, Cardozo L. Symptoms and urethral pressure profilometry for the diagnosis of genuine stress incontinence. J Obstet Gynaecol 1988; 9:168–9.

36. Versi E, Cardozo LD, Studd JWW, Brincat M, O'Dowd TM, Cooper DJ. The urinary sphincter in the maintenance of female continence. Br Med J 1986; 292:166–7.
37. Versi E, Cardozo L, Studd J. Distal urethral compensatory mechanisms in women with an incompetent bladder neck who remain continent and the effect of the menopause. Neurourol Urodynam 1990; (in press).
38. Farquharson DM, Shingleton HM, Orr JW, Hatch KD, Hester S, Soong S-J. The short-term effect of radical hysterectomy on urethral and bladder function. Br J Obstet Gynaecol 1987; 94:341–7.
39. Versi E, Cardozo L. The short-term effect of radical hysterectomy on urethral and bladder function. Br J Obstet Gynaecol 1987; 94:822–3.
40. Mantle J, Versi E. English physiotherapeutic practice: stress incontinence 1989. Neurourol Urodynam 1989; 8:352–3.
41. Tapp AJS, Cardozo L, Hills B, Barnick C. Who benefits from physiotherapy? Neurourol Urodynam 1988; 7:259–61.
42. Versi E, Cardozo LD, Tapp A, Cooper DJ, Brincat M, Studd JWW. The long term effect of hormone implant therapy on the lower urinary tract. J Int Urogynaecol 1990; (in press).
43. Versi E. The menopause. In: Norton P, ed. Urinary incontinence in women, Clinical Obstet Gynecol, Philadelphia: Lippincott, 1990; (in press).
44. Hilton P, Stanton SL. The use of intravaginal oestrogen cream in genuine stress incontinence. Br J Obstet Gynaecol 1983; 90:940–4.
45. Hertogs K, Stanton SL. Lateral bead-chain urethrocystography after successful and unsuccessful colposuspension. Br J Obstet Gynaecol 1985; 92:1179–83.
46. Raz S, Caine M, Zeigler M. The vascular component in the production of intraurethral pressure. J Urol 1972; 93:108.
47. Rud T, Andersson KE, Asmussen M, Hunting A, Ulmsten U. Factors maintaining the urethral pressure in women. Invest Urol 1980; 17:343–7.
48. Zuckerman S. Histogenesis of tissue sensitivity to oestrogens. Biol Rev 1940; 15:231–71.
49. Versi E, Cardozo LD. Urethral vascular pulsations. Proc Int Cont Soc 1985; 15:503–4.
50. Brincat M, Versi E, O'Dowd TM, Moniz CF, Magos A, Kabalan S, Studd JWW. Skin collagen changes in postmenopausal women receiving estradiol gel. Maturitas 1987; 9:1–5.
51. Versi E, Cardozo LD, Brincat M, Cooper D, Montgomery J, Studd JWW. Correlation of urethral physiology and skin collagen in postmenopausal women. Br J Obstet Gynaecol 1988; 95:505–6.

Discussion

Hilton: Dr van Mastrigt's illustration for his diagnostic parameters was in relation to obstructed males. Only 12% of recordings gave absolute readings for v_0 and v_{max}. Does that imply 12% of patients, or 12% of readings on any individual patient?

Van Mastrigt: 12% of patients. This contractility relationship is revealed if there are certain fluctuations in the urethra. I do not think every individual would do that with a certain frequency. Some individuals will do it more often than others: some will probably never do it while others will do it often. The 12% is an average of patient behaviour and numbers of patients.

Hilton: Presumably these fluctuations are something quite different from the urethral pressure variation that was discussed in the non-voiding situation in Section I. Presumably this reflects a degree of dyssynergia to the pelvic floor, and therefore is likely to be something that characterises one group of patients and not another.

Van Mastrigt: It is a kind of an artefact that can be used to detect the contractility relationship. The stop test was the test that was intended to provoke that kind of behaviour in order to use it, and then there were all the problems of invoking other control mechanisms that were not wanted.

Hilton: Any mention of urethral pressure was carefully avoided. Does Dr van Mastrigt have any evidence that will allow him to comment on the correlation between micturitional profiles and his diagnostic parameters in terms of their ability to characterise contractility?

Van Mastrigt: Not with respect to contractility. But I could well imagine that if one did a profile during micturition, one might have some information as to the point where a possible obstruction might be. The urethral resistance relationship sees the urethra as one whole "black box". One can say that overall there is too high a resistance or overall there is a normal resistance, but cannot say where the obstruction might be. A micturitional profile might be of use if there are any doubts about where it is.

Plevnik: Is Dr Versi suggesting that we stop using static UPP measurements for our clinical routines?

Versi: Yes. I do not think there is really any place for them as a routine.

Sutherst: About ten years ago before stress urethral tests were started, some of us made similar measurements, measuring the area under the pressure profile curve and the rate of rise of pressure in the proximal urethra. At the time I constructed an equation of considerable length and it was possible to make some discriminatory type equations out of those measurements. But there was no point, because along came something like a stress urethral pressure profile, or in our case a fluid bridge test, which was somewhat easier to do.

Versi: There is a place perhaps if one could develop it for the full urethral pressure profilometry technique with stress profiles as well. But Mr Plevnik asked specifically about the resting profile and I do not think that has much of a place in clinical practice, although I mentioned strictures and diverticulum.

Stanton: I know of nobody else who has seen a diverticulum on a UP profile.

Versi: I think I have seen one, and certainly Bhatia and Ostergard have.

Stanton: Which is what I mean. Apart from that group and Dr Versi himself. Those are the only three I know.

Can I ask another point? There has been comment in the literature, strangely enough from Ostergard's group, about the low-pressure urethra in incontinent women. People with this diagnosis will invariably do poorly on conventional surgery. What is the feeling about this?

Versi: It strikes me that whether or not someone does well from surgery has a lot to do with the mobility of the urethra and what can be done with it during the surgical procedure. Whether or not there is a low pressure at the beginning is not relevant for genuine stress incontinence because it is the difference in the transmission pressure that will count. I know of published work showing that those who have a low urethral pressure are likely to be more incontinent, but the fact is that they still have genuine stress incontinence. So I really cannot understand what the basis of that analysis is.

Stanton: It is a tempting philosophy that if a patient has a "knackered" urethra, no amount of elevation will make any difference to it and therefore no amount of manipulating pressure transmission ratios will make any difference to those who have a poor urethra with no resistance.

One of the appeals of urethral pressure measurements has always been that there might be some way, using whatever parameters, of identifying the useless urethra.

Versi: So that if, say, a colposuspension works, it will squeeze the urethra up against the symphysis pubis and it does not matter what the resting tone is, as long as it is greater than zero.

Stanton: And if it is not?

Versi: They will leak all the time.

Cardozo: Then they must have a congenital abnormality, or some form of injury which is not a normal urethra. All urethrae have some pressure.

Hilton: That is probably true. Dr Versi is talking about a theoretical rather than a practical concept. Clearly there are patients whose urethral pressures may be greater than zero but are much too low to anticipate that any modification to their transmission will cure them surgically.

There are extremely convincing data in terms of the low-pressure urethra, and our own data accord with them to some extent in that women who fail surgery certainly have lower pressures than those who succeed. But as to the question of whether any individual value can be defined (20 cm H_2O is what they have taken) that allows one to say that a woman has an 80% chance of failing surgery as opposed to an 80% chance of succeeding, it is unrealistic to expect a single measurement parameter to do that. Certainly within our own data no such figure can be identified.

Versi: I would certainly agree. There are elderly women who are actually continent who can manage on 20 cm H_2O as a resting pressure.

Cardozo: Because they never raise their detrusor pressure. But the overlap is far too great, and we do not know what proportion of continence surgery works because it is obstructive rather than because it is repositional. So one cannot say for a given patient whether one should or one should not operate because of low urethral pressure.

Hilton: To a point perhaps one can.

Warrell: I cannot agree with much of what has been said and I would hate it to go recorded without opposition.

I would ask the basic question: how useful is the urethral pressure profile, as Dr Versi described it, as a way of measuring the continence mechanism described in Chapter 4? What one thinks one is doing is measuring the occlusive forces generated by the urethra and by the structures outside the urethra, and the technique that has been described is least likely to do this. What is happening is that something with a parallel diameter is put into the urethra and dilates it and resistance to dilatation is then measured by pulling it through. In other words, once the probe has been inserted into the urethra, the dilatation does not change; it is a set dilatation throughout the test. But if the test is done in some other way rather than pulling it through at a constant speed – say by moving it in 0.5 cm or 1 cm steps down the urethra, so pulling the measuring probe from a dilated to an undilated area – then there is a much better discrimination between patients with stress incontinence and patients with normal control.

Some time ago it was suggested that the resting urethral profile done in steps gave the best discrimination between stress incontinence and normal patterns. Perhaps the question we should be asking is what in the urethra or around the urethra prevents the urethra dilating?

I would sum up by saying that the technique that Dr Versi described is least likely to discriminate the sort of forces which were talked about in the continence mechanism. But I would not criticise the idea. I would criticise the technique rather than the idea. Look, for example, at how heavily dependent cough transmission is on technique. There is a concept that in the rigid catheter withdrawal system that most people use for pressure transmission, the negative transmission was merely the catheter moving into a previously dilated portion of the urethra. And indeed, if a pressure transmission is done in steps, allowing whatever gauge is employed to stop in one part of the urethra, the result is entirely different and quite at variance with the result one gets using the pull-through method.

To illustrate: something of constant diameter will meet with the same occlusive forces throughout. As the gauge is brought into the proximal segment of the urethra it will cause it to dilate and it is the force produced by resistance to dilatation that is measured. If it is done in steps down the urethra, resistance to dilatation is measured by wherever it is caused by the diameter of the gauge. But if a microtransducer is used then once the urethra has been dilated this does not change. I am suggesting that it be more useful to measure something much more akin to the wedge of fluid produced in the urethra by a cough – in other words, the resistance to dilatation.

Versi: If I may answer some of those points.

I certainly would not want to dismiss the urethral pressure profile. What I said was that in the context in which we used it, it was not useful and I think that is still true. The reason why we used it in that context was because that is how most other people use it. What we were doing was to try to evaluate it as a clinical diagnostic tool, and it is not. Maybe the "force" technique will be, but obviously it will have to be assessed. We have looked at 200–300 patients, and could not find a difference. The data using the other techniques, this one included, are from fewer patients.

My point is that whatever the technique, we have to show that it will work in the field. The way we used our technique, it does not work in the field. That is not to say that if we had the patients standing up or if we had the patients with a force gauge, we would not have had a better result. I am only dealing with the data that we have.

Warrell: Perhaps there is a point of agreement, in that case.

Hilton: The major difficulty we have is that we call this parameter that we are looking at "urethral pressure" when quite clearly it is not urethral pressure. What we look at with the microtransducer is probably something more akin to closure force from one particular direction. But clearly it is not intraluminal pressure. Whether we want an intraluminal pressure or not is a separate question, but as long as we are hooked on the idea of pressure, what we find with a microtransducer will not tell us quite what we want to know. That is not to say it is not telling us something that is of clinical value. But it is not what we think it is. And clearly to some extent as well as measuring forces it is also recording something of the distensibility of the urethra; the larger the measuring catheter that is used, the higher the pressure recorded – up to a point, and obviously dependent on distensibility. Maybe more useful information would be obtained by doing a series of urethral pressure profiles with different sizes of catheters or different stiffnesses, but collating all the information that we get from these measuring systems would seem to be beyond us at the moment.

Mundy: But why do it at all?

Versi: The simple question is: can this technique be useful clinically? I have tried to answer that question. Another technique may come along, the same experimental paradigm could be used to assess it, and it might be more useful. That is why we are doing it, to see if it is useful.

Mundy: And for whom is it being done? What is the purpose of it?

Versi: To see if it is possible to demonstrate sphincter incompetence.

Mundy: If a patient comes in who says "Doctor, I leak when I cough", she has no other symptoms, she climbs on the couch and when she coughs, she leaks. What is it that any investigation using multiple discriminatory parameters can show that can do better than that?

Versi: I know. But unfortunately the real world is not as simple as that.

Mundy: The real world is far simpler than complex equations and discriminant parameters. What is the point of doing any sort of investigation if it requires this sort of elaborate detail and it does not contribute either diagnostically or pathophysiologically?

Hilton: With the scenario as Mr Mundy describes it no investigations are needed, but patients like that are few and far between. The majority come in with rather complex medical histories.

Mundy: The majority of patients seen with stress incontinence do not have stress incontinence?

Hilton: Many do not have a clear history of stress incontinence with no other symptoms.

Mundy: Let us stick to stress incontinence on physical examination. If somebody comes in who does not have stress incontinence on physical examination, what should one do?

Hilton: What would I do in clinical practice? That is a slightly different issue from the relevance of urethral pressure profilometry. Personally I would never do a urethral pressure profile to make a clinical decision.

Mundy: But if you saw somebody, what would you do? As far as I can see, none of this provides any information diagnostically, therapeutically or pathophysiologically, and that is why it is a waste of time.

Versi: But Mr Mundy is wrong. The model that I showed using symptoms and UPP analysis gives a correct classification of 93%. That is pretty good for most diagnostic testing.

Mundy: For what purposes? To say it will either be GSI, or normal, or do another test? That is not useful.

Versi: But that is what the answer will be on the basis of that analysis. So one wants to know whether the patient has got GSI. Why do any urodynamic investigation?

Mundy: If somebody comes up, the same conclusion can be reached without doing a test. They have GSI, or they are normal, or they need to have urodynamics.

Versi: I have been misunderstood. It will be one of the three answers, but not all three at once. Each patient would fall into one of those three categories. But the idea is to diagnose the condition, to see whether or not that patient has genuine stress incontinence. And one will get that answer in some patients: that they have not, or that this test cannot tell us.

Mundy: And one can get the same answer by history and physical examination.

Versi: To a degree, but not to the same accuracy. We have analysed that and it is not true.

Mundy: But accuracy does not depend on whether one will get one of those answers in 93% of cases. It is a question of how many percentages will fall into a positive diagnostic group rather than the bucket group at the end. That will vary between the test and history and examination.

Versi: But with history and examination the correct classification is of 80%, compared to 93% when combining UPP data.

Mundy: Yes, but to get from 80% to 93% is it worth all of this?

Versi: Absolutely. A coin would give us 50%: 80% from 93% is only 13% but a very important 13%.

Sutherst: There are some women in whom sphincter incompetence can be demonstrated on urethral tests. They do not have to be as complicated as that. But
there are some women who do not demonstrate stress leakage on examination
for one reason or another, and yet it can be proved during some urethral tests
that they have it. Those might be regarded as minor degrees of sphincter incompetence who perhaps do not need surgical treatment, but nevertheless they are
wet on pad testing perhaps and some sphincter incompetence has been demonstrated. So one has an answer that one did not have before that particular test.
Is that wrong?

Mundy: No. I would agree in that if a patient does not demonstrate it there
is probably a simple explanation. They might have voided five minutes earlier,
or something of that kind. So one can take an extension of the same sort of
investigation and reach a diagnosis which has a practical purpose, and that is
a simple and effective way of doing it without all of this elaboration.

This would be a useful investigation over and above that if it provided some
other information, either prognostic or pathophysiological. But it does neither.
And it only then serves as an alternative, and it seems to me a far more cumbersome
alternative, to doing a physical examination and extending that, for example,
repeating physical examination with a full bladder or doing pad testing.

DeLancey: The basis for the discussion is that we believe that there are two groups
of women, those who have stress incontinence and those who do not have stress
incontinence. We all know that there are many women who have stress incontinence for whom it is not a problem, and I have to agree with Mr Mundy that
if stress incontinence can be demonstrated on physical examination and if a patient
identifies that that is what her problem is, there really is no need for any further
diagnostic test.

At the root of the question though, is that there is a huge group of people
who are in the middle. I am not sure that urethral pressure profiles will discriminate
that because on one day one will be able to see a positive pressure profile and
two minutes later it can be different. We are all agreed that there is a very heterogeneous population out there and that trying to put them on one side or on
the other side is not possible as there is a continuum. There are patients who
have more or less stress incontinence but it is not "yes or no".

Versi: Which is why I have a sigmoid curve.

Stanton: Most of the group would agree on the limited use of the urethral pressure
profile. Certainly we have abandoned this, but I follow these discussions with
interest to see whether there is any aspect of this test, or whether it will lead
on to a better test which will help us to identify that patient who has a urethra
of that so-called low pressure type, over which there is still dispute, because these
are the patients that are failing surgery. I think the issue is not whether we can
diagnose stress incontinence or not – I agree with Mr Mundy that there are simpler
methods of doing it – but whether we can identify beforehand the patient who

will fail conventional surgery and whether we can adapt our surgery to dealing with that kind of patient. The urethral pressure profile at the moment does not seem to be able to do that.

Cardozo: There is another group of patients in whom urethral pressure profile measurements are useful, that is, those women with voiding difficulties in whom one wishes to avoid unnecessary urethral dilatation. We have quite a large number of women who have hypotonic bladders as opposed to urethral strictures or narrow urethras and there is no point in sending them for urethral dilatation when the problem is not in the urethra. And I do think it is a useful test for that.

Mundy: On what basis?

Cardozo: Because we do not have other good ways of determining whether a patient's voiding difficulties are due to her poor bladder or her urethral stricture.

Van Mastrigt: To quantify contractility and urethral resistance.

Mundy: So a "low pressure/low flow" pattern on filling and voiding cystometry is not sufficient?

Cardozo: Not always. If a patient has a low pressure and a low flow, she may have a decompensated detrusor or she may have a detrusor that does not function well to begin with. We cannot necessarily say that she has obstructed outflow due to a urethral stricture because she has low contractility and low flow.

Mundy: If she had low pressure/low flow, I would agree one would not.

Cardozo: If she has high pressure/low flow, that is fine. Obviously she is fighting against a closed urethra. But if she has low pressure/low flow, what do we do?

Mundy: What does the urethral pressure profile tell us in low pressure/low flow?

Cardozo: If a patient has a high urethral closure pressure, it is worth doing urethral dilatation or urethrotomy. But if she does not, then I do not think it is.

Van Mastrigt: And a high urethral closure pressure with a low detrusor pressure?

Cardozo: We do.

Van Mastrigt: If bladder contractility is in order then pressure should be high. If the flow rate through the ureter is low, that is due to some obstruction or functional obstruction or whatever.

Cardozo: But clinically not always.
  I agree that in cases of urethral stricture, a high pressure bladder should go with it. But that is not always the case.

Mundy: But urethral strictures are rare. They are so rare that they are not worth thinking about as a diagnostic group.

Cardozo: They are not common, but we do see some.

Versi: The point was to use the urethral pressure profile to show someone they do not have a stricture and avoid dilating them, which is a common practice in the UK.

Mundy: But why do an unnecessary test to show that they do not have a disease that is so rare in any event?

Cardozo: So that they are not treated unnecessarily.

Sutherst: We are not only discussing urethral strictures. We are discussing stenosis and fibrosis perhaps.

Cardozo: Yes. And not necessarily a stricture de novo.

Hilton: I agree with Mr Mundy, but my argument against using urethral pressure profiles in that situation is that we do not have a normal range from which to work. And to say, therefore, that one urethra is strictured because it has got a high pressure is clearly erroneous.

Plevnik: If we are discussing the continence mechanism, then we are talking about two basic mechanical parameters: the occlusive forces, which have to be high enough to provide closure, and the "washer", the soft tissue of the internal wall of the urethra. The soft tissue has to be sufficiently soft to provide watertight closure. Pressure measurements in the urethra are affected by both the occlusive forces and the washer itself, which means that we can measure high pressures in the urethra, which are mainly due to the rigid washer, and we have no idea what the occlusive forces might be. We are always talking about these two parameters which comprise the pressure being measured, and this may be the main reason why we cannot interpret the results of UPP. Unless we measure we can have no idea of the range of the softness in the urethra. That would probably be the first thing to do, and then we can go further and start to analyse our clinical groups as far as the UPPs are concerned.

Chapter 7

Urethral Electric Conductance

S. Plevnik

The electric conductance of urothelium is considerably lower than that of urine or saline. The amplitude of a weak current passing between two electrodes placed in the urethra will therefore change when fluid enters the urethra from the bladder [1,2]. This new technique which has been further improved and standardised [3] enables the detection of urethral electric conductance (UEC) in one or more points, and allows for the performance of the several standardised static and dynamic UEC tests which have been used in the research and clinical situation.

Measuring Technique

The measuring equipment used for the assessment of urethral electric conductance (UEC) consists of specially constructed 7F probes and battery-powered measuring electronics (Fig. 7.1). The probe consists of two gold-plated brass electrodes, 1 mm in width, mounted 1 mm apart on a flexible silicon rubber tube. A constant sinusoidal voltage with an amplitude of 20 mV peak to peak, and a frequency of 50 kHz, is applied to the electrodes and the amplitude of the current between them is measured. In vitro and in vivo studies revealed the following characteristics of the measuring system:

1. UEC measurements reflect the conductance of a geometrically defined volume corresponding to a cylindrical tube having the inner diameter equal to the outer diameter of the probe, i.e. 2.4 mm; an outer diameter of 6.5 mm; and a length (i.e. axial resolution) of 3.5 mm.

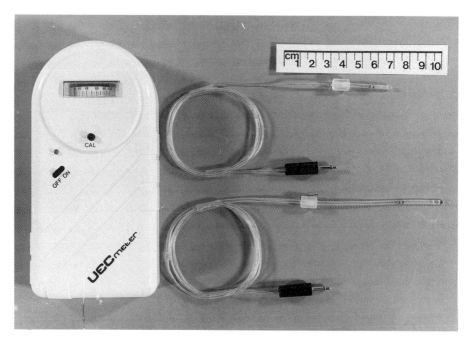

Fig. 7.1. Electronic device for measuring urethral electric conductance (UEC): electronic unit and short and long 7F UEC probes. Note the stabilising collars of the probes (Ormed Ltd, Welwyn Garden City, UK).

2. The conductance measured is independent of the rotation of the probe.
3. The maximum charge is 56 µA.
4. The maximum current density is 5.3 µA mm^{-2}.
5. The temperature effect is 2% per °C.
6. The time response is less than 1 ms.

Two lengths of UEC probe are used for clinical testing: a "short" 50 mm and a "long" 250 mm probe. The special design of the probes allows for stable dynamic recording of UEC by means of a cylindrical collar (Fig. 7.1). As the probe is inserted, the proximal face of the collar meets the external meatus, while the labia minora stabilise the collar and the catheter respectively. In the short probe, the collar is fixed on the probe. The fixed distance between the electrodes and the collar allows for a standard placement of the electrodes 15 mm from the external urethral meatus, i.e. in the distal urethra (in the majority of cases). Thus any fluid which is detected by the short UEC probe would previously have passed the zone of maximum urethral pressure in the mid-urethra and therefore represents true urethral incontinence. In the long probe, the collar is movable along the full length of the probe, so the conductance can be measured at any point in the urethra.

Urethral Electric Conductance Profile (UECP)

Static UECP

The static urethral electric conductance profile (static UECP) is measured by pulling the long UEC probe from the bladder through the urethra at constant withdrawal speed (Figs. 7.2 and 7.11). The electrodes measure the conductance of around 120 µA when placed in the bladder filled with normal saline. A steep gradual decrease in conductance occurs at the level of the inner urethral meatus (IUM) as the electrodes pass from the bladder. As the first electrode is brought close to the IUM, the IUM tissue (which is of lower conductance) suddenly enters the electrode field, at the onset of the gradual decrease in the measured UEC. The UEC continues to decrease gradually until both electrodes are surrounded by the walls of the proximal urethra as the electrodes are further withdrawn through the IUM. This has been confirmed photographically, radiologically and by simultaneous measurement of static urethral pressure profile (UPP) (Fig. 7.2). The UEC is thereafter much lower than that of saline in the bladder and represents the closed (sealed) part of the urethra until the distal 5 mm. This has been shown by simultaneous perfusion with saline and distilled water [3]. When the electrodes are withdrawn through the external urethral meatus a sudden decrease of conductance occurs as the first electrode reaches air. The external urethral meatus can be thus precisely determined on UECP. This allows for an accurate superimposition of UECPs or simultaneously measured UPPs and thus their accurate comparison [4]. The static UPPs are very reproducible and independent of the catheter stiffness, except at the IUM where variations are occasionally seen. The urethral length estimated from UECPs occasionally decreases with bladder volume. Static UECP represents the basis for understanding of other UEC measurements although its clinical value has not yet been explored.

Stress UECP

Stress urethral electric conductance profile (stress UECP) is performed similarly to the static UECP except that the patient is asked to cough at regular intervals during the time of catheter withdrawal. Similarly to the stress urethral pressure profile (UPP)[5], which demonstrates fluid leakage indirectly (at zero urethral closure pressure), stress UECP provides direct information on fluid leakage along the full length of the urethra.

Cough produces closure of the internal urethral meatus (IUM) in younger normal women, i.e. sudden decreases of UEC while the rest of the urethra remains closed since no changes of conductance occur on coughing (Fig. 7.3). In older normal women coughing usually produces an opening of the IUM as well as entry of fluid into the proximal urethra, seen as cough-provoked increases of UEC, while the rest of the urethra remains closed. In genuine stress incontinent female patients, the incontinence is demonstrated by increases of electric conductance in the distal urethra during coughing (Fig. 7.3).

UEC Cystometry

UEC cystometry can be defined as a continuous measurement of the urethral electric conductance at any point in the urethra at the time of the provocative manoeuvres during conventional filling cystometry. After the bladder is filled to maximum capacity and the filling catheter withdrawn (leaving the intravesical pressure catheter and intrarectal pressure catheter), the long UEC probe is inserted and UEC measured at the IUM, and the proximal and distal urethra during coughing and handwashing with cold water, in both supine and erect positions of the patient (Fig. 7.4). For a reliable demonstration of incontinence during cystometry, the short UEC probe is recommended because it allows for a standard placement of the electrodes in the distal urethra, i.e. distal to the point of maximum urethral pressure.

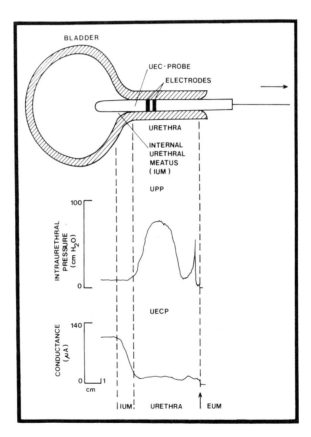

Fig. 7.2. Simultaneously measured static urethral electric conductance profile (UECP) (lower trace) and static urethral pressure profile (UPP) (upper trace) using a specially constructed 7F catheter which allows for a concurrent measurement of Brown and Wickham perfusion UPP. The UECP recording shows high conductance in the bladder, decrease of the conductance at the internal urethral meatus (IUM), low conductance in the urethra, and decrease of conductance to zero at the external urethral meatus (EUM) as the electrodes reach air.

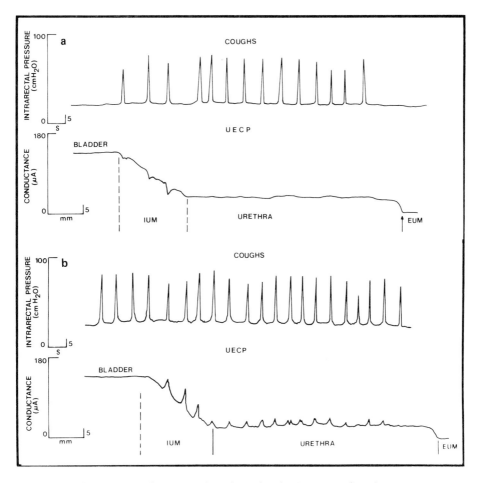

Fig. 7.3.   (a) Stress UECP of the normal continent female. Decreases of conductance are seen at the internal urethral meatus (IUM) while conductance in the urethra remains unchanged during coughing (lower trace). (b) Stress UECP in a patient with genuine stress incontinence showing increases of conductance throughout the full length of the urethra, indicating urethral incompetence (lower trace). Intrarectal pressures are simultaneously measured to show pressure rises during coughing (upper traces on a and b).

A provocative filling cystometry allows: (a) diagnosing genuine stress incontinence (GSI) either by visual observation of fluid leakage at the level of the external urethral meatus or by the presence of a wet perineal pad during absence of detrusor contraction (at stable detrusor pressure); and (b) diagnosing spontaneous and/or provoked detrusor instability (DI) by detecting involuntary detrusor pressure increases. There are two disadvantages of conventional cystometry: (a) urinary leakage cannot always be accurately seen by visual observation (or measured by pad test); and (b) when demonstrated, it can be accurately related to detrusor pressure only when the former is obviously stable. Thus, for example, when leakage is visually seen, or demonstrated by pad test, during cough-provoked detrusor contraction (cough-provoked detrusor pressure rise), it is not possible to say what

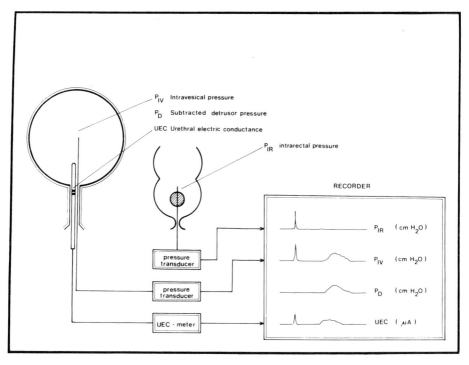

Fig. 7.4. UEC cystometry: diagram of simultaneous measurement of urethral electric conductance (UEC) and conventional provocative cystometry.

is the real cause of incontinence – the increased intravesical pressure during the cough, the detrusor pressure rise which follows immediately after the cough, or both.

UEC cystometry, however, allows accurate assessment of detrusor and urethral function at the time of urethral leakage, which improves the urodynamic diagnosis of the incontinent female patient.

Normal UEC Cystometric Findings

UEC cystometry performed in the normal female shows: (a) a stable detrusor on coughing or handwashing regardless of the patient's position; (b) negative UEC deflections during coughing, indicating internal urethral meatus (IUM) closures, and stable UEC at IUM during handwashing; and (c) continence, i.e. a closed urethra during provocation (Fig. 7.5) in 100% of young asymptomatic females (age 5 to 29 years). However, in 55% (age from 30 to 50 years) and 75% (age from 51 to 80 years) of the older normal female population, cough-provoked increases of conductance are seen at the level of the IUM and proximal urethra, indicating fluid entry into these parts of the urethra, the remaining part of the urethra staying continent regardless of the type of provocation and position of the patient [6,7] (Fig. 7.5).

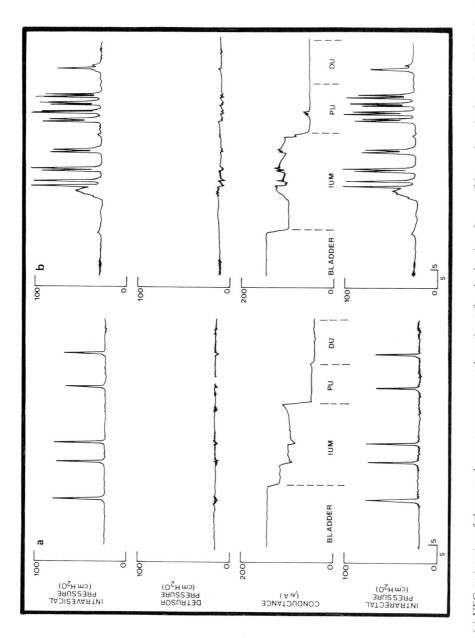

Fig. 7.5. (a) UEC cystometry of the normal young premenopausal continent female showing closure of internal urethral meatus (IUM), i.e. decreases of conductance; and showing competent urethra, i.e. unchanged conductance in the proximal urethra (PU) and distal urethra (DU) during coughing and handwashing in the absence of detrusor contraction. (b) UEC cystometry of an elderly normal continent female showing an incompetent proximal urethra, while the distal urethra is continent, i.e. no changes in UEC are seen in DU during coughing and hand washing in the absence of detrusor contraction.

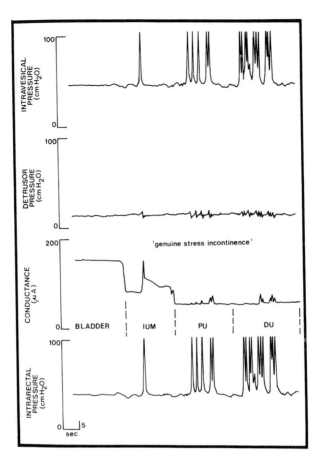

Fig. 7.6. UEC cystometry in a patient with GSI. Increases of the conductance can be seen throughout the full length of the urethra during coughing in the absence of detrusor activity. IUM, internal urethral meatus; PU, proximal urethra; DU, distal urethra.

Genuine Stress Incontinence (GSI)

GSI has been defined by the International Continence Society (ICS) as "a fluid leakage at the external urethral meatus in the absence of detrusor activity". A typical UEC cystometric recording in the GSI patient (Fig. 7.6) shows the upward deflections of conductance during coughing at the level of IUM as well as in the proximal and distal urethra in the absence of detrusor activity, indicating IUM incompetence and urethral leakage.

UEC cystometry, as compared to conventional cystometry, increases the GSI pick up rate by 80% which improves the overall urodynamic diagnosis by 26% [8].

Objective diagnosis of GSI represents one of the most important findings in deciding on treatment, so the 80% increase in the pick-up rate of GSI (alone or associated with DI) as shown on UEC-cystometry further confirms the need for routine UEC measurement in the standard urodynamic work-up of the incontinent woman.

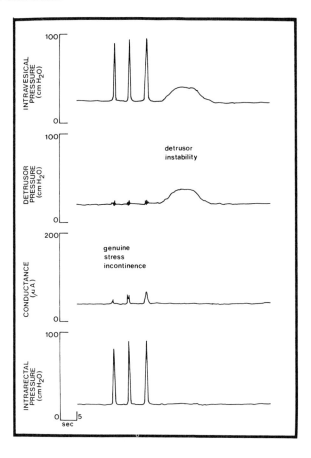

Fig. 7.7. UEC cystometry in a patient with genuine stress incontinence and detrusor instability. Increased distal urethral conductance is observed in the absence of detrusor contraction during coughing with the subsequent involuntary detrusor contraction during which fluid leakage does not occur on a conductance trace, i.e. distal UEC remains unchanged. Note that in such a case only the detrusor instability would be reliably diagnosed from conventional provocative cystometry.

Mixed GSI and DI

The UEC cystometric trace in Fig. 7.7 shows that the intravesical pressure rise during a cough is immediately followed by detrusor contraction, seen as a prolonged increase of detrusor pressure. Urinary leakage which is simultaneously measured by UEC is seen to be present during the cough only, and not during the unstable detrusor contraction, thus revealing the urodynamic diagnosis of mixed GSI and DI. This represents an example when only detrusor instability is diagnosed from conventional cystometry, because urinary leakage, even if observed visually or on pad test, could not be reliably assigned to GSI.

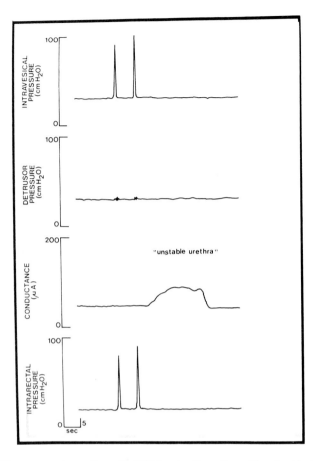

Fig. 7.8. UEC cystometry in a patient with GSI showing the pattern of "urethral instability". Involuntary fluid leakage, i.e. increased distal UEC, occurs in the absence of detrusor contraction as well as in the absence of intra-abdominal pressure rise.

Unstable Urethra

Unstable urethra is, according to the ICS definition, among the GSI patterns and can be recognised as a spontaneous or provoked involuntary urethral leakage (involuntary decrease of urethral closure pressure to zero) which occurs in the absence of the intra-abdominal pressure rise and in the absence of detrusor contraction (Fig. 7.8). The pattern of "unstable urethra" which is sometimes seen on UEC cystometry cannot be recognised from conventional cystometry alone. Only five out of 104 patients were found to have unstable urethra on UEC cystometry and they all also had detrusor instability [8].

Detrusor Incontinence

Detrusor incontinence can be defined as fluid leakage through the urethra detected as an increase in distal urethral conductance at the time of cough-provoked or

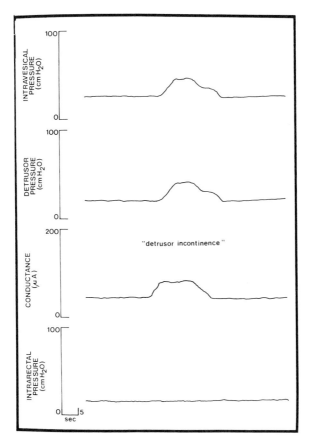

Fig. 7.9. UEC cystometry in a patient with detrusor incontinence showing urinary leakage, i.e. increase in distal UEC during involuntary detrusor contraction.

hand washing-provoked involuntary detrusor contraction (Fig. 7.9). UEC cysto-metry allows for an accurate objective demonstration of detrusor incontinence as defined above, which is not possible when using conventional cystometry. A total of 68% of patients having cystometrically proven detrusor instability were found to have detrusor incontinence on UEC cystometry [8]. The clinical relevance of the objective demonstration of detrusor incontinence remains to be elucidated.

Distal Urethral Electric Conductance (DUEC) Test

Measurement of distal urethral electric conductance per se using the short UEC probe (DUEC test) during provocation proved to be a sensitive means for the demonstration and diagnosis of female urinary incontinence.

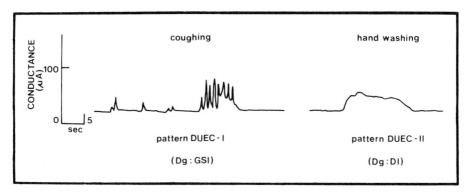

Fig. 7.10. Distal urethral electric conductance (DUEC) test – characteristic patterns. DUEC-I pattern, associated with a diagnosis of genuine stress incontinence (GSI), shows short conductance rises lasting no more than 2 s which occur during coughing; they can also be superimposed on the prolonged conductance rise. DUEC-II pattern is usually associated with a diagnosis of detrusor instability and shows long conductance rises lasting more than 3 s which occur during handwashing with cold water or spontaneously.

Demonstration of Incontinence

The DUEC test performed during standardised provocative manoeuvres such as coughing, hand washing etc., allows rapid and accurate demonstration of incontinence in 75% of symptomatic females. Visual examination and pad test (performed simultaneously with the DUEC test) demonstrated incontinence in 39% and 44% of patients respectively [9] (fluid loss of 1 g was taken as a cut-off point for pad test). A positive DUEC test has been found in 96% of a group of female patients [10] who all had positive simultaneously measured pad tests, taking 0.1 g as the cut-off point.

Diagnosis of Incontinence by the DUEC Test

Two characteristic patterns which can be identified from DUEC traces [9] have been shown to correlate well with the cystometric diagnosis [11]. These two leakage patterns which occur during standardised provocation with coughing and hand washing in cold water are described as follows:

1. DUEC-I pattern: occurs during provocation with coughing and is typically characterised by short rises in conductance which last no longer than 2 s (Fig. 7.10). These can also be superimposed on a prolonged conductance rise and have been shown to occur at the time of the cough and in the absence of detrusor contraction.
2. DUEC-II pattern: usually occurs during provocation with handwashing. It is characterised by a prolonged conductance rise (without superimposed short conductance spikes), lasting for more than 3 s. These rises have been shown to occur during provoked or spontaneous detrusor contraction, and sometimes also in the absence of detrusor activity (Fig. 7.10).

With a full bladder a highly significant association was found between the DUEC-I pattern and a normal detrusor pressure (absence of detrusor contraction during coughing) and similarly, between the DUEC-II pattern and a raised detrusor pressure (detrusor contraction) [11]. This allows a diagnosis of GSI to be made from the DUEC-I patterns and diagnosis of detrusor instability (detrusor incontinence) to be made from the DUEC-II pattern. Furthermore, in relating the patient's symptoms to the urodynamic diagnosis, the DUEC patterns proved to have significantly higher diagnostic sensitivity (higher pick-up rate) than conventional cystometry.

It may be concluded that DUEC diagnosis of GSI and/or DI is sufficient if patients are considered for conservative treatment. However, if operative treatment of GSI is contemplated, more precise diagnosis is required, at least in some patients, since operation should not be undertaken on DI patients. Conventional cystometry or UEC cystometry is still needed in those cases where surgical treatment is being considered. Comparison of the cystometric diagnosis with the DUEC diagnosis suggests a more reliable guideline towards making a decision for operative treatment: using symptoms and DUEC patterns in combination allows correct treatment in 47% of patients without recourse to cystometry. Patients who require further evaluation with cystometry are those complaining of urge incontinence without a DUEC-II pattern.

Internal Urethral Meatus Conductance (IUMC) Test

Detrusor pressure and urethral electric conductance, when measured simultaneously with the electrodes placed at the internal urethral meatus (IUM), i.e. in the middle of the steep portion of the static UECP (Fig. 7.11), have shown variations of IUM conductance in the presence and in the absence of detrusor contractions. These conductance variations (also called "bladder neck mechanism" conductance variations) are caused by IUM movements which are alternately bringing the IUM wall into and out of the electrodes' electric field. Marked increases of IUM conductance which have been shown to occur before (and during) detrusor contraction as well as in the absence of detrusor contraction are due to the opening of the IUM. IUM conductance has also been measured simultaneously with maximum urethral pressure [3], and it has been reported that a reduction in urethral pressure is usually associated with an increase in IUM electric conductance [12]. A highly significant correlation was found between subjective grading of symptoms of urgency (and urge incontinence) and maximum peak to peak IUM conductance variations measured during three minutes with 250 ml of saline in the bladder [13–15]. Thus the IUMC test allows objective grading of urgency (and urge incontinence) and has a place in their diagnosis and follow-up.

UEC-Controlled Stamey Procedure

It has been reported that an intraoperative UEC test during increased intra-abdominal pressures is predictive of failure and success in GSI surgery, i.e. the Stamey procedure, fascial sling, and vaginal repair [16].

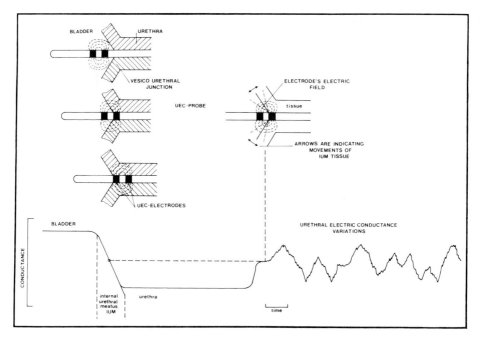

Fig. 7.11. Schematic diagram showing UEC time variations measured with the electrodes placed in the middle of the steep portion of conductance slope at the internal urethral meatus (IUM). The variations are due to the IUM movements (or closures) which are alternately bringing the IUM wall into and out of the electrodes' electric field; and the anatomical locations of the UEC electrodes at the corresponding points of the conductance trace measured during electrode withdrawal through the IUM.

   The Stamey procedure was further intraoperatively controlled by UEC measurement and was assessed objectively and subjectively [17] with the aim of increasing the accuracy of placement of sutures at the vesicourethral junction (VUJ), and of restoring urethral competence at minimum elevation of the VUJ, i.e. at minimum tension of suspending sutures.
   During the UEC-controlled Stamey procedure, the patient is placed in the lithotomy position under epidural anaesthesia and the long UEC probe is introduced. As the electrodes are manually withdrawn from the bladder, the internal urethral meatus (IUM) can be easily recognised on the UEC meter (or on the recording trace) at the middle of the steep portion of the static UEC profile. Similarly, by further withdrawing the probe to the point where conductance stops decreasing, the placement of the electrodes in the proximal urethra is verified. By marking the catheter at the point of the external urethral meatus (EUM) the distance between the catheter demarcation and the electrodes is used to control where the sutures are placed on either side of the VUJ.
   After placement of the suspending sutures the long UEC probe is introduced again, and the electrodes are placed at the level of IUM (Fig. 7.12). With the sutures left untied, the patient is asked to cough, and the positive deflection of IUM conductance is observed on the UEC meter (Fig. 7.13). The sutures are then pulled just enough to be sure that they are straightened and then bilaterally

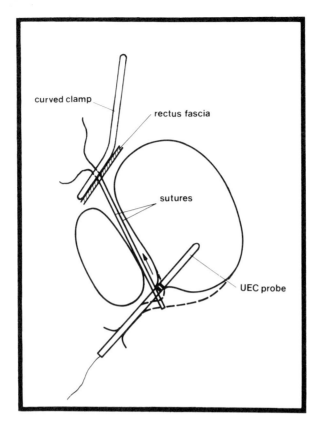

Fig. 7.12.   Diagram of the UEC-controlled Stamey procedure.

temporarily clamped at the rectus fascia, without producing any elevation of the
VUJ. The competence of the IUM and proximal urethra is then checked again
and the sutures are tied so that competent UEC patterns are obtained during
coughing (negative deflection at IUM and unchanged conductance in the proximal
urethra; Fig. 7.13). If urethral incompetence is still present during coughing, the
VUJ is gradually elevated by incremental pulling, i.e. by incremental shortening
of the suspending sutures, until competent patterns are obtained on coughing;
then the sutures are tied. Incremental shortening of suspending sutures can be
most easily performed by re-clamping the sutures, using the third clamp just below
the site where the sutures have been previously clamped. The length of the "elevation increment" thus corresponds to the width of the "holding" part of the curved
clamp. To keep the previously accurately determined "optimum" suture lengths
after the procedure, notches must be made at the level of the curved clamps
before unclamping.

   Fifty female patients with a urodynamic diagnosis of GSI were treated by the
UEC-controlled Stamey procedure [17]. Their mean age was 39 years, range from
34 to 67 years. Pre- and postoperative objective assessment included combined
UEC cystometry and pad testing.

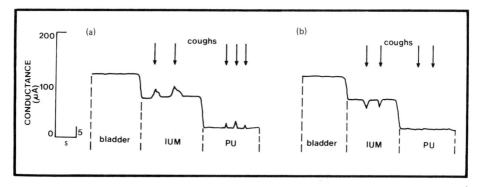

Fig. 7.13. Recordings of the intraoperative measurement of UEC during the Stamey procedure showing (a) opening of the internal urethral meatus (IUM) and proximal urethra (PU) during coughing before fixation of suspending sutures; and (b) closure of the IUM and PU during coughing after fixation of elevating sutures.

In the majority of patients intraoperatively assessed urethral competence was obtained by tying the previously straightened sutures with only minor elevation of the VUJ. In 86% (43 patients) subjective and objective cure was found at the 6–24 months follow-up period. Thirty-nine patients were cured (dry on pad testing, UEC testing and subjectively) while in two patients the catheter was removed after 7 and 14 days respectively. All patients had residual volumes of less than 50 ml prior to catheter removal.

These results permit the conclusion that the UEC-controlled Stamey procedure allows:

1. An accurate placement of elevating sutures.
2. Restoration of urethral competence at minimum elevation of the VUJ and therefore minimum tension in the suspending sutures, thus reducing the possibility of
   a) rupture of the suture through the tissue,
   b) tearing of the sutures,
   c) delayed voiding and postoperative voiding difficulties.
3. Performance of the standardised Stamey procedure by any urogynaecological surgeon.

References

1. Plevnik S, Vrtačnik P, Janež J. Detection of fluid entry into the urethra by electric impedance measurement: electric fluid bridge test. Clin Phys Physiol Meas 1983; 3:309–13.
2. Plevnik S, Brown M, Sutherst JR, Vrtačnik P, Janež J. Tracking of fluid in urethra by simultaneous electric impedance measurements at three sites. Urol Int 1983; 38:29–32.
3. Plevnik S, Holmes DM, Janež J, Mundy AR, Vrtačnik P. Urethral electric conductance (UEC) – a new parameter for evaluation of urethral and bladder function: methodology of the assessment of its clinical potential. In: Proceedings of the Fifteenth International Continence Society Meeting, London, 1985; 90–1.
4. Plevnik S, Janež J, Vrtačnik P. Superimposition of urethral closure pressure profiles using urethral electric conduction measurements. Neurourol Urodynam 1985; 4:129–34.

5. Asmussen M, Ulmsten U. Simultaneous urethrocystometry and urethral pressure profile measurement with a new technique. Acta Obstet Gynecol Scand 1975; 54:385–6.
6. Janež J, Plevnik S, Tršinar B, Mihelič M. Bladder neck and urethral behaviour during stress in continent female: an age stratified study. In: Proceedings of the Sixteenth International Continence Society Meeting, Boston, 1986; 433–4.
7. Janež J, Plevnik S, Vrtačnik P. Assessment of bladder neck mechanism during coughing by urethral electric conductance measurement: UEC-metry. Neurourol Urodynam 1987; 3:179–80.
8. Peattie AB, Plevnik S, Stanton SL. Is the bladder really an unreliable witness? Neurourol Urodynam 1989; 8:303–4.
9. Holmes DM, Plevnik S, Stanton SL. Distal urethral electric conductance (DUEC) test for the detection of urinary leakage. In: Proceedings of the Fifteenth International Continence Society Meeting, London, 1985; 94–5.
10. Mayne CJ, Hilton P. The distal urethral electric conductance test: standardization of method and clinical reliability. Neurourol Urodynam 1988; 7:55–60.
11. Peattie AB, Plevnik S, Stanton SL. Distal urethral electric conductance (DUEC) test: a screening test for female urinary incontinence? Neurourol Urodynam 1988; 3:173–4.
12. Hilton P, Mayne CJ. Urethral pressure variations: the correlation between pressure measurement and electrical conductance in genuine stress incontinence. Neurourol Urodynam 1988; 3:175–6.
13. Holmes MD, Plevnik S, Stanton SL. Bladder neck electrical conductivity in female urinary urgency and urge incontinence. Br J Obstet Gynaecol 1989; 96:816–20.
14. Peattie AB, Plevnik S, Stanton SL. Assessment and treatment of sensory urge incontinence using the bladder neck electric conductance (BNEC) test. Neurourol Urodynam 1987; 3:256–66.
15. Peattie AB, Plevnik S, Stanton SL. The use of bladder neck electric conductance (BNEC) in the investigation and management of sensory urge incontinence in the female. J R Soc Med 1988; 81:442–4.
16. Janež J, Plevnik S, Vrtačnik P. Prognostic value of urethral electric conductance (UEC) stress test performed during surgery of stress incontinence. In: Proceedings of the Fifteenth International Continence Society Meeting, London, 1985; 92–3.
17. Janež J, Plevnik S. UEC-controlled Stamey procedure. Neurourol Urodynam 1989; 8:338–9.

Chapter 8

Vaginal Ultrasound and Urinary Stress Incontinence

M. J. Quinn

Vaginal ultrasound is a new technique for the investigation of the lower urinary tract in women with urinary incontinence. High frequency endoprobes with reduced external dimensions permit dynamic assessment of the bladder outlet in recumbent, sitting and erect positions [1]. Previous radiological techniques have included bead-chain cystourethrography (BCUG) [2] and video-cystourethrography (VCUG) [3]. The dynamic aspects of BCUG are limited to the displacement of the bladder neck during a Valsalva manoeuvre. Synchronous VCUG, with concurrent pressure measurements, permits the nature and timing of leakage of contrast media to be imaged with the result that it has been adopted, in some quarters, as the "reference standard" for the diagnosis of urinary stress incontinence [4]. Both techniques, however, require exposure to X-rays, urethral catheterisation, established radiological facilities and experienced staff.

Ultrasound has been suggested as a suitable alternative to conventional radiological techniques and abdominal, perineal and rectal routes have been proposed [5–7]. Impaired resolution of the image, distortion of the anatomical features and lack of acceptability to patients have limited the development of these techniques. Vaginal ultrasound, using equipment with appropriate technical specifications, is a reproducible technique for imaging the bladder outlet, and provides high resolution images without distortion of the anatomical features or discomfort to the patient. Other contributors to this book have indicated the controversies surrounding the investigation of symptoms of the lower urinary tract and the difficulty of choosing the appropriate surgical operation: this chapter will outline the potential of vaginal ultrasound in both of these situations.

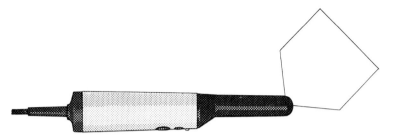

Fig. 8.1. The endoprobe is a mechanical sector scanner operating at a frequency of 7 MHz with an offset field (45 degrees) that scans over a focal range of 1–6 cm through an arc of 112 degrees.

Equipment

In this description, a 7 MHz mechanical sector scanner (Bruel and Kjaer 8537, Fig. 8.1) has been used in conjunction with its parent unit (Bruel and Kjaer 1846). Key features of the endoprobe include its high frequency (7 MHz), offset field (45 degrees), wide field angle (112 degrees) and high frame rate (18 frames s^{-1}). These specifications ensure that a saggital section of the anterior pelvis in the plane of the symphysis pubis may be conveniently obtained by placing the endoprobe 1–2 cm inside the introitus, without distortion of the anatomical features (Fig. 8.2). The high frame rate enables dynamic events such as the response to a cough to be consistently imaged.

Technique

Full assessment includes history, examination, and ultrasound scanning in both recumbent and sitting positions with a "comfortably full" bladder. Explanation of the technique and correct positioning on an adjustable couch are essential preliminaries to successful ultrasound examination. The patient should be horizontal with her head placed on a pillow to permit viewing of the ultrasound screen. The endoprobe is placed in the finger of a sterile, disposable, plastic glove, lubricated with coupling gel and placed one to two centimetres inside the introitus. The position of the full bladder is immediately identified by its hypoechoic appearance. Rotation of the endoprobe around its longitudinal axis identifies a saggital plane in which both the bladder neck and proximal urethra may be imaged.

Examination in the recumbent position permits an accurate assessment of the relative positions of the bladder neck and the inferior border of the symphysis pubis. Assessment in the sitting position is a more sensitive technique to demonstrate opening of the bladder neck with a cough. The ultrasound examination is concluded by the patient voiding to completion so that the bladder volume may be recorded.

Potential problems during the examination include significant prolapse of the anterior vaginal wall and distortion of the anatomical features by the endoprobe.

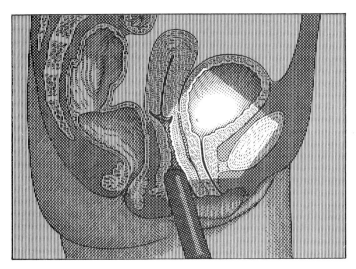

Fig. 8.2. The anatomical field is a sagittal section of the anterior pelvis in the plane of the symphysis pubis. The important landmarks are the urethrovesical junction and the inferior border of the symphysis pubis.

Moderate or severe prolapse of the anterior vaginal wall makes ultrasound examination in the sitting position difficult. Examination in the recumbent position is usually possible, though "ballooning" of the anterior vaginal wall with a cough may prevent satisfactory assessment of the dynamic features during a cough. Minor degrees of prolapse do not restrict ultrasound examination. The technical specifications of the endoprobe, with the transducer mounted at 45° to the horizontal and a maximum diameter of 22 mm, ensure the endoprobe can be placed within the introitus without distortion of the anatomical features. The precise effect of the endoprobe is visible throughout the examination since its position and effect on adjacent tissues may be visualised on the ultrasound screen. Re-orientation of the endoprobe will avoid any distorting effect. The reduced dimensions of the endoprobe and the fact that the patient can see the ultrasound image ensure a high degree of patient acceptability. In a comparison with digital vaginal examination, 48 of 50 women preferred ultrasound examination with this equipment, to traditional pelvic examination.

The Ultrasound Features of the Lower Urinary Tract

Ultrasound appearances of the lower urinary tract depend on the differing acoustic impedances of urine, muscle, ligament, cartilage, and trabecular and cortical bone. Additional information may be gained by introducing materials with a different acoustic pattern, e.g. catheters or pressure transducers.

The symphysis pubis is a secondary cartilaginous joint with ultrasound appearances that are determined by the pad of cartilage connecting the pubic bones. Cartilage appears as a dense, homogeneous, echogenic pattern similar to the

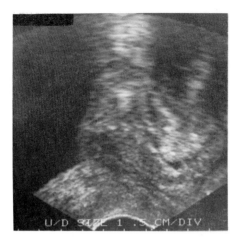 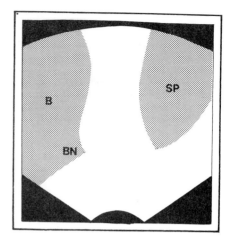

Fig. 8.3. a and b, The cartilage of the symphysis pubis appears as a hyperechoic feature in contrast to the hypoechoic appearance of the stored urine. B, bladder; BN, bladder neck; SP, symphysis pubis.

surrounding connective tissue (Fig. 8.3). The shape of the inferior half of the symphysis and its immobility during a Valsalva manoeuvre or a cough differentiate it from other structures. The pubis adjacent to the symphysis is composed of trabecular bone with a dense inferior cortex so that it appears as a hypoechoic structure (trabecular bone) with a hyperechoic, inferior border (cortical bone). Rotation of the endoprobe around its longitudinal axis identifies both pubic bones and intervening cartilaginous pad.

The Bladder and Urethra

The "bladder neck" may refer to a number of different structures. Radiologically it is the junction of urethra and bladder whereas urodynamically it may denote a gradient in urethral pressure. In the context of vaginal ultrasound the term refers to the junction of the urethra and the bladder. The position of the bladder is identified by the echolucent properties of the stored urine whereas the urethra is usually closed at rest. The course of the urethra may be identified by the echolucent features of its blood supply. The position of the bladder neck is determined by the contrast in echogenicity between the stored urine and the urethra. In women without urinary symptoms, a cough is associated with minor displacement of the bladder neck in the direction of the sacrum, with prompt return to the resting position.

The pubovesical ligaments (PVL) appear in an oblique plane as dense, echogenic structures lateral to the midline, extending between the bladder neck and the inferior border of the symphysis (Fig. 8.4). Rotation of the endoprobe between 10 and 2 o'clock identifies both pubovesical ligaments. The integrity of the PVL may be determined by a Valsalva manoeuvre. Continent women have intact PVL that permit rotation of the bladder neck through an arc that has a fixed radius centred at the pubic insertion. Disruption of the anterior suspensory mechanism

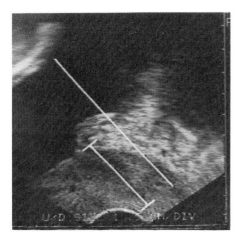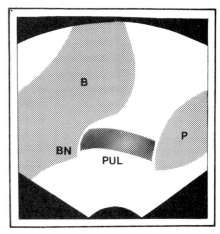

Fig. 8.4. a and b, The pubovesical ligament is seen as a broad echogenic band extending from the posterior surface of the pubis to the bladder neck and adjacent structures. In all the scans illustrated, the longitudinal axis of the patient extends from the top left corner of the image (head) to the bottom right corner (feet). B, bladder; BN, bladder neck; P, symphysis pubis; PUL, pubovesical ligament.

is occasionally seen in women following traumatic vaginal delivery with urinary stress incontinence dating from early in the puerperium.

The Ultrasound Appearances Associated with Lower Urinary Tract Disorders

Ultrasound examination in the sitting position establishes the presence or absence of genuine stress incontinence. Bladder neck opening and urinary leakage concurrent with a cough confirms the diagnosis (Fig. 8.5). The endoprobe is prepared, and is placed at the introitus by the patient. The examiner identifies the position of the bladder neck, selects a minimum frame rate of 18 Hz and asks the patient to cough. Urinary leakage is often directly visible and is accompanied by concurrent opening of the sphincteric mechanism.

Opening of the bladder neck resulting from detrusor activity is associated with a configuration markedly different from that of stress incontinence (Fig. 8.6) and occurs under different circumstances. Detrusor activity may be provoked by bladder filling, by a change in position, or by an increase in intra-abdominal pressure that may provoke subsequent urinary leakage. The differentiation between detrusor activity and sphincter weakness as causes of leakage has not proved to be a practical problem since there is a clear interval between the increase in intra-abdominal pressure and the events that precede urinary leakage in detrusor activity (opening of the bladder neck and proximal urethra) – in contrast to the direct and immediate effects on the sphincteric mechanism in women with urethral sphincter incompetence. Lesser degrees of detrusor instability may produce bladder neck opening without incontinence, or definite "twitches" of the bladder neck. Whether vaginal ultrasound can reliably detect the effects of detrusor instability remains to be established.

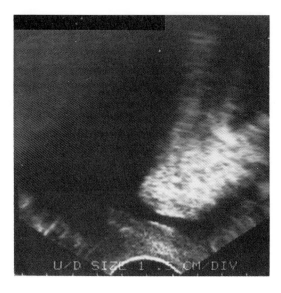

Fig. 8.5. Opening of the bladder neck and proximal urethra with urinary leakage concurrent with a cough establishes a diagnosis of urinary stress incontinence.

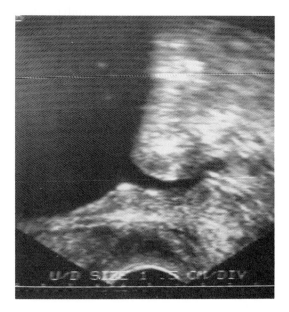

Fig. 8.6. The nature, timing and provocation of bladder neck opening differ in patients with detrusor instability compared to those with urinary stress incontinence.

A Prospective Comparison of Urodynamic Investigations and Vaginal Ultrasound in the Diagnosis of Urinary Stress Incontinence

A prospective comparison of urodynamic investigations and vaginal ultrasound has been conducted to determine whether vaginal ultrasound is a sensitive technique for the diagnosis of genuine stress incontinence and whether it discriminates satisfactorily between stress incontinence and detrusor instability.

A total of 124 women with lower urinary tract symptoms have been consecutively assessed by conventional urodynamic investigations and vaginal ultrasound. Patients were assessed by conventional urodynamic investigations in one of two urodynamic units and referred for vaginal ultrasound without the results of the preceding investigation. All patients underwent vaginal ultrasound and the urodynamic investigations included:

   124/124 women underwent symptomatic enquiry
   124/124 women underwent physical examination
   124/124 women underwent filling and voiding cystometry
    80/124 women underwent urethral pressure profilometry
    25/124 women underwent synchronous videocystourethrography

Both techniques were compared in respect of the presence or absence of genuine stress incontinence. The final diagnoses following the respective investigations were:

	Urodynamic investigation	Vaginal ultrasound
Stress incontinence ($\pm$ detrusor instability)	90/124	93/124
Other conditions (normal; detrusor instability)	34/124	31/124

Discordance between the two investigations in the diagnosis of stress incontinence occurred in 9/124 women (Kappa value = 0.82). The sensitivity of vaginal ultrasound in the diagnosis of stress incontinence was 96% with a specificity of 82%.

Part of the discrepancy arises from the all-embracing urodynamic definition of stress incontinence that includes those women who have a history of stress incontinence in the absence of detrusor instability. Women with relatively minor symptoms, such as stress incontinence during aerobic exercise or on the squash court, are defined as having genuine stress incontinence after negative filling cystometry. Ultrasound, however, demonstrates downward displacement of the bladder neck and no conclusive diagnosis is established. Despite the loss of sensitivity and specificity in patients with minor symptoms, it is clear that for the vast majority of patients with stress incontinence, vaginal ultrasound in the sitting position offers a new method of establishing a positive diagnosis of urethral sphincter incompetence that is simple and convenient when compared to previous methods of urodynamic investigation.

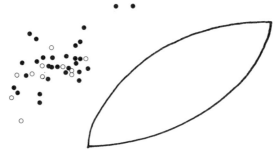

Fig. 8.7. The relative positions of the bladder neck and inferior border of the symphysis pubis in 40 women after colposuspension. ●, successful; ○, unsuccessful.

The Anatomical Consequences of Suprapubic Operations for Stress Incontinence

With the decline in use of vaginal operations, three types of procedure account for the majority of surgical options for urinary incontinence:

1. Retropubic urethropexy, e.g. colposuspension [8] or the Marshall–Marchetti–Kranz procedure [9]
2. Needle-suspension procedures, as described by Pereyra [10], Stamey [11] or Raz [12]
3. Sling procedures with artificial or autologous material.

Despite the redefined surgical repertoire, it is by no means clear which operation is appropriate for which patient, nor is it agreed as to the optimal technique for each type of procedure. Part of the reason stems from the lack of objective assessment of the results of incontinence operations in many series. Symptomatic enquiry is clearly insufficient and many patients find repeat urodynamic investigation an unreasonable proposition. In addition, newer variations of needle suspension procedure have yet to be evaluated over the medium and long term. Comparability between studies is not assisted by variations in patient groups, and variations in technique and in the experience of the surgeon.

Despite these omissions, suprapubic operations have high rates of success in both primary and recurrent incontinence [13,14] and achieve their effect, in part, by elevating and supporting the bladder neck [15,16]. Vaginal ultrasound, under validated conditions, permits the relationship of the bladder neck and inferior border of the symphysis pubis to be reliably assessed. It is therefore a simple and convenient technique to assess the anatomical consequences of different suprapubic operations.

Two consecutive series of patients have been evaluated by vaginal ultrasound after colposuspension or Stamey bladder neck suspension. Operations were performed with a variety of techniques by a number of different surgeons, though no anatomical result appeared to be attributable to technique or seniority. All patients have been scanned in the recumbent position with the endoprobe maintained in a horizontal position using a spirit level fixed to the needle biopsy guide.

Postoperative Results of Colposuspension

Overall 29/40 (72.5%) women had a successful result after colposuspension and 11/40 (27.5%) had persistent or recurrent symptoms. The final position of the

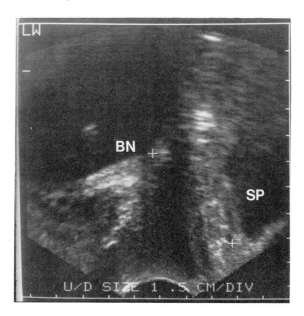

Fig. 8.8. Successful colposuspension. The bladder neck is elevated and supported above the inferior border of the symphysis pubis. The hyperechoic features of non-absorbable suture material are visible at their insertion in the vaginal fornices and iliopectineal ligament. BN, bladder neck; SP, symphysis pubis.

radiological bladder neck relative to the inferior border of the symphysis pubis is shown in Fig. 8.7. Different anatomical configurations are associated with successful and unsuccessful outcomes. Successful outcomes are associated with elevation and support of the bladder neck (Fig. 8.8), whilst unsuccessful results (early and late recurrent stress incontinence, persistent stress incontinence and frequency–urgency syndrome) occurred in 11/40 patients and were associated with different anatomical configurations.

Recurrent stress incontinence occurred at two times: early in the postoperative period (one woman), or later with the onset of menopausal symptoms (four women). Early recurrent stress incontinence in the postoperative period was diagnosed with ultrasound examination. The initial postoperative scan showed an elevated bladder neck but repeat ultrasound at four weeks confirmed a clinical diagnosis of recurrent stress incontinence. The diagnosis of stress incontinence in four peri- and postmenopausal women was established by vaginal ultrasound, where despite evidence of an "intact" colposuspension by digital examination there was opening and descent of the bladder neck with a cough. Recurrent stress incontinence was confirmed by urodynamic investigations in three of the four women.

Inaccurate positioning of the supporting sutures at colposuspension gave rise to either frequency and urgency or persistent stress incontinence, depending on the precise position of the sutures [17]. In the one patient with persistent stress incontinence, no elevation of the bladder neck was achieved and the vaginal shelf indented the bladder base (Fig. 8.9) whilst in the patients with persistent frequency and urgency the vaginal shelf underruns the trigone and may result in the worsening

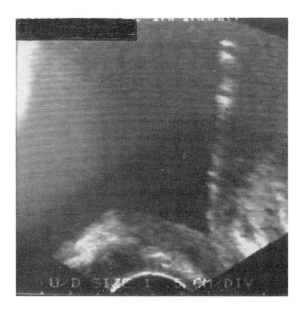

Fig. 8.9. Persistent stress incontinence following colposuspension. The vaginal shelf underruns the bladder base and no elevation or support of the bladder neck has been achieved.

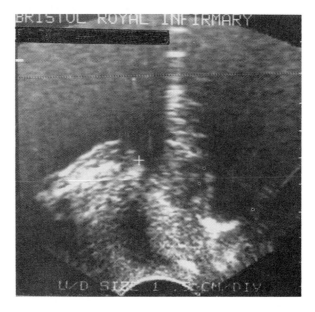

Fig. 8.10. Persistent frequency and urgency following colposuspension is associated with the vaginal shelf indenting the trigone.

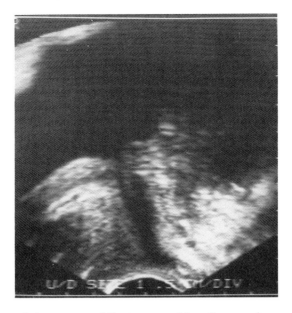

Fig. 8.11. The anatomical appearances following successful needle suspension procedure are similar to those of colposuspension.

of symptoms associated with pre-existing detrusor instability or the onset of de novo detrusor instability following colposuspension (Fig. 8.10).

It is often stated that "suprapubic surgery may worsen detrusor instability" [18] although in many cases a well-executed operation may cure symptoms of stress incontinence and detrusor instability [19]. It is apparent from the above observations regarding the anatomical consequences of surgery, that factors other than the preoperative existence of detrusor instability may produce irritative symptoms following colposuspension. A re-examination of the postoperative causes of worsening irritative symptoms seems necessary, since if the effects of preoperative instability are less significant than was originally thought, there seems little benefit in establishing its presence or absence prior to surgery.

Postoperative Results of Stamey Bladder Neck Suspension

Similar studies have been performed in 30 patients undergoing Stamey bladder neck suspension [11]. Successful results are associated with similar appearances to that of colposuspension (Figs 8.11 and 8.12). Three methods have been used to identify the vaginal attachment of the Stamey suture: a Dacron sleeve, an inert button [20] and serial bites of the paraurethral tissues [12]. Overall 10 of 31 patients in the postoperative period reported recurrent stress incontinence that was confirmed by vaginal ultrasound. In three patients it was clear that one of the two sutures had failed, so that although the position of the bladder neck was maintained at rest there was downward displacement and opening of the bladder neck with a cough. Only one patient complained of persistent frequency and urgency following the operation. Failures occurred irrespective of the surgical technique, but further controlled studies may establish an optimal technique to avoid the prohibitive early failure rate.

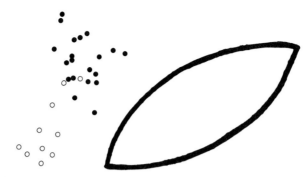

Fig. 8.12. The relative positions of the bladder neck and inferior border of the symphysis pubis in 30 women following bladder neck needle suspension. ●, successful; ○, unsuccessful.

Conclusions

Vaginal ultrasound, with the appropriate equipment, is a simple, non-invasive technique for the dynamic assessment of the lower urinary tract. Objective assessment of the relative positions of the bladder neck and the inferior border of the symphysis pubis permits a comparison of the effects of different suprapubic operations in the treatment of urinary stress incontinence. Examination in the sitting position is a sensitive and specific technique for the diagnosis of stress incontinence and can detect opening of the bladder neck associated with detrusor instability. Should the technique be able reliably to detect the effects of detrusor instability on the continence mechanism, it would obviate the need for many of the invasive techniques that are used for the investigation of urinary incontinence in women.

References

1. Quinn MJ, Beynon J, Mortensen NJMcC, Smith PJB. Transvaginal endosonography: a new method to study the anatomy of the lower urinary tract in urinary stress incontinence. Br J Urol 1988; 62:414–18.
2. Green TH. Development of a plan for the diagnosis and treatment of urinary stress incontinence. Am J Obstet Gynecol 1962; 83:632–48.
3. Bates CP, Whiteside CG, Turner-Warwick R. Synchronous cine/pressure/flow/cystourethrography with special reference to stress incontinence. Br J Urol 1970; 42:714–23.
4. Versi E, Cardozo L, Anand D. The use of pad tests in the investigation of female urinary incontinence. J Obstet Gynecol 1988; 8:270–3.
5. Brown MC, Sutherst JR, Murray A, Richmond D. Potential use of ultrasound in place of X-ray fluoroscopy in urodynamics. Br J Urol 1985; 57:88–90.
6. Richmond DH, Sutherst JR, Brown MC. Screening of the bladder base and urethra using linear array transrectal ultrasound scanning. J Clin Ultrasound 1986; 14:647–51.
7. Bergman A, McKenzie CJ, Richmond J, Ballard CA, Platt LD. Transrectal ultrasound versus cystography in the evaluation of anatomical stress urinary incontinence. Br J Urol 1988; 62:228–34.
8. Burch JC. Urethrovaginal fixation to Cooper's ligament for correction of stress incontinence, cystocele and prolapse. Am J Obstet Gynecol 1961; 81:281–90.

9. Krantz K. Marshall–Marchetti–Krantz procedure. In: Stanton SL, Tanagho E, eds. Surgery of female incontinence. Heidelberg: Springer, 1980; 47–54.
10. Pereyra AJ. A simplified surgical procedure for the correction of stress incontinence in women. West J Surg Obstet Gynecol 1959; 67:223–7.
11. Stamey T. Endoscopic suspension of the vesical neck. In: Stanton SL, Tanagho E, eds. Surgery of female incontinence. Heidelberg: Springer, 1980; 77–90.
12. Raz S. Modified bladder neck suspension for female stress incontinence. Urology 1981; 17:82–5.
13. Stanton SL, Cardozo LD. Results of the colposuspension operation for incontinence and prolapse. Br J Obstet Gynaecol 1979; 86:693–7.
14. Freeman RM, Malvern J. Colposuspension for genuine stress incontinence. J Obstet Gynecol 1987; 8:161–5.
15. Hodgkinson CP, Stanton SL. Retropubic urethropexy or colposuspension. In: Stanton SL, Tanagho E, eds. Surgery of female incontinence. Heidelberg: Springer, 1980; 55–68.
16. Hertogs K, Stanton SL. Lateral bead-chain urethrocystography after successful and unsuccessful colposuspension. Br J Obstet Gynaecol 1985; 92:1179–83.
17. Quinn MJ, Beynon J, Mortensen NJMcC, Smith PJB. Vaginal endosonography in the post-operative assessment of colposuspension. Br J Urol 1989; 63:295–300.
18. Cardozo LD, Stanton SL, Williams JE. Detrusor instability following surgery for genuine stress incontinence. Br J Urol 1979; 51:204–7.
19. McGuire EJ. Clinical evaluation of the lower urinary tract. Clin Obstet Gynecol 1985; 12:311–18.
20. Handley Ashken M, Abrams PH, Lawrence WT. Stamey endoscopic bladder neck suspension for stress incontinence. Br J Urol 1984; 56:629–34.

Chapter 9

Role of Electrophysiological Studies

R. S. Kirby and I. Eardley

The bladder is unusual in that it is autonomically innervated, but functions under voluntary control. Three sets of nerves innervate the bladder and urethral sphincter: sympathetic, parasympathetic and somatic, and each of these transmits both motor and sensory information. The system is integrated through connections in peripheral ganglia, sacral spinal cord and in the medulla and pons. Higher centres, including the basal ganglia, hypothalamus and frontal cortex, act to super-impose voluntary control, mainly by inhibition, on the pontine micturition centres of Barrington.

Ideally, electrophysiological tests should be capable of assessing the integrity of each of these sets of nerves, as well as examining the function of the pontine and cortical controlling centres. In practice this ideal has yet to be achieved, partly because we still lack the ability to investigate the sympathetic and para-sympathetic innervation of the bladder electrophysiologically. However, some more indirect tests can provide valuable information about the integrity of the autonomic innervation while it is now possible to assess completely the somatic innervation of the striated urethral sphincter.

Overall Electrophysiological Assessment of Sphincter Activity

Much of the early work on urethral sphincter electromyography (EMG) focused on the overall sphincter activity recorded during urodynamic studies. The record-ings were usually made from catheter-mounted electrodes or hooked needle elec-

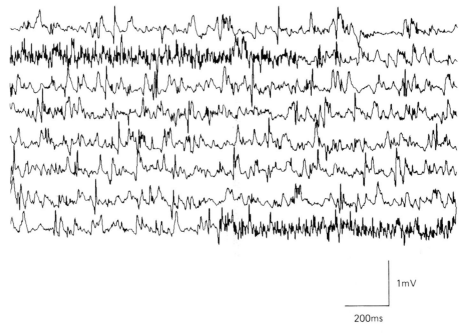

1mV

200ms

Fig. 9.1. Complex repetitive discharges recorded from a patient with chronic urinary retention (continuous EMG tracing).

trodes. Spontaneous sphincter activity can be recorded at rest, even during sleep, and this activity increases with bladder filling. Relaxation of the muscle, characterised by electrical silence, normally occurs only during micturition. Failure of relaxation of the sphincter in these circumstances is termed detrusor sphincter dyssynergia (DSD) [1]. This phenomenon occurs in diseases which affect the suprasacral spinal cord, such as multiple sclerosis, and also in injuries to the cervical and thoracic spinal cord. By contrast, neurological diseases affecting the innervation of the bladder above the level of the pons, such as cerebrovascular accidents, do not result in DSD.

Apart from confirming the presence of DSD, recordings of overall EMG activity seldom provide much clinically useful information. One exception to this is in a group of young women who have long-standing urinary retention; in a proportion of these abnormal EMG activity can be recorded from the urethral sphincter and these so called complex repetitive discharges may result in a failure of sphincter relaxation and ultimately urinary retention may ensue (Fig. 9.1). The cause of these discharges is still uncertain, but many of the patients appear to suffer from the polycystic ovary syndrome, and it is possible that a hormonal imbalance may be a contributory factor [2].

Individual Motor Unit Analysis

More precise quantitative information about the somatic innervation of the urethral sphincter, pelvic floor or anal sphincter may be obtained by EMG studies

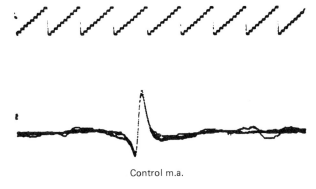

Control m.a.

Fig. 9.2.   A normal motor unit recorded from a control patient.

using a concentric needle introduced percutaneously. The needle is introduced 1 cm lateral to the urethral meatus and advanced anteriorly until the characteristic tonic EMG activity of the striated sphincter is encountered. Using a technique known as "signal triggering and delay" individual motor units may be isolated and their various parameters – amplitude, duration and polyphasicity – may be recorded (Fig. 9.2). Criteria of normality have been established by studies in control patients [3]. In any condition where the peripheral innervation of the pelvic floor has been damaged, abnormal motor units can be recorded which are polyphasic and of abnormally increased amplitude and duration (Fig. 9.3) [4]. This technique provides a sensitive means of identifying lower motor neuron lesions of the pelvic floor and may also be useful as a predictor of eventual recovery of bladder and urethral function in such cases.

Sacral Reflex Latency

The sacral reflex latency (SRL) may be elicited by electrically stimulating either the dorsal nerve of the clitoris or the urethral mucosa and recording the evoked contraction of the pelvic floor musculature. The interval between the application of the stimulus and the onset of pelvic floor contraction is taken as the reflex latency (Fig. 9.4). Prolongation of the latency (or absence of the response) suggests a neurological deficit of either the motor or sensory limbs of the reflex arc (both of which are carried by the pudendal nerve) or a disorder affecting the second to fourth sacral segments of the spinal cord. If the stimulating electrode is placed at the bladder neck the latency is somewhat longer than following clitoral stimulation, and this is thought to reflect slow conducting non-myelinated sensory fibres which probably carry the afferent impulses from this region. Although considerable claims have been made for this method, the technique is of limited value in the female subject because the clitoral branch of the pudendal nerve is smaller and therefore much less readily stimulated than the analogous nerve in the male, and as a consequence, absence of the reflex is commonly encountered in female control subjects. Nonetheless, prolongation of the response may provide clinically useful evidence of a disturbance of conduction in the sacral reflex arc.

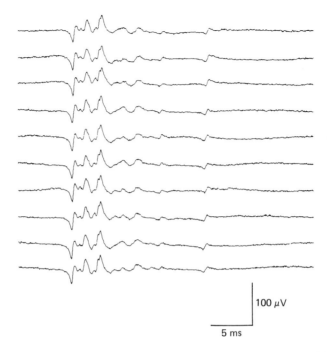

100 μV

5 ms

Fig. 9.3. An abnormal motor unit recorded from a patient with a pelvic nerve injury. Note the prolonged duration and polyphasic appearance of the motor unit.

Cortical Evoked Responses

Repetitive stimulation of the pudendal nerve at an intensity about two and a half times the sensory threshold produces afferent impulses which ascend via the dorsal columns to the cerebral cortex, where they may be measured with scalp electrodes and a neurophysiological averaging unit. If a series of responses is averaged electronically a cortical evoked response (CER) can be measured, and the latency of this response provides information about the integrity of the somatic sensory pathways from the urethra to the motor cortex (Fig. 9.5). Diseases which affect either peripheral or central sensory conduction through the nervous system will produce either prolongation or absence of this response. Unlike the SRL, the CER is reliably elicited in control subjects and often present when the SRL cannot be elicited.

Terminal Pudendal Motor Latency

Stimulation of the pudendal nerve may be achieved using an electrode mounted on a finger stall which is introduced per rectum. Stimulation of the pudendal nerve at the level of the ischial spine will evoke a direct contraction of the pelvic

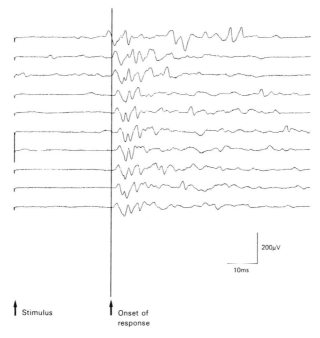

Fig. 9.4. A sacral reflex latency response recorded in a female patient (falling leaf display).

floor and of the anal and urethral sphincters. The latency between stimulation and contraction will be prolonged in any condition causing a slowing of motor conduction within the pudendal nerve. As with the other tests described above, this technique reflects conduction in fast-conducting large diameter myelinated fibres.

Motor Evoked Potentials

Electrical Stimulation

The motor cortex, the cervical spinal cord and the sacral nerve roots can be stimulated transcutaneously by using an electrical stimulator and this results in contraction of the pelvic floor [5]. By this means, the descending motor conduction pathways from the brain to the pelvis can be assessed. The main drawback of this method is the discomfort induced by the stimulating electrode, particularly following cranial stimulation.

Magnetic Stimulation

Recently we have been evaluating magnetic stimulation of the brain as a means of producing contraction of the pelvic musculature. This technique has the considerable advantage of being painless and responses can be reliably elicited in

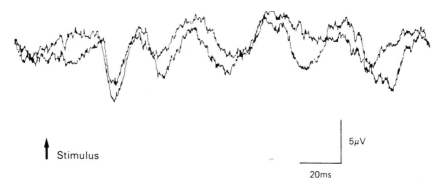

Stimulus

5µV

20ms

Fig. 9.5. The cortical evoked response from repetitive pudendal nerve stimulation in a control subject.

the pelvic floor with this technique in control subjects. A large capacitor is discharged through a low impedance coil placed over the head of the subject. The time varying magnetic field produced results in the formation of an action potential within the corticospinal tract and the pudendal nerve. Diseases affecting the motor pathways, such as multiple sclerosis (MS), result in either delay or absence of the response [6].

Clinical Situations in Which Neurophysiological Tests are of Value

Diseases Affecting the Lower Motor Neurons

Cauda Equina Lesions

Lesions of the cauda equina may be clinically obvious or occult. Early diagnosis is essential if restoration of function of structures innervated by the sacral segments is to be achieved. Neurophysiological testing, especially individual motor unit analysis, and to a lesser extent SRLs may provide the first objective evidence of cauda equina injury and indicate the need for myelography or scanning by magnetic resonance imaging (MRI). Repeated studies in established lesions may be of prognostic value since the process of re-innervation by nerve regrowth can be monitored.

Pelvic Nerve Injuries

The pelvic nerves may not only be injured by radical pelvic surgery but even by simple hysterectomy [7] although minor postoperative disturbances of micturition are more common than complete loss of continence. Following pelvic nerve injury, urodynamic investigations reveal loss of compliance and arreflexia, whereas urethral sphincter EMG with motor unit analysis will reveal pathological motor units and the SRL may be delayed or absent. These findings may be of diagnostic significance [4].

Multiple System Atrophy

The condition of multiple system atrophy (MSA), formerly known as the Shy–Drager syndrome, is characterised by selective neuronal degeneration of central autonomic neurons. In addition, the anterior horn cells of Onuf's nucleus, which innervate the striated muscle of anal and urethral sphincters, are also selectively affected. As a consequence patients afflicted by this disease suffer postural hypotension and disabling urinary incontinence [8]. The diagnosis should be suspected if a middle-aged patient presents with severe incontinence and a history of syncope. Urodynamic investigations usually reveal a loss of bladder compliance and an absent micturition reflex, while the bladder neck is characteristically open on an upright cystogram. Urethral sphincter EMG reveals pathological motor units which are of polyphasic and of prolonged duration indicating that denervation and re-innervation of the sphincter has occurred. The SRL may be prolonged and there may also be abnormalities of central motor and sensory conduction [9].

Diabetes Mellitus

Diabetes mellitus is the commonest cause of a generalised peripheral neuropathy, but bladder symptoms in this condition are surprisingly uncommon. Urodynamic evaluation may reveal a bladder which empties poorly, while urethral sphincter EMG often confirms the presence of a greater than normal number of motor units. These findings should alert the clinician to the risks of incontinence if urethral dilatation or urethrotomy are considered. Instead, patients should be instructed to void regularly by the clock and to pay great attention to complete bladder emptying. These simple measures, together with the eradication of urinary tract infections may be all that is needed in the management of the diabetic bladder.

Stress Urinary Incontinence

The concept has arisen of late that stress urinary incontinence in females is due to a peripheral neuropathy affecting the motor innervation of the pelvic floor and striated urethral sphincter. The cause of this neuropathy is presumed to be either birth injury or neuronal damage resulting from prolonged abdominal straining. There is evidence from the work of Allen and Warrell [10] that childbirth results in pathological changes in the urethral sphincter EMG, reflecting some degree of denervation and reinnervation and furthermore these changes are also influenced by the duration of labour and the weight of the baby. In patients with stress incontinence muscle biopsies taken from the pelvic floor at the time of colposuspension demonstrate changes consistent with a process of denervation [11] and individual motor unit analysis of the pelvic floor in such women also shows a greater than normal predominance of pathological motor units. Furthermore, Snooks et al. [12] have reported significantly prolonged terminal pudendal motor latencies in patients with stress incontinence compared with age and parity matched controls. However, Barnick and Cardozo [13] have recently reported no difference in motor unit duration between women with stress incontinence and controls matched for age and parity with no urinary symptoms. Thus it seems although denervation may be a factor in stress urinary leakage, other factors such as ligamentous injury at childbirth and smooth muscle function at the bladder neck may also play a role.

Meningomyelocoele

Patients with spina bifida often have a profound denervation of the pelvic floor which results in both urinary and faecal incontinence. The urodynamic findings usually demonstrate a loss of bladder compliance, with or without unstable bladder contractions. The sphincter is profoundly weak and often fails to relax during voiding attempts (which may result in upper tract dilatation and progressive renal impairment). Urethral pelvic floor or anal sphincter EMG shows a pattern of profound denervation, in that motor units are difficult to detect, and if present are abnormal. Fibrillation potentials characteristic of denervation are commonly present, while the SLR and CER are generally absent. As the infant with spina bifida grows, the abnormalities in the pelvic floor and bladder may deteriorate, probably as a result of cord tethering, and this may also contribute to progressive urodynamic deterioration and upper tract dilatation, which is often seen.

Diseases Affecting the Upper Motor Neurons

Multiple Sclerosis

More than 100 000 patients in the United Kingdom suffer from multiple sclerosis (MS), and of these more than 78% will have symptoms of bladder dysfunction. Difficulties of diagnosis have been eased by the development of magnetic resonance imaging (MRI) which can demonstrate the plaques of demyelination that occur anywhere within the central nervous system.

Patients commonly suffer from either incontinence or retention of urine and the urodynamic abnormalities vary from detrusor hyperreflexia with DSD to hypotonic arreflexic bladder. The latter finding has been attributed to S2–S4 cord segment involvement, producing a lower motor neuron bladder. However, urethral sphincter EMG in these patients reveals motor units of normal configuration, although there is often a profound reduction in the overall striated sphincter tone. This suggests that there is a loss of facilitatory sensory input to the anterior horn cells of Onuf's nucleus, due to damage to both ascending and descending spinal pathways, rather than direct damage to the lower motor neuron. In some patients with neurogenic bladder due to MS there is a marked prolongation of the SRL, suggesting that a proportion of patients do have occult sacral cord demyelination. However, most of the urodynamic abnormalities in MS reflect disruption of the connections between the pontine and sacral micturition centres. Accordingly it is not surprising that patients with hyperreflexia and dyssynergia commonly have delayed or absent cortical evoked responses and motor evoked potentials (MEPs) [6].

Parkinson's Disease

Idiopathic Parkinson's disease is due to basal ganglia degeneration and is characterised by tremor, akinesia and rigidity. Bladder dysfunction results from the loss of basal ganglia inhibition of the pontine micturition centre and the urodynamic abnormalities seen in this disease consist of marked hyperreflexia together with some degree of pelvic floor spasticity. Urethral sphincter EMG reveals normal motor units [14] and the CERs and MEPs are also normal [15]. In clinical terms these results offer a means of differentiating between patients with idiopathic

Parkinson's disease and those with multiple system atrophy (who may also present with parkinsonism); the ability to distinguish between these disorders may be of value both in terms of response to levodopa and other medications and in providing the patient and relatives with a prognosis of the condition [15].

Cerebrovascular Accidents

Bladder dysfunction is common following cerebrovascular accidents (CVA). The defect is probably due to loss of cortical input to the pontine micturition centre, as well as impaired cortical awareness of bladder distension. Because the neuronal pathways between the bladder and the pons are intact, a co-ordinated micturition reflex occurs normally, but at lower bladder volumes than usual and without voluntary control. In patients with this condition urethral sphincter EMG reveals normal motor units and, when present, the SRL is of normal duration.

Conclusions

Electrophysiological studies of the incontinent patient are at an early stage of development. Urodynamic evaluation is still the mainstay of investigation in that it characterises the end organ abnormality and dictates lines of pharmacological or surgical management. What it often fails to do, is to identify with any certainty the cause and location of any neural defect and it is here that neurophysiological testing has a role to play. Identification of an abnormality of urethral sphincter or lower motor neuron function in a patient with urinary retention is not uncommon in women whose problems have been labelled "psychogenic". Abnormalities of CERs or MEPs in patients with detrusor hyperreflexia may lead the clinician to suspect early MS. Finally neurophysiological studies are a potent research tool with which to explore the neural mechanisms controlling continence and micturition both in disease and in health.

References

1. Blaivas JG, Sinna HP, Zayed AAH, Lahib KB. Detrusor sphincter dyssynergia: a detailed electromyographic study. J Urol 1981; 125:545–8.
2. Fowler CJ, Christmas TJ, Chapple CR, Parkhouse HP, Kirby RS, Jacobs HS. Abnormal activity at the urethral sphincter, voiding dysfunction and polycystic ovaries. Br Med J 1988; 279:1436–8.
3. Fowler CJ, Kirby RS, Harrison MJG, Milroy EJG, Turner-Warwick RT. Individual motor unit analysis in the diagnosis of disorders of urethral sphincter function. J Neurol Neurosurg Psychiatry 1984; 47:637–41.
4. Kirby RS, Fowler CJ, Gosling JA, Milroy EJG, Turner-Warwick RT. Bladder muscle biopsy and urethral sphincter EMG in patients with peripheral nerve injury to the bladder. J R Soc Med 1986; 79:270–3.
5. Swash M, Snooks ST. Motor conduction velocity in the human spinal cord. J Physiol 1985; 390:50.
6. Eardley I, Kirby RS, Nagendran C, Fowler CJ, Macdonald WI. Where are the lesions which cause the neurogenic bladder in multiple sclerosis. Neurourol Urodynam 1989; 8:9–10.

7. Parys BT, Haylen BT, Woolfended KA, Parsons KF. Vesicourethral dysfunction after simple hysterectomy. Neurourol Urodynam 1989; 8:14–15.
8. Kirby RS, Fowler CJ, Gosling JA, Bannister R. Urethrovesical dysfunction in progressive autonomic failure and multiple system atrophy. J Neurol Neurosurg Psychiatry 1986; 49:554–62.
9. Eardley I, Quinn NP, Kirby RS, Marsden CD, Bannister R, Fowler CJ. The neurophysiology of the urethral sphincter in multiple system atrophy. Electroenceph Clin Neurophys 1989; 73:91P–62P.
10. Allen RE, Warrell DW. The role of pregnancy and childbirth in partial denervation of the pelvic floor. Neurourol Urodynam 1987; 6:183–4.
11. Smith ARB, Hosker GL, Warrell DW. The role of pudendal nerve damage in the aetiology of genuine stress incontinence in women. Br J Obstet Gynaecol 1989; 96:318–19.
12. Snooks ST, Badenoch DF, Tiptatt RC, Swash M. Perineal nerve damage in genuine stress incontinence – an electrophysiological study. Br J Urol 1985; 57:422–6.
13. Barnick CG, Cardozo LD. Electromyography of the urethral sphincter in genuine stress incontinence: a useless test. Neurourol Urodynam 1989; 8:318–19.
14. Fitzmaurice H, Fowler CJ, Rickards D et al. Micturition disturbances in Parkinson's disease. J Urol 1985; 57:652–6.
15. Eardley I, Quinn NP, Fowler CJ, Kirby RS, Parkhouse H, Marsden CD, Bannister R. The role of the urethral sphincter EMG in the differential diagnosis of parkinsonism. Br J Urol (in press).

Discussion

Hilton: These three chapters relate to very different tests which all represent adjuncts to conventional urodynamics, or potential adjuncts.

Van Mastrigt: The three authors showed the specificities and sensitivities of their methods in detecting genuine stress incontinence. What was the "gold standard"?

Kirby: I stated mine as videocystourethrography (VCU).

Plevnik: Mine was the ICS pad test.

Quinn: A final urodynamic diagnosis which may have included VCU.

Van Mastrigt: Is there any uniformity? Dr Plevnik showed that the sensitivity of the pad test, for instance, was not 100% as compared to VCU.

Plevnik: To demonstrate incontinence by using urethral electric conductance (UEC) we showed that in 75% we can demonstrate it taking the 1-hour ICS pad test as the gold standard. It was positive in 100% of them on pad test.

Cardozo: But the ICS 1-hour pad test is not a good gold standard. It has already been shown to be inferior to other pad tests.

Hilton: The other problem with the pad test is not just its ability to detect leakage, which is what it is aimed to do, but its ability as a diagnostic test of GSI, which is what we are discussing here.

Sutherst: I do not think we need a sensitivity test with something like a UEC probe. A test is either positive or negative. There is no argument about that.

Plevnik: We were just saying it is much more accurate and objective as compared to visualising.

Versi: One cannot say that no gold standard is needed to compare it against. There will be false positives and false negatives, for whatever reason; electrical, or discharge, or whatever.

Sutherst: The only false positive in that test is from movement of a catheter perhaps at the bladder neck.

Plevnik: But that is not so.

Sutherst: You cannot get false positives?

Plevnik: In the normal course of events we do not find them.

Sutherst: A negative result means that the bladder neck has not opened. There is no reason for a change in conductance unless there is some fluid present. So there can be no false results.

Plevnik: We can always talk about some infinitesimally small drops which we may pick up with a 3-hour pad test and not with a UEC.

Cardozo: So what. If urine enters the urethra it has to come from the bladder.

Van Mastrigt: The point is most interesting. Urine can enter the urethra from the bladder but not exit it. But do we call it incontinence when somebody has fluid in their urethra?

Sutherst: We have to distinguish between a proximal test and a distal test.

Plevnik: We have a distal test for showing incontinence in the distal urethra, which means the distal part of the UPP. So it has to, according to the laws of physics, move down the pressure gradient, and exit the meatus.

Kirby: The other variable is the volume of the bladder at which leakage occurs. In the few hundred urodynamic investigations that I did there was quite marked variation in the tendency to leak according to the bladder volume, and I guess that the fuller the bladder is, the more reflex activity there is in the pelvic floor and perhaps in the sphincter as well. Should we not standardise for bladder volume before doing these tests?

Peattie: We did it at maximum cystometric capacity.

Kirby: Is that the optimum time at which to look for stress incontinence? My observation is that people leak not when they are ultra full, but when they are mid-full.

Plevnik: We say 250 ml or more is the best volume for our purposes.

Quinn: I do all mine with them comfortably full, but they void after the examination. I would use any patient who had more than 200 ml in the bladder. That does not include everybody but they have to have 200 ml in order to reliably assess the position of the bladder neck.

Cardozo: Is any other group using urethral electric conductance either clinically or for research, and if so what are their experiences?

Stanton: It is a complicated test and there are people who may not yet have grasped it!

Hilton: It is a beautifully simple test, and it is one that we have used quite a bit in Newcastle over the last couple of years, but unfortunately have not been able to replicate any of the results that Dr Plevnik has described.

We have used it during the course of physiotherapy as a means of providing biofeedback to patients to see if it encourages them to contract the pelvic wall better, and we found it no better than standard perineometry. We have used it preoperatively in patients having Stamey procedures and found it no better than a simple clinical assessment of suture tension either in terms of success or failure of the operation, nor any different in terms of postoperative voiding problems. So as a clinical test we have not found it to be in any way useful.

Plevnik: Those two examples are new studies that we have not yet done.

Hilton: You have looked at surgery?

Plevnik: Not during general anaesthesia. We were talking of surgery under epidural anaesthesia and we took the internal meatus as a reference. That is different.

Secondly, we never did exercise. We have used biofeedback on patients with sensory urgency and unstable bladders where the UEC showed quite good clinical values. So you cannot compare these.

Hilton: I would not want to compare them directly, but in relation to the question of sensory urgency our results do not accord with yours. We have certainly found patients who have marked variation in UEC at the bladder neck. In fact those patients correlate quite well with urethral pressure variation. But we do not find any link between those variations either in pressure or UEC and the sensation of urgency. In fact all the readings we have done have been specifically in patients without any desire to void at the time.

Kulseng-Hanssen: We have been asked if somebody uses it. I use it with ambulatory recording and it is extremely useful. When the patient leaks we can see what happens.

Sutherst: That is an advantage.

With regard to bladder neck testing, and testing for sphincter incompetence, we still use the fluid bridge test, which was the forerunner of Dr Plevnik's test.

Cardozo: That is not the distal urethral?

Sutherst: No, but we use it routinely as part of our urodynamic investigations to pick up the people who have some evidence of sphincter incompetence who cannot demonstrate it on clinical examination, without doing UPPs.

Cardozo: We use VCU for that. If one has a technique for doing it, it does not much matter what it is. I just wondered if anyone was using distal urethral electric conductance, and if not, then why not.

Plevnik: The apparatus has only been available for about eighteen months, which is quite a short time. One has to decide to buy it and get the funds for it, and that can take at least a year.

Mundy: Do people generally use VCU as the gold standard for the objective demonstration of genuine stress incontinence of urine?

Cardozo: We do.

Hilton: We have already heard that people use widely differing gold standards.

Sutherst: The pad test is an objective measurement of urine loss, but it does not differentiate between stress leakage and other types of leakage unless it can be shown at the same time that a woman has got a stable bladder.

Peattie: But that is where distal UEC is so useful.

Sutherst: But the pad test is a lot cheaper than the DUEC machine and at the end of the day the bottom line must surely be how wet the woman is when she is pottering around.

Mundy: If VCU is the gold standard, is that because of some belief that if they do not get visible stress incontinence on VCU the patients do not have stress incontinence?

Cardozo: We cannot say that.

Versi: Not at all. The gold standard is not the perfect test, but it is the best available. If it is not demonstrated on VCU they may still have it but we do not have another way of detecting it.

Cardozo: Except that two tests are better than one. If we do not diagnose it on the first test we may do so on the second.

Mundy: When you say that they do not have it demonstrably, it is my experience that if I ask a patient if she has wet herself she will quite often say that she has done, but that it is not actually demonstrable on the fluoroscopy screen. So it is actually demonstrable, but it depends on how the patient is viewed. It depends on whether one accepts what one sees on the screen, what one sees at the meatus or what the patient says as part of the VCU.

Versi: If it can be seen on the VCU but not on the floor or on a pad, then the VCU surely is more sensitive. We see it with the VCU better than with any other test.

Mundy: The question I asked was: is your gold standard the demonstration of it fluoroscopically, or do you also include whether the patient says she leaks during a study, or visual observation of the meatus?

Versi: Fluoroscopy alone.

Cardozo: Can I answer from data. This year we compared 150 VCUs with 150 cystometries and eyeball tests done on the same patients consecutively. Half had

VCU first and the other half had cystometry and eyeball test first, done by independent observers. As far as diagnosing GSI or detrusor instability were concerned, there was no difference between VCU or cystometry and the eyeball test.

The interesting thing was that we made far more diagnoses by doing two tests than just one, and it was not always the same test which picked up more abnormalities than the other.

The only difference made by doing VCU as compared to cystometry and eyeball test was that morphological abnormalities were picked up that would not have been diagnosed on cystometry alone.

Mundy: Does that mean that you would regard the gold standard as doing VCU or two separate investigations or eyeballing during a VCU?

Cardozo: It depends what one is trying to diagnose. If we are trying to provide a urodynamic service to cover all patients who come in complaining of a variety of different things, then yes, we would do VCU first, and if we did not make a diagnosis and the patient still had complaints then we would do other adjunctive tests. And that would mean perhaps a cystoscopy or various other tests. There are several tests that one might want to do.

But yes, we ask the patient what happens to her, and we also visualise if we do not see anything on the VCU. And we do all of those things as part of our VCU.

Mundy: So what then is the gold standard? VCU plus eyeballing the meatus?

Cardozo: The best available is more than one test. So the best available is the VCU plus another test if that is what is needed, and if no diagnosis has been made.

Hilton: The gold standard as far as Versi's and Cardozo's studies are concerned is VCU fluoroscopy. That is what they are saying.

Cardozo: It is what we use.

Hilton: In terms of making a clinical diagnosis aside from their research studies, then they use as many tests as appears appropriate for that individual patient.

My own gold standard, whether it is in a research sense or in a clinical sense, is simply seeing urine leakage from the meatus. And I would put that always above anything that I saw on a fluoroscope screen.

Mundy: That is what I was interested to know.

DeLancey: The other point that we should not neglect is the identification by the patient that that is her problem. Someone with detrusor instability who has a little bit of stress incontinence may well say that this happens but that that is not why she has been referred. She has been referred because when she feels cold air and she feels the urge to urinate, water runs down her leg.

Mundy: I do not wish to labour the point, but if people who are talking about their tests are comparing them against a gold standard, it is nice to know what the gold standard is. I do not think fluoroscopic appearance is a very good gold standard.

Cardozo: But one has to choose a standard test to compare another one against. One test cannot be compared against a variety of other tests. It would not be possible to analyse the results satisfactorily saying that urethral pressure profile was compared against VCU or cystometry or cystometry and eyeball, or the patient's history or clinical demonstration on the couch. The analysis would be impossible.

Hilton: We are talking about a very important principle and I would hate to limit discussion, but we need to direct our questioning to some of the other topics that have been discussed.

Sutherst: We have done a fair bit of work on linear array scanning, and only recently I compared the two using two machines on the same patient at different times. I still get better pictures with the linear array scanner.

Quinn: I have tried such a scanner. In fact I have tried several. I agree that linear arrays can in some patients provide nice pictures. For those patients that have well-supported bladder necks and when we want a focal range of more than 5 cm – maybe 3–8 cm – the 5 MHz is absolutely fine. But the problem with the linear array is that the arrangement of the crystals in the head is such that they are either perpendicular fields or end-firing fields. There are a few with offsets but the spatial arrangements of the arrays and the asymmetry of the end of the probe means that they are often 4–5 cm long, and I think they interfere with the anatomy in many patients. Not all, but some. Therefore, in terms of using them for the wide range of patients that come in I think there would be difficulties with some of them, but I do not have a very wide experience.

Sutherst: We are certainly not using a linear array scanner transrectally, because of that potential problem. But we have recently used it transvaginally without any apparent disturbance in either urodynamic tests or anatomical change.

Quinn: That is fair enough. I do not have enough experience with them to be that definite, but I do find that the resolution we can get in the near field with the 7 MHz mechanical sector scanner is very good.

Sutherst: There is one advantage. We used the small portable linear array scanner which we thought at the time might be very useful for intraoperative measurements. Mr Quinn talked about pre- and postoperative testing. But his machine would be too big to use intraoperatively. The small machine can be carried into the theatre.

Quinn: We can use it. I have used it for preoperative measurements, but one could probably gain as much by looking at one's own results pre- and post-operatively and one would see how tight one was tying them.

I would reinforce Dr Plevnik's point that most people do tend to tie the needle suspension procedures a little too tightly, and one can see that with the way that they are so very high postoperatively.

Murray: Mr Kirby showed a slide of an abnormal sphincter EMG after radical Wertheim hysterectomy, "showing that nerve damage occurred at the time of operation". That statement has medicolegal implications – perhaps he would rephrase that statement?

Kirby: That was one motor unit. But in that scatter diagram of the 10 or so patients that we looked at, every single unit that we were able to identify – and we would usually look at 10 or more – was abnormal in those patients. As soon as a needle is put into the sphincter we have absolutely glaring evidence that every unit is abnormal. It is the same with the patients with autonomic failure. It is an unmistakable EMG appearance, and after a bit of experience one can find it. It is quite different from the sorts of things one sees in patients who have had several children. In those cases we find abnormal motor units, and I agree one abnormal motor unit is not evidence of denervation. But if the whole sphincter muscle is denervated, that is definite evidence of nerve damage at the time of operation.

Murray: Definite evidence of nerve damage, but not as to when it arose.

Kirby: I accept that. But with a history of someone who is unable to void following a hysterectomy and some incontinence as well there is good circumstantial evidence to back it up.

Murray: The problem is that too many of these patients never had a decent history taken before they had their Wertheim's hysterectomy and a significant proportion of them may have had urological abnormalities prior to that.

Kirby: That may be true. But a significant proportion of them do incur nerve injury at the time of Wertheim's hysterectomy.

Cardozo: It is not necessarily the hysterectomy. It may be their bladder aftercare, which is very deficient in some cases.

Kirby: But we would not expect urethral sphincter or pelvic floor abnormalities with that. I agree that women can get a detrusor overstretching phenomenon and that is very important.

Cardozo: It happens quite often.

Kirby: But what we pick up on needle EMGs is the same as after an AP-resection. It is exactly the same. And none of the male patients after AP-resection have had childbirth as a complicating factor.

Hilton: I stand by Mr Murray's implied point that longitudinal studies are what are required to prove the point.

Voiding Difficulties

Chapter 10

Pathophysiology of Voiding Disorders

P. J. R. Shah

Introduction

Normal voiding appears to be a simple process and normal individuals probably do not even consciously consider the dynamics of micturition. However, the process of normal micturition depends on a multitude of complex factors which must be working in a co-ordinated way in order for bladder emptying to take place without disturbance. Voiding consists of a combination of bladder contraction and outlet relaxation such that emptying is rapid and without retention of residual urine.

The neurological connections involved in the process of micturition are complex. Any disturbance in any of the connections within the voiding mechanism will produce a disorder of micturition. Factors that may disturb micturition will therefore include psychological factors, neurological factors, abnormalities of detrusor muscle and other extrinsic factors to the bladder and sphincters which influence micturition. Tables 10.1 and 10.2 list the many causes of voiding disorders in the female.

Normal female voiding is rapid, at relatively low intravesical pressure and occurs without the retention of residual urine, except when the female does not sit to void but crouches, when bladder emptying is less efficient and may not be completed [1].

Bladder contraction occurs at a lower pressure in the female than the male as there is a lower outflow resistance in the shorter, straighter female urethra. Female voiding pressure may be very low or unrecordable in spite of rapid and efficient voiding. This is due to the fact that detrusor muscle contraction is occurring efficiently but pressure does not rise because the resistance is low. Thus,

Table 10.1. Causes of acute retention in the female

Postoperative
   Rectal surgery
   Hysterectomy
   Surgery for stress incontinence
   After any surgical procedure
Neurological
   Multiple sclerosis
   Myelitis
   Diabetes mellitus
Gynaecological
   Uterine prolapse
   Cystocele
Urethral calculus
Urethral stricture
Acute cystitis
Constipation
Psychogenic
Idiopathic

low pressure voiding tends to occur in patients with stress urinary incontinence in view of their low outflow resistance. This is of no consequence until outlet surgery takes place for stress incontinence when voiding becomes inefficient or impossible. Pressure flow studies prior to surgery should help to predict those patients in whom the outcome may not be entirely satisfactory after surgery.

Aetiology and Pathophysiology

It is important to diagnose the cause of a voiding disorder in the female. The aetiology may be clear, as occurs in neuropathy, or unknown, as in some cases of retention of urine. Even though the treatment of many conditions is similar, the primary diagnosis should be sought.

Neurological Disorders

Lesions in the nervous system tend to produce specific types of voiding abnormality.

1. Lesions in the brain which affect voiding function may occur in the frontal lobes, internal capsule, reticular formation of the pons and cerebellum. These abnormalities will tend to vary according to the severity of the lesion, the age of the patient and whether dementia forms part of the neurological process. Voiding disorders that are associated with confusional states in the elderly often right

Table 10.2. Causes of voiding difficulties and retention

1. *Neurological disease*
   As a result of spinal injury – spinal shock phase
   Upper motor neuron lesion – spinal injury, multiple sclerosis
   Lower motor neuron lesion – spinal injury, multiple sclerosis
   Autonomic lesion, e.g. after pelvic surgery
   Local pain reflex after surgery

2. *Pharmacological*
   Tricyclic antidepressants
   Anticholinergic agents
   a-adrenergic stimulating agents
   Ganglion blocking agents
   Epidural anaesthesia

3. *Acute inflammation*
   Acute urethritis
   Acute cystitis
   Acute vulvovaginitis
   Acute anogenital infection (including herpes)

4. *Obstruction*
   Distal urethral stenosis
   Acute urethral oedema of surgery
   Chronic urethral stenosis
   Foreign body or calculus in the urethra
   Impacted pelvic mass
       Retroverted gravid uterus
       Haematocolpos
       Uterine fibroid
       Ovarian cyst
       Faecal impaction
   Urethral distortion with cystocele
   Ectopic ureterocele
   Uterine prolapse
   Leiomyoma of the bladder

5. *Endocrine*
   Hypothyroidism
   Diabetic neuropathy

6. *Psychogenic*
   Anxiety or depressive illness
   Hysteria

7. Overdistension

8. *Iatrogenic*
   After transtrigonal phenol injections
   After surgery for stress incontinence
   After anal surgery
   After hysterectomy

9. Idiopathic

themselves once the confusional state is corrected; urinary incontinence which includes a normal voiding event to completion but at inappropriate times and places, is a feature of dementia. Urinary retention may result from acute lesions such as cerebrovascular accidents, whereas more chronic lesions such as multiple sclerosis and Parkinson's disease, may be associated with detrusor hyperreflexia and as a consequence, urinary frequency, urgency and incontinence.

2. Lesions in the spinal cord are caused by trauma, tumours, prolapse of an

intervertebral disc or spina bifida. If the lesion is above the level of the sacral parasympathetic reflex arc, after a period of spinal shock, the bladder becomes autonomous and its urodynamic dysfunction is represented by hyperreflexic detrusor behaviour combined with detrusor sphincter dyssynergia. This combination almost invariably leads to urinary incontinence in the female, often combined with the retention of varying degrees of residual urine due to the unco-ordinated relationship between detrusor and sphincter function. Urinary incontinence of this type is often difficult to control. If the affecting lesion is in the cervical cord, intermittent catheterisation becomes difficult if not impossible, even if hyperreflexic contractions can be suppressed with anticholinergic agents.

3. Lesions which occur below the reflex arc, at or below the level of the outlet of the sacral root, tend to produce bladder acontractility. This type of bladder dysfunction produces a bladder that does not contract (acontractile) with an associated non-relaxing sphincter mechanism. These patients tend to void by straining, often leaving a residual urine. Incontinence may be a feature due to chronic retention with overflow.

4. Pelvic plexus injuries occur as a result of damage during surgical procedures in the pelvis, such as abdominoperineal excision of the rectum or radical hysterectomy. The neurological lesion may be incomplete and produces a disorder of bladder function which is unpredictable. A bladder with reduced compliance, urinary incontinence and incomplete emptying may result.

A pelvic nerve injury may also rarely follow the transtrigonal injection of the pelvic plexus nerves with phenol for the treatment of detrusor instability [2].

Pharmacological Causes

Anticholinergic agents are used for weakening detrusor contraction in patients with detrusor instability or hyperreflexia. If they produce reduced voiding ability this may be gratefully accepted, especially in neuropathy; these agents may, however, produce voiding dysfunction. The most commonly prescribed agents are atropine (used in premedication), probanthine, oxybutynin, terodiline, flavoxate, imipramine and other tricyclic antidepressants. During the taking of the clinical history a knowledge of current and previous drug treatment should be obtained.

Ganglion blocking agents produce similar effects to the anticholinergic drugs, whilst α-adrenergic stimulants increase outflow resistance and may cause voiding dysfunction.

Epidural anaesthesia may produce temporary retention by interruption of the reflex arc.

Acute Inflammation

Acute inflammation of the urethra, vulva, vagina or bladder may be associated with urinary retention or abnormalities of bladder emptying with frequency of micturition, obstructed flow and incomplete bladder emptying. The acute inflammatory process produces oedema which if it affects the urethra will increase the outflow resistance.

Genital herpes affecting the anogenital region [3] and the cervix or vulva [4,5] have been shown to cause acute urinary retention. The urinary effects are thought to be due to central nervous involvement with the likeliest lesion being a lumbo-sacral meningomyelitis, though painful inflammation of the vulval area must contribute to voiding dysfunction.

Obstruction

Bladder outflow obstruction in the normal female is usually a consequence of failure of relaxation of the urethral sphincter mechanism which may be voluntary or involuntary (as would occur in neuropathic conditions). In the female with neuropathy this tends to be due to detrusor sphincter dyssynergia.

The diagnosis of urethral stenosis in the female is uncommon; a urologist may expect to see very few true urethral stenoses each year. It is usually the result of urethral scarring following chronic urethral inflammation, in association with surgery around the urethra, or as a consequence of instrumentation. Typically the condition occurs in the postmenopausal woman and there is no obvious aetiological cause. Occasionally a urethral caruncle may be associated with urethral stenosis or its surgical treatment may cause stenosis. The diagnosis of urethral stenosis is made at the time of urethral catheterisation, at the time of cystometry or cystography, or at the time of endoscopy for the diagnosis of voiding difficulty. Urethral stenosis is treated by urethral dilatation either by means of graduated urethral dilators or the Otis urethrotome.

Other causes of urethral obstruction include urethral oedema secondary to premenstrual fluid retention and foreign bodies within the urethra including urethral calculi.

A "hypersensitive female urethra" or a catheter sensitive urethra will produce a voiding disorder with low voiding flow rate and raised voiding pressure [6]. This is associated with the symptoms of frequency, nocturia and urgency. If a female with those symptoms is seen and the urethra is sensitive to the passage of the catheter, the diagnosis is made. The primary cause is inflammatory, though no infective agent has yet been implicated.

Impaction of a retroverted gravid uterus, uterine fibroids and ovarian cysts or haematocolpos may all cause retention of urine, and an ectopic ureterocele may be a rare cause of voiding dysfunction in children.

A large cystocele with descent of the bladder neck may cause urethral distortion or "kinking" which may produce a functional obstruction. Repair of the cystocele may then be all that is necessary to restore the normal line of the urethra and normal voiding. This underlines the importance of vaginal examination in all females with voiding difficulties.

Surgery for stress incontinence is associated with abnormalities of bladder emptying. Although repositioning of the bladder neck into an intra-abdominal environment is the primary aim of the modern surgical treatment of stress incontinence in the female, there is evidence to suggest that voiding difficulty is a consequence of both vaginal and abdominal procedures [7]. The Burch colposuspension elevates the bladder neck and stretches the urethra especially if the vaginal sutures are tied closely to the ileopectineal ligament. It should be expected that these patients may experience voiding problems after surgery [8,9]. Those patients with preoperative low pressure voiding are particularly likely to run into difficulty with bladder emptying in the early postoperative phase. All but a small percentage of these patients will recover normal bladder emptying but usually with reduced flow rates.

Iatrogenic Causes

As well as those iatrogenic causes mentioned above which may be partly or entirely responsible for voiding dysfunction, anal surgery [10] and other factors listed in Table 10.2 may be involved and should be carefully considered in the aetiology if the primary cause is not immediately obvious.

Overdistension

Bladder overdistension should never be overlooked as a cause of voiding disturbance. After surgical procedures such as hysterectomy, or during delivery, if retention occurs it should be relieved immediately. Even after a single episode of urinary retention patients may never recover normal voiding function and are left with hypocontractile or acontractile bladders. If a female patient cannot void it is far better to pass a small bore catheter to relieve the retention as soon as possible. If the retention is relieved quickly the patient is very grateful and a long-term voiding problem may be avoided. The patient may void in a hot bath or shower which does assist pelvic floor and general relaxation but if the bladder is significantly overdistended this may not be successful. Drugs to stimulate bladder contraction are not usually successful and carry their own risks and side effects.

Psychogenic Retention

This diagnosis should only be made when, after a careful process of exclusion, no abnormalities have been discovered. The occasional late neurological abnormality may turn up in an initially apparently normal patient. A careful history and examination is necessary along with a neurological examination performed by a neurologist. The majority of patients suffering from psychogenic retention of urine are females between 15 and 45 years. There is usually a relationship between the onset of the retention and a stressful event such as childbirth, marital discord, surgical treatment or rape. Hysteria, depression, and schizophrenia may all be causes of this problem. However, once a psychiatric diagnosis is made the treatment remains as in those with defined organic pathology. Return to normal voiding function may be expected in the majority [11] although the use of clean intermittent catheterisation may be satisfactory management.

Presentation

Symptoms

Many females are infrequent voiders, only voiding once or twice a day. Some patients with disorders of voiding function may not be aware that they have a problem until they develop urinary tract infection or retention. Young females often develop "cystitis" which is related to sexual activity. Questions related to voiding ability, however, should be asked.

Lower urinary tract infection in an older female should be investigated more completely as abnormalities of bladder function are more likely.

Females will admit to the symptom of poor stream. Straining to void is associated with reduced contractility of the detrusor. A feeling of incomplete emptying may be associated with retained residual urine. Urinary incontinence may be a consequence of chronic retention of urine but again this is uncommon in the female.

A general history with particular reference to past medical and surgical treatment is very important as many voiding problems stem from or are temporarily related to previous pelvic and abdominal surgery and childbirth. A drug history should also be obtained.

Signs

Careful abdominal examination should be performed in all patients. The kidneys should be carefully palpated and are usually felt in all but the very obese. Abdominal masses should be noted. It is not always easy to palpate the full bladder during abdominal examination. Bimanual examination will often confirm one's suspicions of bladder fullness as the bladder may be more easily palpable. Gentle percussion in the suprapubic region will reveal the characteristic dullness which is present when the bladder is full or when other pelvic masses are present. The wheelchair-bound patient must always be examined even though this may be particularly difficult because of immobility and deformity.

The urethra should be examined for its appearance, position and tenderness, (the normal female urethra is not tender). The vulva and vagina should be observed for signs of atrophy and inflammation in addition to prolapse and scarring in association with childbirth and previous surgery. A careful bimanual examination should also be made.

A general neurological examination should be performed, although if a neurological abnormality is suspected a neurologist's opinion should be sought. The patient's general demeanour should also be observed.

Investigation

Investigations should be used sensibly. The patient should be investigated according to the suspected abnormality. As these patients' symptoms are related to the lower urinary tract, it is not always necessary to perform urography. A free flow rate, abdominal radiograph (to look for calcification and soft tissue masses) and pelvic and renal ultrasonography are primary investigations. The demonstration of a reduced flow and a residual urine on bladder ultrasound will confirm a diagnosis of voiding difficulty and the next step will be to perform urodynamic studies.

The Frequency/Volume Chart or Urinary Diary

A weekly voiding diary should be sent to the patient prior to the outpatient appointment and the patient given instructions as to how to fill it in. A record of fluid intake, volumes voided and the timing of voids, episodes of incontinence and any other relevant features may then be discussed with the patient at her first consultation.

Infrequent Voiding

Normal voiding frequency, accepted as less than seven times daily, is determined by fluid intake, habit, anxiety and stress, and the presence of abnormalities of bladder function which may be motor or sensory. Infrequent voiding, i.e. the passing of urine less than two or three times a day with a normal fluid intake, is abnormal. Patients who void infrequently should be investigated with a frequency/volume chart and advised about their normal requirements of intake and the frequency of voiding. Infrequent voiders should be recommended to void every 3 to 4 hours during the day. Infrequent voiding with normal bladder volumes should not lead to long-term harm to bladder function, whereas the holding on to large volumes of urine tends to lead to overstretching of bladder muscle fibres and may result in hypocontractile bladder dysfunction. This problem is seen in females who are reluctant to void in public places or who have busy occupations which do not easily allow them time to spend in bladder emptying.

The Flow Rate

A free urine flow rate, as in the male with prostatic outflow obstruction, is a valuable first urodynamic investigation; several abnormal patterns may be discovered.

Urethral Pressure Profilometry

Urethral pressure profilometry does not usually aid in the diagnosis or treatment of voiding disorders and should be reserved for complex abnormalities and research purposes.

Cystometry

Cystometry will provide the most clinically useful information in this group of patients and should always be used where there is doubt about the diagnosis or where neuropathy is present. Filling and voiding cystometry may be all that is necessary for the majority of patients, however combined synchronous videocystometry is preferable where available, particularly where neuropathic disorders are known or suspected. Videourodynamics enables radiological examination of the voiding process and will provide information about the bladder appearance – the presence or absence of trabeculation, diverticula and reflux, and the behaviour of the bladder neck and urethral mechanisms. External striated sphincter function should be carefully examined during videocystometry. Abnormalities of sphincter function are seen in some normal patients who have inhibited voiding and in neuropathic disorders where detrusor sphincter dyssynergia gives rise to obstructed voiding. Table 10.3 describes the features which may be encountered in the urodynamic investigation of voiding dysfunction.

Table 10.3. Classification of voiding difficulty

Condition	Symptom	Urodynamic data
Occult voiding difficulty	Frequency, urgency due to urinary infection or No symptoms	Obstructed flow Elevated, normal or reduced voiding pressure ± Residual urine or large capacity with low pressure voiding
Symptomatic voiding difficulty	Poor stream Incomplete emptying Straining Frequency	Flow $<15\,ml\,s^{-1}$ Elevated voiding pressure $>50\,cm\,H_2O$ ± Residual urine
Acute retention	Painful or painless sudden onset	Residual urine
Chronic retention	Reduced sensation Hesitancy Straining to void Frequency, nocturia Urgency, incontinence Urinary tract infection	Flow $<15\,ml\,s^{-1}$ Residual urine High pressure or low pressure voiding
Acute-on-chronic retention	Painful or painless History of chronic retention Incontinence	Residual urine

Electromyography (EMG)

EMG is useful for the diagnosis of neurological disorders of micturition but is a specialised investigation which should be performed in conjunction with urodynamic studies. Videourodynamic studies will often obviate the need for EMG.

Endoscopy

Cystourethroscopy should not be used as a primary diagnostic investigation. It does, however, become important once the diagnosis is made as part of treatment, e.g. for the purpose of urethral dilatation, to obtain a true measure of bladder volume, or to assess mucosal appearance and take biopsies.

Prophylactic Measures

Many voiding problems may be avoided by the early recognition of potential problems. Therefore if urinary retention is suspected or imminent after surgical procedures, the early use of catheterisation before overdistension has occurred will prevent many long-term bladder problems. If a patient complains of urinary difficulty after surgery, or cannot void, the institution of a programme of intermittent catheterisation until the time of recovery of bladder function is highly acceptable. If the patient will not accept this regime and voiding problems are likely to be prolonged a suprapubic catheter is recommended.

Difficulty with resuming normal micturition after surgical treatment may occur in over 60% of patients undergoing surgery for stress incontinence (slings, colposuspension and endoscopic bladder neck suspension), and in 45% of patients undergoing radical pelvic surgery for gynaecological malignancy or rectal surgery [12,13], and after epidural anaesthesia for childbirth or gynaecological procedures.

Indwelling catheters should therefore be used prophylactically after any surgical procedure which may through a direct or indirect effect be associated with voiding problems. If the catheter is to be placed for only a short period of time, a urethral catheter of small calibre should be used. However, if a catheter is required for longer periods or if trials of voiding and assessment of bladder emptying are necessary, a self-retaining suprapubic catheter is preferable.

A clear explanation of the possibility of voiding difficulty should be given to all patients who are to undergo any surgery which carries with it this risk. Those patients who express dissatisfaction with surgical outcome are those who have not received an adequate preoperative explanation of the potential problems. It is also very helpful where indicated, to teach the female patient the art of self-catheterisation preoperatively. If it is not later needed the patient is very pleased, if it is found necessary she is not aggrieved.

The process of intermittent catheterisation should be part of the training of both medical and nursing staff involved in the management of these patients.

Conclusion

The female patient with urinary difficulty or incontinence may have voiding dysfunction. A careful history and examination should precede investigations. Acute retention should never be overlooked or trivialised. Surgical treatment of voiding disorders is usually the last resort after urodynamic investigation and conservative measures have been tried first.

References

1. Moore KH, Richmond D. Crouching over the toilet seat: prevalence, and effect upon micturition. Neurourol Urodynam 1989; 8:422–4.
2. Cox R, Worth PHL. Chronic retention after extratrigonal phenol injection for bladder instability. Br J Urol 1986; 58:229–30.
3. Oats JK, Greenhouse PRDH. Retention of urine in anogenital herpetic infection. Lancet 1978; i:691–2.
4. Hemrika DJ, Schutte MF, Blecker OP. Elsberg syndrome: a neurologic basis for acute urinary retention in patients with genital herpes. Obstet Gynecol 1986; 68:37S-39S.
5. Ryttov N, Aagaard J, Hertz J. Retention of urine in genital herpetic infection. Urol Int 1985; 40:22–4.
6. Shah PJR, Whiteside CG, Milroy EJG, Turner-Warwick RT. The hypersensitive female urethra – a catheter diagnosis? Proceedings of the thirteenth annual meeting of the International Continence Society, 1983; 202–3.
7. Coptcoat MJ, Shah PJR, Cumming J, Charig C, Worth PHL. How does bladder function change in the early period after surgical alteration in outflow resistance? Preliminary communication. J R Soc Med 1987; 80:753–4.
8. Stanton SL, Cardozo LD. A comparison of vaginal and suprapubic surgery in the correction of incontinence due to urethral sphincter incompetence. Br J Urol 1979; 51:497–9.
9. Lose G, Jørgensen L, Mortensen SO, Mølsted-Pedersen L, Kristensen JK. Voiding difficulties after colposuspension. Obstet Gynecol 1987; 69:33–8.

10. Lyngdorf P, Frimodt-Moller C, Jeppensen N. Voiding disturbances following anal surgery. Urol Int 1986; 41:67–9.
11. Barrett DM. Evaluation of psychogenic urinary retention. J Urol 1978; 120:191–2.
12. Fraser AC. The late effects of Wertheim's hysterectomy on the urinary tract. J Obstet Gynaecol Br Commonw 1966; 73:1002–7.
13. Smith PH, Turnbull GA, Currie DW, Peel KR. The urological complications of Wertheim's hysterectomy. Br J Urol 1969; 41:685–8.

Chapter 11

Medical and Surgical Management of Female Voiding Difficulty

K. Murray

Under normal circumstances, the lower urinary tract serves both storage and eliminatory functions. For an individual to remain continent and to void at will requires the balance of intravesical pressure and urethral resistance. Voiding difficulty can be said to occur when the balance of these forces is displaced towards "storage" and bladder emptying becomes inefficient. The bladder is an unreliable witness and nowhere is this more evident than in the setting of the female with voiding difficulty. In men, the cardinal symptoms of bladder outflow obstruction with a complaint of voiding difficulty are hesitancy and a poor stream [1], to which may be added a sensation of incomplete emptying postmicturition. However, symptoms of voiding difficulty are relatively uncommon in women. Versi and Cardozo [2] reported an incidence of a complaint of a poor stream or incomplete emptying in 5.6% to 13% of peri- and postmenopausal women attending a menopause clinic. In a broader age range of 600 women referred for urological rather than climacteric symptoms, Stanton et al. [3] described voiding difficulties in a third of their patients. These figures for the incidence of voiding symptoms in different patient populations must then be compared with the objective demonstration of an imbalance in micturition function as measured by urodynamics. The Dulwich [2], Tooting [3] and Bristol [4] groups have all reported a low (3%–8%) incidence of voiding difficulty. The results of all three groups are broadly comparable despite different populations and slight differences in the criteria for diagnosing voiding difficulty. Only Shepherd et al. [5] differentiated those patients with low detrusor pressure/low flow voiding (8.1%) and those with classical high pressure/low flow obstructed voiding (3.7%). Furthermore, although hesitancy was a common symptom, only 7% of women complaining of this problem were found to be objectively obstructed and the sensitivity of the urological history alone in diagnosing outflow obstruction was only 18% [5]. It is against this rather

Table 11.1.   Causes of female voiding difficulty

Immobility: Postoperative overdistension of the bladder

Urinary tract infection and "the urethral syndrome"

Constipation

Neuropathy
    Multiple sclerosis
    Transverse myelitis
    CVA
    Diabetes mellitus

Drugs
    Anticholinergic, e.g. tricyclic antidepressants, anti-Parkinsonian medication
    Sedatives, e.g. long-acting benzodiazepines
    ? Adrenergic agonists, e.g. ephedrine, phenylpropanolamine

Surgery obstruction following surgery for stress incontinence or radical pelvic surgery

Gynaecological causes
    Enlarged retroverted uterus
    Gross cystocele
    Ovarian cyst

Urological causes
    Urethral diverticulum
    Bladder calculi
    Urethral stenosis/stricture
    Urethral carcinoma

uncertain background that the management of female voiding difficulty must be viewed.

Aetiology of Voiding Difficulty

The causes of voiding difficulty are well reviewed in Chapter 10. Table 11.1 lists the common and some of the less common causes to provide a framework for the discussion of management.

Investigations

Although a symptomatic history can be misleading, as previously noted, it is important not to underestimate this stage of the investigation. A history of infrequent voiding, the "camel bladder" is not uncommon and 33% of women who are subsequently shown to have bladder outflow obstruction give a history of episodes of acute urinary retention either postoperatively or postpartum [4]. The pattern of bowel activity should be determined and a menstrual history taken. A careful drug history should be elicited to exclude the possibility of iatrogenic impairment of detrusor function. Clinical examination should include vaginal examination to exclude pelvic mass lesions and this can be combined with a cervical and vaginal smear if indicated. A full neurological examination is essential and must include assessment of perineal sensation and anal reflexes. If the clinical history suggests demyelinating disease, fundoscopy may reveal the pale discs of optic neuritis. A history of diabetes mellitus should raise the possibility of autonomic neuropathy and measurement of a patient's blood pressure lying and standing may demonstrate postural hypotension.

All patients should provide an MSU to exclude urinary tract infection. A plain full-length abdominal film performed after micturition will exclude the presence of bladder calculi and may reveal an enlarged bladder soft tissue shadow. Intravenous urography is unhelpful in the routine case, but if indicated by a history of associated haematuria can be usefully modified to provide information about voiding efficiency by performing an "intravenous urodynamogram" [6]. The simplest non-invasive screening test is to perform a flow rate followed by a post-micturition pelvic ultrasound scan to assess residual urine and to exclude masses arising from the pelvic viscera. Various diagnostic criteria have been suggested to confirm a diagnosis of voiding difficulty: a peak urine flow rate (PFR) of less than $15 \, \mathrm{ml \, s^{-1}}$ with a residual urine greater than $100 \, \mathrm{ml}$ on two occasions [2] or any two of the following: flow rate less than $12 \, \mathrm{ml \, s^{-1}}$, peak flow detrusor pressure (PFP) greater than $50 \, \mathrm{cmH_2O}$, urethral resistance (PFP/PFR^2) greater than 0.2 and "significant" (sic) residual urine in the presence of a raised PFP or urethral resistance [7]. The latter set of diagnostic criteria depend on the use of full pressure/flow urodynamic studies and this author reserves this form of invasive investigation for patients who have had previous urogynaecological surgery, usually for sphincter weakness incontinence or for those in whom simple treatment modalities have failed to resolve the patient's symptoms. I find urethral pressure profilometry unhelpful.

A number of other investigations may be useful in specific situations. Acute urinary retention may represent the first presentation of neurological disease [8] and if the symptoms and signs suggest the diagnosis of multiple sclerosis (MS), confirmation requires the demonstration of pathology in at least two separate sites in the nervous system. Measurement of visual evoked responses (VERs) provides a useful method of demonstrating covert pathology in the central nervous system (CNS). Abnormal VERs are found in 70%–97% of definite cases of MS and up to 40% of patients investigated for possible demyelination [9]. Where access to such facilities is available, magnetic resonance imaging provides a sensitive diagnostic tool in the assessment of MS [10]. In women with otherwise unexplained urinary retention, urethral sphincter electromyography may demonstrate abnormal activity in the form of decelerating bursts and complex repetitive discharges, similar to the findings in pseudomyotonia [11].

Treatment

Acute Urinary Retention

Painful retention of sudden onset and yielding less than a litre of urine occurs most commonly in the immediate postoperative or postpartum period [8]. The majority of these cases resolve after a single "in and out" catheterisation or a short period of indwelling catheter drainage. Short acting, powerful cholinergic agonists such as carbachol are unpleasant for the patient, often causing intestinal colic and are not recommended. Some authors have recommended intravesical instillation of prostaglandin F_{2a} to reduce the incidence of postoperative urinary retention following vaginal hysterectomy [12] and stress incontinence surgery [13]. If confirmed in fully double-blind, placebo-controlled trials this would be a useful addition to the armarmenterium. Specific treatment of a gynaecological pelvic mass or procidentia should also result in restoration of normal voiding. In the absence of a demonstrable cause, patients should be taught clean intermittent self-catheterisation. Voiding function can recover as mysteriously as it failed and in the interim the patient is in control of her urinary destiny. Phenytoin has been reported to restore spontaneous micturition in a single woman with an abnormal urethral sphincter EMG [11].

Chronic Voiding Difficulty and Chronic Retention

General measures such as the treatment of significant bacteriuria with an appropriate course of antibiotic and the correction of constipation should always be considered before offering specific therapies.

Drugs Acting on the Bladder and Urethra

Parasympathomimetic Agents. Bethanechol chloride is a cholinergic agonist and has been used on an empirical basis for over 30 years. However in a urodynamically controlled study of "normal" women and women with idiopathic detrusor failure [14], 5 mg of bethanechol subcutaneously had no effect on flow rate or residual urine. In paraplegic patients with neuropathic voiding difficulty, oral bethanechol has no significant effect [15]. There is no indication for the use of this drug in women with voiding difficulty.

Anticholinesterase Agents. Distigmine bromide is an acetylcholinesterase inhibitor which has been reported to prevent postoperative retention [16]. Philp and Thomas [17] were unable to demonstrate any improvement in voiding efficiency in patients with neuropathic bladders using oral distigmine. It is the author's experience that long-term oral distigmine has nothing to offer in the management of voiding difficulty in women.

Prostaglandins. In addition to the reported use of PGF_{2a} in acute retention (vide supra), intravesical PGE_2 has been used to stimulate detrusor contraction. Bultitude et al. [18] and Desmond et al. [19] reported improved voiding efficiency after a single instillation of prostaglandin in women with detrusor failure and claimed that this response was maintained for up to 3 months. Delaere and his colleagues were unable to achieve any success with this treatment [20]. It is difficult to understand how such long-term responses could be obtained in view of the short half-life of the prostaglandins.

a-Adrenergic Blocking Agents. Unlike men, women have no evidence of adrenergically innervated circular bladder neck sphincter. There is, therefore, no theoretical indication for the use of drugs such as phenoxybenzamine and prazosin to decrease urethral resistance and this is born out in clinical practice.

Hormone Replacement Therapy (HRT)

Roberts and Smith [21] suggested that the rigid atrophic urethra of the patient with an inadequate level of endogenous oestrogens is a common cause of voiding difficulty after the menopause. They reported a prolonged remission of symptoms after oestrogen therapy in cases resistant to simple dilatation. This group subsequently presented findings clearly demonstrating the cytological changes in distal urethral epithelium [22] and showed that it paralleled the oestrogen-dependent changes in the vaginal epithelium and that it could also be changed by exogenous oestrogen therapy. Given the common embryological origin of the distal urethra and the vestibule of the vagina from the caudal part of the urogenital sinus, there is a solid ontological basis for these findings. Furthermore, the demonstration of the presence of oestrogen receptors in the female lower urinary tract adds to the rationale for the use of oestrogens in postmenopausal voiding symptoms [23]. In the presence of abundant circumstantial evidence that urinary tract function is oestrogen dependent, it is disappointing that there are few published data on the effect of HRT on voiding function. Hilton and Stanton [24] have reported an improvement in the symptoms of voiding difficulty in a small group of patients using intravaginal oestrogen cream. Versi and Cardozo used oestradiol implants in an uncontrolled trial in symptomatic peri- and postmenopausal women and found a significant improvement in all voiding symptoms except urgency [2].

In the presence of the plethora of preparations available for postmenopausal hormone replacement including tablets, creams, pessaries, subcutaneous implants and transdermal patches the responsible physician requires a rationale for planning treatment. The author uses intravaginal unconjugated oestrogen cream as the first line of treatment in women in whom simple urethral dilatation has failed, as it often does, to relieve symptoms. In addition to its appeal – "The cream; apply to the affected part as directed" – there is sound experimental evidence that this preparation produces physiological plasma oestrogen levels [25] which result in demonstrable oestrogenisation of the urethrovaginal epithelium. The additional advantages of using a "natural" preparation delivered systemically are that, not requiring "first-pass" liver metabolism, the thrombogenic effects are minimised [26] as is the diabetogenic effect [27]. Systemically absorbed preparations also produce a more physiological oestradiol/oestrone ratio. Some women find the use of intravaginal cream distasteful and messy and it has been known to produce gynaecomastia in their sexual partners [28]. In patients who cannot tolerate vaginal cream, the author uses oral oestrogens in the form of a combination calendar pack in women with an intact uterus and oestradiol implants in women who have undergone hysterectomy. Cyclic regimens are to be avoided if possible as endometrial hyperplasia occurs in 7%–15% of women [29] and long-term therapy requires the addition of progestogens. Any woman with a history of postmenopausal or irregular bleeding requires endometrial biopsy either by dilatation and curettage or Vabra suction curettage as 1%–2% of postmenopausal women may have premalignant endometrial changes [30]. All patients are re-assessed after 3 months and if their voiding symptoms have responded to HRT then those women with an intact uterus should have progestogen replacement for days 1–11 each month with, for example, norethisterone 1 mg daily. This confers protection against endometrial hyperplasia during long-term therapy but frequently results in some degree of withdrawal bleeding. Patients may require years of treatment as the vaginal cytology and so presumably urethral cytology reverts to its atrophic state within 2 weeks of withdrawing therapy. If requested by the patient, withdrawal of HRT should be gradual to reduce the incidence of climacteric symptoms.

Surgery

Beyond diagnostic cystoscopy, the mainstay of the surgical treatment of women with voiding difficulty has been, and remains urethral dilatation. Bougie-a-boule are no longer used to calibrate the female urethra. Wyndham-Powell, Canny-Ryall or Hegar dilators can all be used but care should be taken to avoid over-dilatation producing urethral bleeding. Especially in woman with bladder neck incompetence it is better to avoid excessive overdistension producing sphincter weakness incontinence. Dilatation to 70 FG ("thumb size") has been recommended in women with total detrusor failure [31] but this is seldom if ever indicated with the introduction of clean intermittent self-catheterisation (CISC). Simple dilatation to 36 FG together with oestrogen replacement if necessary resolved voiding difficulty in 76% of women with "intramural" (sic) problems [32]. Urethral recalibration with the Otis urethrotome serves the same purpose as simple dilatation. In this technique the instrument is expanded in the sagittal plane until it is gripped by the urethra. It is then further expanded by 10 FG to produce a recalibration. The knife blade is not required. Otis urethrotomy/sphincterotomy with the blade has a place in producing a selective sphincterotomy in separate stages to 35, 40 and 45 FG in the management of neuropathic sphincteric obstruction. Endoscopic bladder neck incision and incision under direct vision using a small nasal or urethroplasty speculum has been used in the past to relieve female bladder neck obstruction. Any incision should be in the 12 o'clock position to avoid the risk of urethrovaginal fistula. However less than 50% of patients in one study obtained a satisfactory response from the procedure [33] and the author does not recommend it. There is no indication for reduction cystoplasty by partial cystectomy or Hamilton–Russell vesicoplication.

Clean Intermittent Self-Catheterisation

Lapides et al. [34] developed the concept of CISC from the use of sterile intermittent catheterisation in paraplegics and the excellent results in their patients of long-term follow-up has led to the widespread acceptance of this technique for the management of both children and adults. The Bristol group [35] reported the first large group of patients treated by CISC in the UK. They found it useful in female chronic retention, multiple sclerosis, acute retention and for self-dilatation of urethral stricture.

The eyesight, manual dexterity and motivation of patients for CISC should be carefully assessed and counselling may be helped by the introduction of a patient already using this technique as in stoma care. Patients use a 12 FG simple short plastic catheter (Nelaton type) and use one per week, cleaning it in warm clean soapy water after use. Some patients feel happier using a mild sterilising solution such as Milton though this is not necessary. Significant bacteriuria ($>10^5$ colony counts ml^{-1}) can be expected in 40–50% of patients but in the absence of symptoms this does not require antibiotic therapy as this will only select out resistant organisms. Patients should attempt to void before passing the catheter. By giving the patient control over their own bladder again many patients show a marked improvement in morale and general self-confidence. CISC is the treatment of choice for the management of iatrogenic obstruction following suspensory surgery for sphincter weakness incontinence and all patients undergoing this form of surgery should be warned of the possible need for CISC if their condition is "overcorrected". However, measurement of maximum voiding pressure ($> 20\,cmH_2O$) and peak flow rate ($> 25\,ml\,s^{-1}$) may allow better prediction of those patients likely to develop postoperative voiding problems [36].

If chronic retention of urine is complicated by symptomatic stress incontinence and is not relieved by CISC alone, a number of further surgical options are open. Stamey, bladder neck suspension [37] has particularly helped those patients with a neuropathic aetiology. Transvulval urethral closure [38] to which this author adds a Martius labial fat pad interposition can be combined with either a permanent suprapubic Foley cystostomy or a Mitrofanoff continent stoma for self-catheterisation. A small number of patients may find that ileal conduit diversion is the only answer to their intractable problems.

Conclusion

Massey and Abrams have elegantly summarised the management of this often difficult problem [32]:

Aggressive measures in the management of female outlet obstruction are rarely applicable in modern practice. Radical surgical procedures carry a significant risk of producing incontinence. Drugs are largely ineffective, except perhaps for hormonal replacement. We recommend a logical progression from cysto-urethroscopy and urethral dilatation via Otis sphincterotomy to intermittent self-catheterisation.

Acknowledgements. My thanks go to Miss Vanessa Garlinge for kindly typing this manuscript.

References

1. Abrams PH, Feneley RCL. The significance of symptoms associated with bladder outflow obstruction. Urol Int 1978; 33:171–4.
2. Versi E, Cardozo LD. Oestrogens and lower urinary tract function. In: Studd JWW, Whitehead MI, eds. The menopause. Oxford: Blackwell Scientific Publications, 1988; 76–84.
3. Stanton SL, Ozsoy C, Hilton P. Voiding difficulties in the female: prevalence, clinical and urodynamic review. Obstet Gynecol 1983; 61:144–7.
4. Abrams PH, Feneley RCL, Torrens M. Urodynamics. Berlin: Springer-Verlag, 1983.
5. Shepherd AM, Powell PH, Bass AJ. The place of urodynamic studies in the investigation and treatment of female urinary tract symptoms. J Obstet Gynaecol 1982; 3:123–5.
6. Turner-Warwick R, Whiteside CG. Milroy EJ, Pengelly AW, Thompson DT. The intravenous urodynamogram. Br J Urol 1979; 51:15–18.
7. Massey JA, Abrams PH. Obstructed voiding in the female. Br J Urol 1988; 61:36–9.
8. Doran J, Roberts M. Acute urinary retention in the female. Br J Urol 1976; 47:793–6.
9. Sokol S. Visual evoked potentials. In: Aminoff MJ, ed. Electrodiagnosis in clinical neurology. New York: Churchill Livingstone, 1986; 441–66.
10. Ormerod IEC, Miller DH, McDonald WI et al. The role of NMR imaging in the assessment of multiple sclerosis and isolated neurological lesions. A quantitative study. Brain 1987; 110:1579–616.

11. Fowler CJ, Kirby RS. Abnormal electromyographic activity (decelerating burst and complex repetitive discharges) in the striated muscle of the urethral sphincter in 5 women with persisting urinary retention. Br J Urol 1985; 57:67–70.

12. Jaschevatzky OE, Anderman S, Shalit A, Ellenbogen A, Grunstein S. Prostaglandin $F_{2\alpha}$ for prevention of urinary retention after vaginal hysterectomy. Obstet Gynecol 1985; 66:244–7.

13. Tammela T, Kontturi M, Käär K, Lukkarinen O. Intravesical prostaglandin $F_{2\alpha}$ for promoting bladder emptying after surgery for female stress incontinence. Br J Urol 1987; 60:43–46.

14. Wein A, Malloy T, Shofer F, Raezer D. The effects of bethanechol chloride on urodynamic parameters in normal women and in women with significant residual urine volumes. J Urol 1980; 124:397–9.

15. Philp NH, Thomas DG, Clarke SJ. Drug effects on the voiding cystometrogram: a comparison of oral bethanechol and carbachol. Br J Urol 1980; 52:484–7.

16. Cameron MD. Distigmine bromide (Ubretid) in the prevention of post operative retention of urine. J Obstet Gynaecol Br Commonw 1966; 73:847–8.

17. Philp NH, Thomas DG. The effect of distigmine bromide on voiding in male paraplegic patients with reflex micturition. Br J Urol 1980; 52:492–6.

18. Bultitude MI, Hills NH, Shuttleworth KED. Clinical and experimental studies on the action of prostaglandins and their synthesis inhibitors on detrusor muscle in vitro and in vivo. Br J Urol 1976; 48:631–7.

19. Desmond AD, Bultitude MI, Hills NH. Shuttleworth KED. Clinical experience with intravesical prostaglandin E_2. Br J Urol 1980; 53:357–66.

20. Delaere KPJ, Thomas CMG, Moonen WA, Debruyne FMJ. The value of intravesical prostaglandin E_2 and $F_{2\alpha}$ in women with abnormalities of bladder emptying. Br J Urol 1981; 53:306–9.

21. Roberts M, Smith P. Non malignant obstruction of the female urethra. Br J Urol 1968; 40:694–702.

22. Smith P. Age changes in the female urethra. Br J Urol 1972; 44:667–76.

23. Iosif CS, Batra S, Ek A, Astedt B. Estrogen receptors in the human female lower urinary tract. Am J Obstet Gynecol 1981; 141:817–20.

24. Hilton P, Stanton SL. The use of intravaginal oestrogen cream in genuine stress incontinence. Br J Obstet Gynaecol 1983; 90:940–4.

25. Whitehead MI, Minardi J, Kitchin Y, Sharples MJ. Systemic absorption of estrogen from Premarin vaginal cream. In: Cooke ID, ed. The role of estrogen/progestogen in the management of the menopause. Lancaster: MTP Press, 1978; 63–75.

26. Studd JWW, Dubiel M, Kakkar W, Thom M, White PJ. The effect of hormone replacement therapy on glucose tolerance, clotting factors, fibrinolysis and platelet behaviour in post-menopausal women. In: Cooke ID, ed. The role of oestrogen/progestogen in the management of the menopause. Lancaster: MTP Press, 1978; 41–59.

27. Thom MH, Chakravarti S, Oram DH, Studd JWW. Effect of hormone replacement therapy on glucose tolerance in post-menopausal women. Br J Obstet Gynaecol 1977; 84:776–84.

28. Di Raimondo CV, Roach AC, Meador CK. Gynaecomastia from exposure to vaginal oestrogen cream. N Engl J Med 1980; 302:1089–90.

29. Sturdee DW, Wade-Evans T, Paterson MEL, Thom M, Studd JWW. Relations between bleeding pattern, endometrial histology and oestrogen treatment in menopausal women. Br Med J 1978; 1:1575–7.

30. Whitehead MI, Campbell S. Endometrial histology, uterine bleeding and oestrogen levels in menopausal women receiving oestrogen therapy and oestrogen/progestogen therapy. In: Brush M, Taylor RWT, King RJB, eds. Endometrial cancer. London: Bailliere Tindall, 1978; 65–80.

31. Farrar DJ, Osborne JL. Voiding dysfunction in women. In: Mundy AR, Stephenson TP, Wein AJ, eds. Urodynamics – principles, practice and application. Edinburgh: Churchill Livingstone, 1984; 242–8.

32. Massey JA, Abrams PH. Obstructed voiding in the female. Br J Urol 1988; 61:36–9.

33. Deane AM, Worth PHL. Female chronic urinary retention. Br J Urol 1985; 57:24–6.

34. Lapides J, Diokno AC, Silber SJ, Lowe BS. Clean intermittent self-catheterisation in the treatment of urinary tract disease. J Urol 1972; 107:458–61.

35. Murray K, Lewis P, Blannin J, Shepherd A. Clean intermittent self-catheterisation in the management of adult lower urinary tract dysfunction. Br J Urol 1984; 56:379–80.

36. Norton P, Stanton SL. Isometric detrusor tests – a predictor of post-operative voiding difficulties. Proceedings of the eighteenth annual meeting of the International Continence Society. Neurourol Urodynam 1988; 7:287–8.

37. Lawrence WT, Thomas DG. The Stamey bladder neck suspension operation for stress incontinence and neurovesical dysfunction. Br J Urol 1987; 59:305–10.

38. Feneley RCL. The management of female incontinence by suprapubic catheterisation, with or without urethral closure. Br J Urol 1983; 55:203–7.

Discussion

Sutherst: There are times when we find difficult cases, perhaps after incontinence surgery, when the patient gets some obstruction afterwards. We go through all the machinery of urethral dilatation and it does not work, and we go through intermittent self-catheterisation. But I have a number of patients who still cannot empty their bladders, and still have high residuals. Where do we go from there? What is the next step? Should we go on to aggressive surgery at that stage or should we try to get by with intermittent self-catheterisation?

Murray: There are two points. In the past it has been suggested that the p-iso stop test would help us predict which of our patients would have difficulties. I know that Mr Stanton feels that the p-iso is not so good and we should take more notice of the peak voiding pressure and the peak flow rate as better discriminants. So perhaps we could pick our patients better.

I personally feel that we should be prepared to warn all patients undergoing GSI surgery that clean intermittent self-catheterisation (CISC) either in the immediate postoperative period, or possibly even long term, may be necessary.

Shah: But it does not answer the question. Even in spite of those recommendations and in spite of being open with the patients and training them in CISC before they go for surgery, some of them reject it eventually. Patients who have large residual urines were mentioned. If this is the case they are not catheterising effectively and one must ensure that they are emptying effectively. But if that fails and the patient is still wet, is having problems with emptying and does not want to catheterise, we are in trouble. It is a very rare occurrence, but in those that I have come across I tend to put suprapubic catheters into them. I tell them that I shall leave them on permanent suprapubic drainage, and do.

Shepherd: And close off the urethra?

Shah: Not always. If they are dry with a suprapubic catheter there is no point in closing the urethra. If they are wet with a suprapubic catheter then either one can close the urethra (which I have done but only in multiple sclerosis (MS) patients) or one can do a urethrocleisis, which I have also done with success in patients who have not had MS.

Sutherst: The patients I am talking about are sometimes quite young women who have had two or three operations on the urethra for stress incontinence and who have a fairly fixed nasty urethra. I suppose that certain urologists would go on to an artificial sphincter.

Mundy: I am certainly not in the habit of doing urethrocleisis and bladder neck closure in a permanent suprapubic.

Shah: We are seeing a different group of patients.

Mundy: In genuine stress incontinence?

Shah: In multiple sclerosis. But the patients that have been described are really quite extreme. What would Mr Mundy do?

Mundy: It depends on age, on the state of the urethra and on the state of the bladder, whether their bladders are normally functioning and how much the residual urine is. As Mr Shah says, it would be very surprising for somebody to be catheterising competently and having a residual urine > 50 ml. I have seen people emptying down to 50 ml but no less, but anything other than that suggests they are not catheterising properly.

If they had had recent incontinence surgery, I would be prepared to suggest they wait for up to 12 months after that operation before concluding that they would never again void spontaneously. They have to be given adequate time before deciding what to do next. If they are still not emptying then, they are better off on long-term self-catheterisation than any other alternative. If they are emptying and they are still incontinent there are only two options: to implant an artificial sphincter, assuming they are emptying reasonably well, or to do some other form of reconstructive surgery. The choice between the two really depends on the state of the urethra.

Sutherst: That is what I was getting down to. In my practice the most difficult patients to deal with are those that have a mixture of obstruction and perhaps some residual stress incontinence. The bladder is not completely empty, the detrusor is not working, and they have very poor flow rates and very high residuals. Some of them do self-catheterise very frequently and I believe them when they tell me they are doing it properly.

Mundy: I am sure that is absolutely right. These are the ones with the most rigid urethras who have the particular problem of incontinence and residual urine. Many of them tend to be older. In those elderly patients a case can be made out for doing something to bypass the urethra if the urethra is hopeless. It can be done either by permanent suprapubic catheterisation in the very elderly, or in the not quite so elderly with a Mitrofanoff type of procedure. And that is particularly applicable when somebody has done that ghastly gynaecological practice of putting in a sling. If anything can be guaranteed to foul up the urethra totally, a sling can, and in those where the urethra is uncatheterisable and they have those problems, that may be the only alternative. But otherwise I would have thought the option is a urethral reconstruction or an artificial sphincter, depending on the state of the urethra.

Sutherst: What would be involved in a urethral reconstruction?

Mundy: The most likely technique if the urethra is seriously damaged would be with a bladder flap and a urethroplasty. That requires excision of the urethra. A bladder neck reconstruction cannot just be dropped on top of a urethra of normal length; it will concertina and the closure will just fall apart. The urethra has to be excised, a bladder flap rolled down and reconstructed around a 12 gauge catheter. And that is really quite a large undertaking.

Stanton: Mr Shah used the blanket term "hysterectomy causing voiding disorders". That is probably a trifle unfair. If he had said vaginal hysterectomy plus vaginal surgery I would agree, but the average abdominal hysterectomy should not cause voiding disorders.

Shah: I agree.

Stanton: On a more serious note, there was a report that after about a year, any urethral closure would tend to fall apart. Is that the general experience?

Mundy: The problem with urethral closure is that it tends to hold for three months or so, particularly in patients with severe spinal injury and multiple sclerosis, and then it breaks down again. I prefer the method by which the whole urethra is mobilised and inverted into the bladder so it stands up like a stump with two or three ligatures around it and there is no suture line to break down.

The problem is that in my experience, (and that includes also talking to other people with similar experience) the bladder neck is only really used in urethral closure in people who have terrible bladders, e.g., the bedbound, bedbound spinal injury and multiple sclerotic patients. But if they are done in the situation I described a moment ago of a relatively normal bladder but a worn out urethra, and something like suprapubic catheterisation or a Mitrofanoff is done as an alternative to reconstruction because of the patient's age or circumstances rather than because of their neurological disability, then the technique holds up rather better.

Shah: I would agree that the method of doing a bladder neck closure, using a skin flap which is put in on a vascularised flap and sutured into the open bladder base is an illogical one. In fact good bladder closure which does not break down provided the catheter does not block can be produced very successfully. The problem with breaking down, is, I am sure, related to postoperative problems with catheter management. Of course if it blocks then leakage will occur in the early postoperative phase. But inkwelling back in, which can be done without opening the bladder at all, is a very good way and those that I have done have all been effective.

Mundy: A stitch can be dropped down from the bladder through the urethra, mobilising the urethra up tight around the external meatus and it can just be hauled back in.

Shah: But there is no need to do that. By dissecting below the pelvic floor the urethra can be easily dissected up from its base, and then just eased back in. Then with several layers of sutures as it is closed into the bladder, probably about three or four layers of sutures, it should hold.

Stanton: That is the one that I like. I think I have had one that broke down. But I thought that there had been bad experiences of that technique as well.

Mundy: I have had bladder neck repairs break down. I am probably more cautious and I do them from above.

Shepherd: Mr Murray mentioned briefly women with high-pressure bladders and women with low-pressure bladders and I wondered whether the management should be different.

Murray: It is the women who have the high pressure/low flow and appear to have some form of demonstrable obstructive element who will do better with urethral dilatation. Urethral dilatation for the low pressure/low flow is empirical, and it may be no more than letting out the evil spirits.

Hilton: The high pressure ones are much less common. Within our clinic there are ten times as many low pressure/low flows as high pressure/low flows.

Stanton: But high pressures become low pressures.

Cardozo: Some high pressures become low pressure, but not all. But I have far more low pressure/low flow than high pressure/low flow cases.

Shepherd: High pressure/low flow in women is very rare.

Kirby: Clearly we are in need of a useful pharmacological agent. The problem is quite a common one whatever the cause and it is a most frustrating problem for the patient and for the surgeon. I wonder whether the drugs Mr Murray quoted and rejected have been tested properly. There are so few papers on any of those agents, and the papers that I have read on them are useless.

It is not very easy to study because we see such patients only occasionally and it is not an easy thing to build a clinical trial on. But in my experience some of these agents work in some patients, maybe a subcategory. In pharmacological terms, is there any evidence that they work at all?

Andersson: Sandocal is the only drug that has been thoroughly investigated and it has been shown that it does not produce contractions that can effectively empty the bladder per se. But because it increases tension in the bladder wall, it might evoke reflex emptying of the bladder, and that is believed to be the mechanism, based on animal experiments.

But this is a discussion of postoperative voiding difficulties. It is routine at several centres in Sweden at least to give carbachol to prevent urinary retention, but there are no systematic studies on whether or not it helps the patients and nobody knows if it is really effective for emptying the bladder.

I have seen a series of studies on α-blockers used postoperatively and some of these studies report positive results. But the theoretical basis for using α-blockers postoperatively is not very well founded. Even if intraurethral pressure or outflow resistance in these patients can be decreased, in the absence of active detrusor contraction the bladder cannot be emptied and most of these patients postoperatively have no active contraction of their bladder. In those cases it would be preferable to give, say, naloxone. I do not think the studies done so far with muscarinic receptor stimulating agents or α-blockers, convincingly show anything.

Kirby: I have seen patients with neurological bladder deficit, some of the rather unusual ones with parasympathetic denervation, who have a very dramatic response to carbachol; not only an increased pressure rise, but actually voiding as well as getting this terrific sensation.

I personally think carbachol has a place, but there is no objective scientific evidence to prove it.

Mundy: I think it is a total waste of time. I am a little bothered about the logic of giving a drug with a 4–6 h half-life for an event with a 1-minute half-life.

Kirby: I accept that.

Mundy: If there was an agent that we could give, when a patient has an indwelling catheter, for example, a suprapubic catheter after a colposuspension, and they are having difficulty voiding, if the carbachol could be given intravesically to help them to get going, that might be a nice idea.

Cardozo: Given subcutaneously?

Mundy: I am suggesting that some drug could be given intravesically.

Cardozo: But it works quite quickly subcutaneously.

Mundy: If we could give a subcutaneous agent like people have been trying for voiding dysfunction in multiple sclerosis, that is fine, but I cannot see that any oral agent would ever give a very satisfactory result.

Kirby: That is probably right. What is wanted is something that will reactivate the sensory system. That is why it would be logical to go back and look again at prostaglandins, because they might just do that. They might give more sensation. I am sure that the main reason these women do not void is they have no sensation of bladder fullness. They cannot tell when they are full and therefore they do not get the neurophysiological feedback.

Stanton: We have spent a lot of time giving prostaglandin (PG) E_2 to patients who had had colposuspensions and had catheters in place. I think we gave some PG F, but principally PG E_2.

Cardozo: These were tried for a long time, and it did absolutely no good. But we also gave them valium and various other things. What works best is subcutaneous carbachol, just anecdotally, and we started a trial of it at King's College Hospital, London. But the ward sister stopped it because she said it made the patients vomit. She thought the reason they were passing water was because they were nauseous, and not because it was having any effect on the bladder.

Stanton: But they get diarrhoea too.

Cardozo: They get diarrhoea and they vomit.

Mundy: Total evacuation.

Kirby: What is interesting is that the patients will put up with the side effects.

Cardozo: I gave them myotonine orally as well, to take home with them.

I agree there have been no good drug trials and I think we are being somewhat negative because there is not much else to offer.

Mundy: But just because there is nothing else to offer it does not mean that that is necessarily any good.

Cardozo: We spent time giving patients substandard drugs for detrusor instability. Why do we feel that we should not give them drugs?

Murray: I should like to come back to the discussion about naloxone. I am disappointed in it. The work we did at Bristol shows that naloxone has an effect by its encephalinergic blockading action, but the percentage changes are very small. Work has been done on bladder strips showing that the actual degree of modulation that might be achieved with naloxone is really very small.

Andersson: My concept is that pain, for example, causes endogenous release of encephalins in the spinal cord, and that blocks transmission in the efferent branch of the reflex. I do not know if anyone has shown that there is atony of the bladder and an acontractile bladder as the reason for the voiding dysfunction. It might well be that because of pain and because of the operation the introduction of encephalins would block the micturition reflex, and that breaking it at some place, perhaps by injecting naloxone, could wake it up.

I know of no trial but this would be a reasonable way to proceed. The bladder has to have a contraction to be able to empty and I do not think that this can only be done with a-receptor blockade.

Hilton: But the functions of contraction of the bladder and relaxation of the sphincter are so intimately co-ordinated that surely there is some logic behind a-blockade in that having achieved urethral relaxation, detrusor contraction may follow as a natural consequence.

Mundy: There is a flaw in that argument, that a-blockade produces urethral relaxation.

Kirby: It does probably drop urethral pressure slightly. I accept that that is not quite the same thing.

Mundy: But surely the crucial factor is more a question of rhabdosphincter opening, and if we could do that, that would be a different matter.

Hilton: A striated muscle blocker might be expected to be more effective if we are pursuing that line of argument.

Andersson: What is crucial is to evoke the micturition reflex, and any pharmacological approach that can achieve that – to try to contract the bladder or to relax the urethra – is to be preferred. It is better to micturate normally if that is possible.

Mundy: Would it be theoretically possible to use one of those machines to stimulate the pons and cause the patient to micturate directly?

Kirby: We have not actually measured bladder pressure when we stimulate the pons. But neurosurgeons now are talking about microsurgical techniques whereby they could implant microtubules into the pons and stimulate that effectively. They know now the agents in the rabbit, the rat and the cat that cause micturition centres to fire; dopamine and various other things will do it and theoretically one could use that. But that is to talk about the next century; 100 years from now.

Mundy: But theoretically could it be done electrically, as a sort of stereotactical impulse?

Van Mastrigt: There are two centres, a micturition centre and a continence centre, and they are very close together. This has been shown in a number of studies. It might be very difficult to stimulate one and not the other.

Sutherst: We have yet to discuss postoperative voiding problems. Is there any consensus on how we might avoid those? Apart from slings?

Shah: That is an important point. Probably the most important preventive method of avoiding these disorders is to ensure that nurses are aware that many patients cannot micturate following surgery, and they should prevent retention from taking place.

Sutherst: I was thinking more about the preoperative dynamics that might demonstrate or identify the patients who might have postoperative voiding difficulty.

Shah: The majority of patients that I see with postoperative voiding dysfunction were normal before. What has happened is they have been left in retention for 24 hours or more and not had that retention relieved. They have been sat in the bath, they have been medicated, and nothing has worked, and they have been left with over-distended bladders for a long time. Education is the key.

Hilton: It is certainly a major difficulty in surgery throughout our hospitals, and most important of all on our postnatal wards. The situation that Dr Sutherst is discussing is postoperatively following incontinence surgery where a patient has a catheter in from operation.

Sutherst: Postcolposuspension specifically.

Shah: The postcolposuspensions have suprapubics in, or they have in my practice, and we can assess what their voiding abnormality is and do urodynamics if necessary before they go home.

Sutherst: But they develop voiding dysfunction.

Shah: I suppose those that have low voiding pressure prior to surgery with low isometric pressures tend to do worse than those with normal pressures. But 95% of patients will void normally eventually, even those with higher pressures.

Van Mastrigt: I think contractility should be assessed and not flow rates or pressures. As a remote example perhaps, but nevertheless applicable, in a series of patients who had a transurethral resection procedure, by using the contractility parameters we could predict which of them would have residual urine afterwards, because they had low contractile bladders rather than obstructed urethras. And I think that the same would apply to females.

Mundy: But there is a difference between theory and practice. In theory we may be able to predict things like this, but in practice there are two main aspects. First, is this patient likely to have a voiding problem? In such a case it would be sensible to put in a catheter proleptically to make sure there is no trouble. Second, if the standards of nursing care are of the highest and the patient is regularly asked about voiding the bladder and someone keeps an eye on volume, then there are no problems. But on a busy postoperative ward, nurses have their work cut out to keep track of blood pressures and pulses and, where patients are being given large doses of diamorphine or, more commonly, Omnopon, the patients do not feel pain and even if they could they could not micturate.

Stanton: I think that is not the way to go about it. To have a nurse go about the ward putting her hand on the abdomen every five minutes is just the way to produce anxiety. We run a busy ward, we tend to see patients about once a day, and we usually try to explain, certainly to those who are in for slings, that they may have voiding problems.

The first consideration is to dispel anxiety before operation and to tell the patient that it really does not matter when they void in terms of their ultimate cure rate, and if they are not voiding effectively by six or seven days we try to send them home.

Mundy: We are talking about acute retention problems.

Sutherst: Some of us are talking about postcolposuspension voiding difficulties.

Mundy: If the patient seems likely to run into trouble, I would put in a catheter and not let it happen.

DeLancey: Talking about postcolposuspension voiding problems, I wonder if the concepts that underlie the operations we do are based upon an anatomical concept that the urethra is fixed in place and immobile. Perhaps that is the reason that a certain number of individuals have difficulty voiding afterwards. Maybe the concept behind the operation is one that we should re-evaluate, and perhaps we should be looking at other operations that do not fix it immovably in place.

Stanton: I do not think it is the immobility alone. I am convinced it is the high elevation. This is the trouble with colposuspension, which is a great operation, and if one is enthusiastic one will tie them reasonably tight and some of them will be well elevated. I do not think it is immobility: I think this is one of those things that have been passed down from father to son, and nobody has ever proved to me that it is immobile.

DeLancey: No. Although the different reports of postoperative voiding difficulties, show that in the operations that re-attach the tissues on to the lateral pelvic side wall rather than to bone, there have been virtually no voiding difficulties.

Stanton: I take the point. But is that actually objectified?

DeLancey: No.

Stanton: This is the difficulty. We are talking about a variety of operations.

DeLancey: But it was objective in terms that they looked at how often the patients were catheterised, if they did not have a catheter after the operation. And if there were significant voiding difficulties, I am sure that these people's eyes would have turned yellow before they left the hospital. In fact they did not. This is something that we know very little about and it needs to be studied. But when we look at all the reports over the last 40 years, our continence rates have not improved with retropubic procedures.

Stanton: They have, because they should be more honest. With great respect, the subjective ones always stay at 95% or 98% rising 0.5 a year with inflation! But the objective ones in fact are coming out now and they are being a lot more honest and these are rising. They are still down at about 80%–90% but they are a lot more reliable than the subjective ones.

Hilton: With regard to the question of fixity of the urethra, Mr Stanton suggests that hyperelevation is the problem. But work that Dundas did in about 1982 [1] showed that fixity of the urethra appeared at least as important as superelevation in those patients who had voiding problems postoperatively. They had virtually no bladder base descent on voiding.

Stanton: Most of the good colposuspensions have that anyway. What I was trying to emphasise was that those who got into voiding problems were the ones that were really placed very high.

Hilton: They were high, but they were also more fixed.

Mundy: More fixed in a higher position.

Hilton: They were not only higher at rest, but when a patient attempts to void there is no descent.

Versi: Can I come back to the question of voiding by abdominal strain? What does one do with a patient who has an overelevated bladder neck following colposuspension? What advice should we give her?

Shah: I discourage voiding by abdominal strain, by telling them not to do it.

Cardozo: What should they be told to do instead?

Shah: Use intermittent self-catheterisation.

Mundy: But half the population micturates with abdominal straining as part of their performance.

Cardozo: Most people do abdominal straining.

Shah: It is a matter of what we mean by abdominal straining. I was not referring to a minor push.

Mundy: But the difference is some groan and get their bladders empty and others groan and do not. Usually people who can empty their bladders very well do so without giving themselves subarachnoid haemorrhage every time they empty their bladder. There are a lot of people who, if they are shown the residual urine, can take a breath and squeeze it out in a few seconds.

I agree that if they cannot empty their large residual urine volume without strain they have to use intermittent catheterisation. But if they are shown their residual urine a lot of them can squeeze it out without any difficulty.

Versi: But following bladder neck failure they will have problems.

Shah: They would need to be evaluated urodynamically before coming to any conclusion as to whether they should strain or not.

I use this particularly in respect of spinal injury patients, whom I tend seriously to discourage from straining because they have very weak pelvic floors in any event and they tend to get quite major problems with pelvic floor descent if they strain because they have nothing to oppose that strain.

Kirby: What about the Credé manoeuvre? I have one patient who uses the Credé manoeuvre, so much so that she actually inverts her rectus muscle and rectus sheath, right down into the pelvis. It is a most extraordinary sight.

Hilton: Mr Versi's question was in relation to patients who void by the Valsalva manoeuvre. How do we deal with them after colposuspension or other suprapubic procedures, which is a slightly different issue from simply managing their problem in the first place. If they void by strain and have stress incontinence how do we deal with that? Certainly the studies that we have done in relation to colposuspension suggest that trying to void by strain after such marked elevation of the bladder neck will not allow them to pass urine at all. My own feeling in those patients is that either we do not do a colposuspension but we do a less obstructive procedure, or we must teach them to self-catheterise before we do a colposuspension.

Kirby: So that we do not end on a note of therapeutic nihilism, I wanted to mention that the best method is to implant one of Giles Brindley's anterior root stimulators, just for the sake of completeness.

Mundy: I would qualify that statement. The best way of getting people to void is by implanting a sacral anterior root stimulator.

Kirby: I would go along with that.

Shah: It is only appropriate in people with complete spinal cord injury or in those patients in whom one is prepared to cut the posterior root and make their sensory input absent. Otherwise they get pain when stimulated. It is fine for patients with suprasacral spinal cord injuries, both male and female, complete generally. But if they are incomplete and the sensation they have is not useful to them then we should cut the posterior roots. And if it is useful to them then they will probably have pain.

Mundy: We would want to cut the posterior roots in any event.

Shah: We do want to cut the posterior roots. But in those that have sensation, we want to preserve that sensation and they may elect to have the implant in spite of the fact they may have pain. But it is a relative contraindication.

Murray: Which is why I did not include it.

General Discussion

Hilton: I should like to bring the discussion back to the question of the so-called gold standard, either a gold standard for demonstration and recognition of incontinence or a gold standard for the definition of GSI or other forms of incontinence. Clearly some of us have differing views from others, and yet if we are all to discuss our researches into different therapeutic manoeuvres we should be looking to the same sort of standard.

Stanton: It is a very broad question. Specifically gold standards on what?

Hilton: On the demonstration of incontinence, on the quantification of incontinence and so the diagnosis of GSI, which seems to have been the area where there is most argument.

Stanton: One actually either needs to be able to see it visually, or else a pad test is needed – either an hour's pad test, or as we tend to use, the DUEC. That should take care of most complaints of "I lose urine".

Hilton: As a gold standard only one of those can be allowed, or a combination of them that should be applied to every patient.

Stanton: The combination that we have is cystometry plus DUEC. As an occasional modification I would use pyridium if there is doubt as to whether the woman is having a vaginal discharge or is just prevaricating.

Hilton: To make it a very "gold" standard!

Sutherst: I cannot see a reason for having a single gold standard. One's global appreciation of the problem using various dynamic tests should be the group of tests against which to match another one, surely.

Stanton: But what is the test or the tests that one would use at the end of the day? When one is faced with a panoply of investigations, which is the most useful?

In that situation, I have said what I would go for. If I were asked about urethral function tests I would certainly go for a range of tests because there is nothing that is head and shoulders above anything else and also because there are various urethral defects that one might want to highlight.

Cardozo: There is no range of urethral function tests available.

Stanton: There are. There is the urethral pressure, there is the urethral electroconductance, there is the elastance test produced by Lose et al. [2] that I think is a very serious contender, and there is Mr Warrell's force gauge.

Cardozo: But no one uses all of these.

Stanton: I use some of them. These are a variety of tests that are available and in terms of urethral function there is nothing that is head and shoulders above the rest.

Cardozo: You started by saying that you do not use urethral pressure profiles. The only test that you have mentioned that you use is UEC, yet you say that we should use a range of them.

Stanton: Probably because I am very dissatisfied at the moment with urethral function. I have a totally negative attitude towards urethral pressures, otherwise I would use them. I should like to evaluate elastance in the group of patients that I see because that seems to be an alternative that has not been explored in the UK.

Versi: There is a difference between what one would use for research purposes and what one would use for diagnosis. The question related more to what we should have for research purposes. But we are discussing the different tests and we have to have some standard we all agree on against which we should compare any new technique. That is what I understand by the gold standard. We can argue about what should be the gold standard, but at the end of the day if we are part of society we should agree on the gold standard that people should use for research. And it does not have to be one test: it can be a combination of tests.

Van Mastrigt: And should not the most important property of that test be that if the test does not show stress incontinence then such patients should be told that they have no stress incontinence?

Versi: No, because that would imply that the gold standard was the perfect test, and I do not think that we can possibly come up with that assertion. All we can say is that it is the best available test that we have and one that is reproducible and that others will use to compare their tests with.

Stanton: The gold standard is a fallacy. We can talk about it, but if we take it seriously we are looking at many different parameters and many different symptoms when we evaluate our patients and the concept of one single test is naive.

Versi: Not necessarily.

Mundy: It is not naive. It is perfectly reasonable that one should have a good, reliable, reproducible general screening test which may then point in the direction of something else that might be more appropriate, and it is quite reasonable that that test should serve as a gold standard without being perfect. It does not have to be perfect. It can be improved on by making it more effective. But equally, if it is just as effective, it might be cheaper, it might be simpler, it might be quicker to use.

Stanton: I would not disagree. But I am saying that I do not think there is one test that is the best test and that often several tests might be needed. I would agree that one test might well be chosen first, and if that is what is called the gold standard, then fine. I would go along with that test being used first and there would be several tests that might be used after that.

Hilton: But in the context of trying to evaluate one urethral function test or another, which is the context in which this discussion arose, there has to be something to which we can relate those new tests. The problem is that one group is using VCU, another group is using cystometry, another group is using a pad and another group is using "the patients says". Those may all be in order but we should all use the same one.

Mundy: For most people we see in clinical practice there is one test that we use. We have a urodynamic test, and usually where the facility is available, a video urodynamic test. That is the test we all use, surely. And then occasionally we use the other tests because we are interested in them, because we are investigating them, because there is some problem we want to investigate. But video urodynamics is the basic tool we all use, isn't it?

Cardozo: Mr Stanton uses cystometry and UEC.

Stanton: I use cystometry, and if I do not get the results I then go on to video. I do not think to submit every single one of my women who vary in age and vary in physical disability to video. And I can only get access to video one afternoon a week.

Mundy: If you had unlimited access, might you not use it more often?

Stanton: My last researcher was pregnant and there was no way she would stand in front of an X-ray screen!

Van Mastrigt: There is no reason to say that the gold standard should be the preferred test for each patient who comes in, or that it should be the first test. There is no reason at all to do that.

Mundy: I am not saying that one should. I am saying that we are talking as though we sit down and think about which test to use when we do not. We use one test. That is the routine in real life. We talk about other tests, but the basic test we use is the same for everybody.

Van Mastrigt: There are two different themes here. One might have a preferred test, which is cheap, which imposes a very low load on the patient or whatever, such as the eyeball test. If the majority of patients can demonstrate their stress incontinence on direct examination, that is surely sufficient, and there would be no need to have recourse to the gold standard. That would only be necessary to test a new test, and not for diagnosing every patient that comes in.

Mundy: Whether or not the video appearance is thrown in, the crucial factor is to have filling and voiding cystometry measuring abdominal pressure, rectal pressure and electronic subtraction with the flow rate recorded.

Stanton: Surely all of us must use that as the standard and starting point in the case of any wet patient. We then throw in video, or we then throw in UEC, or we then throw in urethral pressures.

Mundy: There is an advantage in having the gold standard of investigation as the one which is most routinely used.

Van Mastrigt: No. It might involve a very high patient load. It might involve a lot of radiation or whatever.

Cardozo: It makes the research much easier to have it as the routine test. It also makes the research much more meaningful. If what one is doing in practice is what one is researching, then better and more appropriate answers with higher numbers will be obtained.

Stanton: The first commitment is to the patients.

Kirby: On the point about urethral function, and coming back to what tests can be used to predict those women who will not do well from stress incontinence surgery, which is very important, one possible test is the use of neurophysiology. Mr Swash has just reported on the use of neurophysiology in patients with rectal prolapse or for rectal incontinence surgery, and those with severe denervation

on his tests do much worse after surgery. Whilst not all patients with stress incontinence have denervation, some do, and maybe they are the ones who do not do
very well if the bladder base is simply hitched up. I cannot prove that, but it
is a possibility.

Mundy: I think that is right.

Warrell: I am happy to say I shall be able to report on that.

Mundy: Is this a test we can do routinely using needle electrodes?

Warrell: Yes. Pudendal nerve conduction tests are cheap, painless and easy.

Hilton: We should draw the discussion to a close. Quite how one can summarise
in a few short words I am not entirely sure.

Chapter 5 described the application of animal models to cystometry and the
derivation of diagnostic as opposed to symptomatic variables. Van Mastrigt's
data appear to give some clarity to the diagnosis of contractility and urethral
resistance. Perhaps this is the way that cystometric assessment should be moving
in the future as far as the investigation of voiding problems at least is concerned.
Clearly these are very common problems, even in the female population within
specialist clinics at least, and I am sure we do need better methods of evaluating
them. It will require something of a quantum leap to transmit these new parameters
which at the moment lie within the medical physics department. To transmit
those to clinical practice will not be an easy step, but perhaps is the way we
should move. It remains unclear just how these parameters may assist in what
is perhaps the most difficult and controversial area as far as the gynaecologist
is concerned, which lies more within the filling phase of the micturition cycle
rather than the voiding phase.

Mr Versi (Chapter 6) discussed some of the applications of urethral pressure
profiles, and from his own studies came to the conclusion that whilst the UPP
may be useful as a research tool, it has relatively limited clinical application.
From subsequent discussions it seems that at least part of the uncertainty about
the role of UPPs lies in the fact that we are not clear what it is we are measuring
when we talk about urethral pressure. One of the major difficulties we have is
that the tools that can measure urethral pressure, and by that I mean fluid perfusion
catheter techniques, whilst they may tell us urethral pressure at rest are not
adequate to assess the urethra in dynamic situations. Those methods that can
assess the urethra in dynamic situations probably do not tell us pressure; they
tell us something more akin to force. But until we have resolved these issues
it is inevitable that these tools will have relatively limited clinical application.

As far as UEC is concerned, chapter 7 describes the applications of this technique. It is clear that this technique, perhaps more than any other tool, is able
to detect the presence of urine within the urethra – if that is something that
we are interested in. It seems that it also has the ability not only to detect but
also to quantify urine within the urethra. It was suggested that the technique
may be of some diagnostic reliability, although to my own mind, at least, the

evidence for that is not as convincing as it might be. The question of prolonged increases in UEC which Dr Plevnik related to unstable contractions seems to me more to look at large quantities of urine rather than any specific diagnosis, and the evaluation in baseline of UEC is a volume-related phenomenon. It just happens that patients with DI tend to leak large volumes and we therefore have this apparent diagnostic reliability. But I remain rather dubious about that.

As far as other tools are concerned, ultrasound and neurophysiological testing, it is clear that as independent investigations these will not have mileage within urogynaecology. But as an adjunct to urodynamic tools, particularly in those patients who either have pre-existing evidence of a neuropathy or have urodynamic evidence suggestive of the neuropathy, they may give us additional useful information.

References

1. Dundas D, Hilton P, Williams J, Stanton SL. Aetiology of voiding difficulties. Proceedings of the twelfth annual meeting of the International Continence Society, 1982; 132.
2. Lose G, Colstrup H, Saksagar K, Kristensen J. New methods for static and dynamic measurement of related values of cross-sectional area and pressure in the female urethra. Neurourol Urodynam 1988; 6: 465–76.

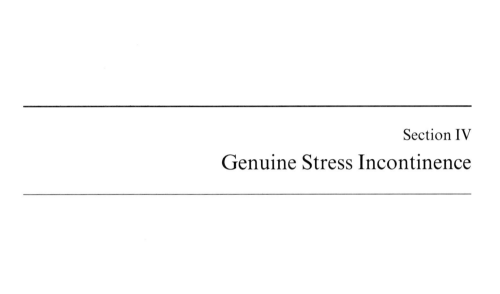

Section IV
Genuine Stress Incontinence

Chapter 12

Pathophysiology of Genuine Stress Incontinence

D. W. Warrell

Chairman's summary of Mr Warrell's contribution:

Mr Warrell talked about the pathophysiology of genuine stress incontinence and explained two studies that he had carried out in Manchester. He said that stress incontinence mainly occurs in multiparous women with bladder neck prolapse and that oestrogen deficiency has an adverse effect but there are exceptions. He then went on to describe a study in which they looked at 69 controls, both nulliparous and multiparous, and compared them to 105 women with genuine stress incontinence and/or prolapse. The women were investigated by muscle biopsy of the pelvic floor, pudendal nerve terminal latencies and single fibre EMG of the pubococcygeus, and he showed by all three parameters, that there was more evidence of denervation and re-innervation in those women with prolapse and/or stress incontinence than amongst his control group.

He then went on to look at fascial damage among women with genuine stress incontinence. He took a group of 60 women who had untreated genuine stress incontinence (in other words no previous surgery), some of whom had severe prolapse, some moderate prolapse and some no prolapse, and he found that the motor unit fibre density was greater in those without prolapse. He hypothesised that re-innervation had taken place more in those without prolapse than in those with prolapse. He therefore made the hypothesis that both fascial damage and nerve damage are important in the genesis of genuine stress incontinence.

In addition he has looked at collagen in the last group of patients and feels that there may be a weakness of collagen or poor repair of collagen in those who have prolapse, as against those who do not. He summarised that stress incontinence without prolapse may be a denervation problem, but in patients with prolapse there is likely to be less denervation.

His penultimate comment was on posterior vaginal wall effect on women with stress incontinence, and he showed that retracting the posterior vaginal wall has an effect on the maximum urethral closure pressure greater in those who do not have anterior vaginal wall prolapse than in those who do.

His final comment was that there is a multifactorial genesis of genuine stress incontinence.

Discussion

Swash: The problem of the relationship between damage to the nerve supply and other factors is really the nub of the question. Clearly denervation in the pelvic floor and the sphincter muscles is not the only cause of stress incontinence. But there is room for argument as to whether it is a major contributory cause, and if so, what is the relationship between that contributory cause and the other causes.

Something that struck me when I was reading the literature on this subject, not being a gynaecologist and having access to personal experience, was that stress incontinence sometimes begins during the first pregnancy, before delivery, and that therefore there must be factors that are not related to denervation at all but are simply related to a lump, an expanding fetus, in the pelvis that must be related to the development of stress incontinence.

Cardozo: That concurs with what Francis [1] showed many years ago.

Warrell: I guess what one is looking at is the supporting structure, the collagen. But there may be an oestrogen effect on smooth muscle tone.

Cardozo: Our own work shows that stress incontinence is pregnancy related as much as it is delivery related, and therefore innervation cannot be the major factor.

Swash: Not the only factor, but it may be the factor that leads to the continuation of the problem as a chronic problem later.

Warrell: One thing commonly quoted in the name of Winnie Francis, although she has no evidence for it, is that patients who have stress incontinence for the first time during pregnancy are those who develop stress incontinence in later life. That is the quote but I know of no hard evidence in her paper.

Cardozo: It is written in her paper but when we look at her data she has not studied those women 20 years on.

Warrell: We are in the process of following up these 100 women and it is a question which we hope to answer. I am cautioning against accepting that blanket statement.

Sutherst: In the light of present day findings those figures of Winnie Francis would probably be regarded as suspect. She found that 50% of pregnant women when questioned fairly thoroughly admitted to some incontinence, which fits in with figures from a number of other authors that 50% of normal nulliparous women have some incontinence at some stage in their lives. I am not sure that her figures can be entirely relevant now, 30 years on.

Warrell: There is room for a big study of bladder function in pregnancy because the papers that have been written express some quite diverse views on what happens to bladder function in pregnancy.

Cardozo: Not just a big study, but a longitudinal long-term prospective study.

DeLancey: The idea of stress incontinence starting during pregnancy was one that was asked about in the Macer project, which was a community-based survey of about 2000 women – normal women, not women with incontinence. One of the strong correlations with the later development of urinary incontinence was the development of incontinence during pregnancy, and that was a significant correlation. What they were unsure of when the data were analysed afterwards was whether – since these women were recalling events from 40 years before – it was simply that those who continued with incontinence afterwards recalled it during pregnancy and those who did not continue with incontinence did not recall it.

Warrell: There are many women who begin with incontinence for the first time after delivery, as some women in our series did.

Stanton: That happened in the series at St Bartholomews Hospital, London.

DeLancey: It is an intriguing series of observations. One of the things that struck me about the distributions – I cannot remember whether it was latency or fibre density – was the fact that in the stress incontinence group there were a number of people who fell into what would be the normal range and that there was that small amount of overlap. Did those patients seem to be different from the ones who had marked denervation or marked latency? Were they women who had more of an anatomical defect or more of some other factor?

Warrell: The study was flawed because we included patients who had had previous repair. But certainly in our last study, of 60 women who had had nothing of any sort, there is a very clear relationship between stress incontinence, a lot of denervation and no prolapse, and the patients who had prolapse where they have different collagen with less muscle damage.

Cardozo: In view of the fact that Mr Warrell's work is highly respected and will be widely quoted, and the numbers are large would it not be worth re-analysing the data for those who have and those who have not had previous surgery? There are 105 women with stress incontinence and/or prolapse who have been analysed as a heterogeneous group, which is obviously unwise and less valuable than if they had been analysed separately. There must be sufficient within that group to be able to analyse those who have not had surgery.

Warrell: We are in the process of doing that. What we are looking at is how they fare with surgery.

Cardozo: That would be very useful for everyone who quotes the work in the future.

Swash: Might the notion that I put forward earlier, that there might be a dual innervation to what we call the urethral sphincter and musculature, have some importance in view of some of the difficulties in understanding some of these patients?

Warrell: I do not know. We have not tried to assess the perineal supply. All we have done is to measure the pudendal nerve supply.

Cardozo: We have studied the EMG of the actual urethral sphincter, differentiating it from the striated muscle of the pelvic floor, and we have not reproduced Mr Warrell's results. Our women who have stress incontinence as compared to those who have prolapse as compared to controls with neither stress incontinence nor prolapse have no difference in their EMGs of the urethral sphincter, as opposed to the pelvic floor. That would possibly be an explanation for our findings as compared to his.

Stanton: But there is some doubt about the interpretation of the signals in those data.

Cardozo: We have re-analysed our data, and have also looked at amplitude. Although we have not yet reported that we have looked at both duration and amplitude, the results are the same.

Warrell: There is no doubt that having a baby is bad for a woman and that very few emerge without some sort of nerve/muscle damage.

Cardozo: I agree, but the damage may not be to the striated muscle of the urethral sphincter. It may be to the posterior muscle in the pelvic floor. Mr Warrell's biopsies showed that there was greater damage to the posterior part of the pelvic floor than to the anterior part.

Warrell: I accept that. What one cannot get over is this very clear distribution.

If we measure the terminal motor latency of the pudendal nerve there is quite a big difference, and in patients who have prolapse and normal urinary control their pudendal terminal motor latency is normal.

Swash: One must be careful not to draw functional conclusions from latencies and re-innervated measurements such as fibre density, or length duration or amplitude. We have to be careful to recognise that pressure measurements are functional measurements, for example, whereas EMG and nerve conduction criteria are measurements of what the nerve can do electrically they do not necessarily coincide with what force the muscles it innervates can produce.

Versi: We have shown correlations between skin collagen content and urethral pressures, but we were worried about whether the collagen in the pelvic fascia was the same as the collagen in the skin.

Warrell: I think this is the beginning of a whole new avenue of work. Up to now our field of urodynamics has been concerned with measurement and making a diagnosis. We are now starting to ask the fundamental question: why? Just demonstrating that patients with and without prolapse have different sorts of collagen raises a whole avenue of interest.

One speculation, and it is wild speculation, is that having a baby causes damage in the sense that it inevitably extends the vagina, and one of the factors that affects whether or not a woman will get a prolapse is her ability to produce good repair collagen. There is a very respectable hypothesis that genetic disorders of collagen are common. The genetic disorder is not something gross like an indiarubber man, but the ability to produce good or bad repair collagen is what determines whether someone gets arthritis or their joints remain healthy as they get older. It may be that what we are talking about – and this is wild speculation – is involution. In other words, are some patients recovering well after being stretched by vaginal delivery and others not?

The alternative explanation is that it is "egg not chicken", and that the people who have prolapse have different collagen, and that because they have different collagen their prolapse is being stretched. That could be a quite different explanation.

Stanton: One has still to go back to first principles. I think Mr Warrell is right here that people may be very different.

There are a number of nulliparous young girls of 15 or 16 who develop incontinence who have obviously neither been through the insult of pregnancy, nor had some mass in the pelvis which would cause abnormal EMGs in the pelvic floor.

The second point is racial difference. Black women, who may undergo several deliveries, have much much less prolapse than their white counterparts. Presumably this is also collagen.

Warrell: Certainly there is a well-documented difference in the collagen of the skin of black people as opposed to white people.

Stanton: One thing puzzles me. Am I right in assuming that there was more denervation and deterioration in patients who had stress incontinence but no prolapse?

Warrell: I think I take Dr Swash's point, that the pudendal nerve terminal motor latency was greater in patients who had stress incontinence, and the amount of re-innervation was greater. I do not know how justified we are in saying that greater re-innervation necessarily means greater nerve damage beforehand.

Swash: I do not think it does. It could mean only that there has been longer for the re-innervated capacity to be demonstrated.

Warrell: Yet all these groups were identical. This group was a remarkably homogeneous group.

Swash: Given that, one would be prepared to accept that there had been more denervation and therefore more re-innervative capacity demonstrated as a consequence. There is a limit to the re-innervative capacity of the muscle.

Stanton: But one would need to do perineal work. And is it not odd that there almost seems to be less change with prolapse?

Warrell: It did seem odd. We have now come to the conclusion that what we are looking at is the other cause of prolapse and the other cause of stress incontinence, which is support, and which may be related to different collagen as one of the major factors if not the only factor.

References

1. Francis WJA. The onset of stress incontinence. J Obstet Gynaecol Br Emp 1960; 67:899–903.

Chapter 13

Conservative Management

A. M. Shepherd

Introduction

When urinary incontinence is due to pelvic floor dysfunction or urethral sphincter incompetence conservative management involving re-education of the pelvic floor muscles is recognised by many to be one of the methods of regaining continence. The precise alteration in the normal mechanism which causes genuine stress incontinence has not been defined and thus it is difficult to understand the exact mode by which this treatment is effective. The pubococcygeus portion of the levator ani is most closely related to the urethra and the muscle fibres interdigitate, inserting into the lateral walls of the vagina. Because of their proximity to the urethra it is probable that contraction of these fibres increases urethral closure pressure as well as causing an appreciable contraction which can be felt within the vagina. Both slow- and fast-twitch muscle fibres are present giving the muscle the unusual dual role of constant postural tone provided by the slow-twitch fibres, with the fast-twitch fibres being recruited in response to a sudden increase in abdominal pressure on coughing or sneezing.

History

During the course of evolution the animal kingdom has altered its stance from the pronograde to the orthograde position. In order to adapt to the upright posture the contractility of the pelvic floor has been exchanged for tensile strength as fascial tissue has replaced muscle [1]. Hence, the primary functions of maintaining continence of urine and faeces and controlling the expulsive activities of the body in quadrupeds have been replaced in humans. Instead, the pelvic floor acts as a hammock with the important static role of supporting the pelvic organs. As with any other muscle in the body the periurethral muscles can become fatigued or damaged and can atrophy from disuse. Likewise, this is a muscle group which may be re-educated with restoration of function, either partially or completely.

Green-Armytage wrote an article in 1948 entitled "The role of physiotherapy in obstetrics and gynaecology"[2]. He mentioned that 30 years earlier Stacey-Wilson in Birmingham had advocated the use of pelvic exercises in "hyposthenic" girls showing signs of congenital prolapse, incontinence and backache. It is interesting to note that he commented on the work of his French colleagues who put as great emphasis on pelvic floor re-education then as they do now. They expected a well trained "lady" to be able to "casser une noisette" per vaginam! Arnold Kegel [3] in California was another early protagonist of conservative management of stress incontinence. He stated that between 30% and 40% of women lack any appreciable ability to contract the muscles of the pelvic floor. Also, he recognised that few parous women could stop their urinary flow in mid-stream. It was he who first developed a perineometer and used it to monitor pelvic floor contractions before and after treatment [4].

By tradition it has been the physiotherapist who, of all the professional carers, has been responsible for physical rehabilitation. Various methods of management for urinary incontinence are mentioned in reference books from the past; these include the use of baths, douches, light therapy, ionisation techniques and various forms of heat, although none of these has stood the test of time. Although antenatal and postnatal exercises were taught in the 1950s, surgery has been the first line of management for urinary incontinence for many years. Clinicians and most physiotherapists have paid only lip service to the place of pelvic floor re-education. Pioneers like Minnie Randall, Principal of the Department of Physiotherapy at St Thomas' Hospital (1911–1945) promoted the usefulness of postnatal exercises at the request of the obstetrician in charge [5] but even she did not advocate re-education for older groups of women. Few clinicians supported her progressive views and teaching in this area for both doctors and physiotherapists, was universally low key. Women themselves have never understood the function of the pelvic floor muscles nor the part they play in maintaining urinary control.

Through groups such as the Association of Chartered Physiotherapists in Obstetrics and Gynaecology and more recently the Association of Continence Advisors both physiotherapists and nurses are becoming aware of the importance of conservative management. Over the past few years it has been exciting to note the increasing interest of the medical profession. Ten years ago, at the ninth annual meeting of the International Continence Society, there was no mention of conservative management. In 1988 a whole session with 19 presentations was devoted to the topic and in 1989 there were two sessions.

Methods of Conservative Management

Conservative methods of treatment are based on electrical stimulation, exercises, or a combination of both techniques. Evaluation of these methods has been sadly lacking because of failure of objective pre- and post-treatment assessment from most studies. Despite many attempts in recent years there is no satisfactory method of measuring pelvic floor function and of monitoring progress during treatment. Even today the most practical way of assessing a contraction is by digital examination of the vagina.

Electrical Stimulation

The rationale for using electrical stimulation and producing muscle contraction as a method of treatment is fourfold. It increases the local blood supply, it is thought to break down painful adhesions formed during the healing of damaged muscle, it increases the resting tone of the muscle and, most importantly, it restores cortical awareness. This enables those patients with no voluntary control to become aware of a particular muscle or group of muscles and to train themselves to contract those muscles.

Until recently the type of current used most commonly was faradism (low-frequency alternating current) or interrupted direct current. With the latter it is possible to vary the intensity, the pulse duration and the frequency of the current. Treatment can be given using electrodes positioned externally, where at least five different methods have been described, or a vaginal electrode can be used with a large indifferent electrode placed either on the abdomen or under the sacrum. The latter method has been found to be the most effective in stimulating the pubococcygeus muscle [6] and certainly the placing of an electrode within the vagina increases the tactile awareness of these muscles through the proprioceptive nerve endings.

Though effective, this type of current has been criticised because of the discomfort which it causes. Within the last few years interferential therapy has become popular in many centres. This uses two high frequency currents which overcome epidermal resistance at a tolerable intensity. Using two cross-firing currents of slightly different frequency the resulting low frequency current may be used to stimulate the pelvic musculature [7]. Slow- and fast-twitch fibres respond to different frequencies, the former acting between 10 and 20 Hz and the latter between 30 and 50 Hz. Thus for effective stimulation the frequency used should be between 10 and 50 Hz [8].

Results of Electrical Stimulation

In 1981 Brown (personal communication) compared different forms of physiotherapy using a perineometer for objective assessment. He found that electrical stimulation alone was of no particular value. Wilson et al. [9] agreed with his results stating that the addition of interferential therapy or faradism did not appear to give any significant improvement over pelvic floor exercises alone. However, Laycock [7] comparing interferential therapy with pelvic floor exercises concluded that interferential therapy on its own was an effective treatment and she suggested that this should be the method of choice for patients unable to co-operate in an active course of pelvic floor exercises.

Patient-administered electrical stimulation using a portable vaginal device has been used in Europe for over 20 years [8]. It has never gained widespread application due to muscle fatigue, technical faults and poor patient compliance [10]. Initially stimulation was applied for up to eight hours daily but more recently the time has been limited to much shorter periods. In 1989 Bent et al. [11], reported their results, using transvaginal electrical stimulation for 15 minutes daily for six weeks in the treatment of genuine stress incontinence (GSI) and detrusor instability (DI). Of 23 women with predominant GSI 20 had 50% or greater subjective improvement but objective results were disappointing. There were no adverse effects reported but urodynamic parameters showed no consistent change and an extended follow-up was recommended to assess the long-term benefits.

Muscle Re-education

The rationale behind the re-education of muscles includes the reinforcement of cortical awareness of the muscle group, hypertrophy of the existing muscle fibres and a general increase in muscle tone and strength. The pelvic floor needs to be in a constant state of tone and to have the ability to respond immediately to any sudden increase in abdominal pressure. For a scheme of exercises to be effective it must be selected to cover both these aspects and should include simple repetitive exercises and graded resisted exercises. However, the most important ingredient is a proper understanding and the continued motivation of the patient provided by the encouragement and support of the therapist.

A Programme of Re-education

Theoretically pelvic floor re-education can be undertaken by any trained carer although it may be more practical for a physiotherapist who has had a specialised training. The following details of a method which has been found to be effective may be helpful for those wishing to set up a similar programme [12]. On average five treatment sessions are sufficient. The first session lasts for one hour and is followed by four others of 40 min duration within the next two weeks. In those five visits the bulk of remedial therapy will have been undertaken and the patient has one month on her own to consolidate the learning and technique of the pelvic floor re-education before reporting to the clinician.

Explanation

The first session starts with the therapist discussing and assessing the size of the problem with the patient. A grading system of 1 to 10 with 1 being totally wet and 10 being totally dry is convenient for this purpose. This will enable the patient to set her own goal posts. Her aim should be realistic, complete dryness is not always achieved. Few women are never wet. Inspiration and dedication are essential, she must want to help herself and realise that she is responsible for the prevention of subsequent deterioration. An anatomical description helps to set the scene before the first practical lesson.

Demonstration

Teaching active relaxation of all those adjacent muscle groups will prevent trick movements before introducing pelvic floor contractions. Concentrating on the perineal region the patient is asked to "pull up inside" or "try to stop the urine coming". By contrasting this contraction with that of the abdominal or gluteal muscles the anterior and posterior fibres of the levator ani can be brought into action. Digital examination by the therapist and by the patient herself is often the best method of assessing the function of the muscle and can be used to stimulate active contraction – "don't let me pull my fingers out".

Stimulation

If there is no flicker observed or felt then electrical stimulation is the next step. If using faradism or interrupted current the patient is asked to lie in the semi-recumbent position with two pillows under her knees. One electrode is placed in the vagina and a large, indifferent electrode and pad are applied to the abdomen. The patient is able to tolerate a greater intensity of current with the abdominal electrodes than one placed under the sacrum and there is less involvement of the gluteal muscles. The intensity should be increased until the patient is aware of the muscle contracting and then a surged current controlled by the patient is given within this range. It is common for the patient to express surprise and delight when feeling the pelvic floor tighten and she is encouraged to superimpose a voluntary contraction in time with the surge of current.

Facilitation

During the first session the content of the training programme is discussed. Bearing in mind that the periurethral muscles contain both slow- and fast-twitch fibres the exercises taught must be directed to serve both these functions. Thus for the slow-twitch fibres the emphasis needs to be on endurance and repetition. The patient should be encouraged to increase the number of contractions and to prolong the length of each contraction. When concentrating on the fast-twitch fibres the exercise is aimed at increasing the strength of the muscle. To do this the exercise should concentrate on quick contractions of greater amplitude. A programme containing both these elements is easily developed [13]. Reminders are given about the constant repetition of the pelvic floor contractions during daily chores such as washing-up, ironing, queuing in the supermarket and, best of all, while using the telephone. One of the common faults is breath-holding while putting maximum effort into the pelvic floor. This cannot be done while talking! There is little variety in the exercises involved in rehabilitating this muscle group. For the treatment to remain effective their constant use must become a way of life and thus the patient should involve them in every day activities.

Quantification

Before finishing the first session a record of vaginal pressure is made using a perineometer. Watching the gauge often brings home the problem. The muscle can be delayed in its response although a weak increase in pressure is recorded as the slow-twitch fibres contract or, more commonly, there is a quick flicker as the fast-twitch fibres come into action but this cannot be maintained. What is required is a constant state of tone as well as a reflex increase in pressure on sudden increase in abdominal pressure.

As with the rehabilitation of any other muscle group, the patient is usually aware of aches and stiffness after such prolonged effort. The following sessions consolidate the information which has been learnt at the first attendance. Some evidence of improvement is expected immediately and if none is recorded by the third occasion there is little hope of success.

Trials of Pelvic Floor Re-education

When comparing the results of any trials of treatment both subjective and objective findings need consideration. In many therapeutic studies complete cure is not possible and to be successful it is the patient who must be satisfied. Thus it is with conservative management. Complete objective dryness is not always demonstrable and urodynamic parameters are seldom altered.

The success rate of pelvic floor re-education has been reported to vary between 60% and 90% in different trials. In a study of 54 women treated by pelvic floor exercises alone 90% were still satisfied with the results two years later [14]. An interesting presentation by Klarskov et al. [15] compared physiotherapy with surgery. This was a controlled study and showed that after 4–12 months the results of surgery were superior to pelvic floor re-education but that surgery could be avoided in one-third of cases. In 1989 [16] he reported a long-term follow-up of these patients using a questionnaire, a pad weighing test and a urinary diary in his assessment. He found that 80% of those patients who had received pelvic floor training still used the programme at least once a week. He concluded that the long-term results of re-education and surgery were essentially the same as they were after 4–12 months adding that patients with significant incontinence adapt to the situation by altering their lifestyle.

Henella et al. [17] reported the results of two groups of comparable women treated in two different hospitals. Of a total of 58 patients the overall success rate was 67% at a follow-up undertaken three months after treatment; this fell to 50% twelve months later. In contrast to this in 1989 Tapp et al. [18] published the results of a randomised trial comparing pelvic floor physiotherapy with the Burch colposuspension. Of three groups of women one had pelvic floor exercises alone (PFE), one had pelvic floor exercises with faradism (PFE+F) and the third group had a Burch colposuspension (BC). The women all had GSI proven on videocystometry and were randomly allocated to the three treatment groups. At the 6 month assessment of the PFE group 2/21 were cured, 7/21 were symptomatically improved and 12 requested surgery. Of the PFE+F group 2/23 were cured, 8–23 were symptomatically better and 13 requested surgery. Those who had a BC fared very much better with 18/24 having an objective cure and 23/24 noting an improvement. The authors concluded that physiotherapy compares poorly with surgery and pointed out that this method is time consuming for both patient and hospital staff.

Principles Involved in Management

These disappointing results bring into question a number of principles involved in the successful use of conservative management. First it is essential that the instructor, be they physiotherapist, nurse or doctor, has an intimate knowledge of the subject. They must be able to explain the problem in simple terms and describe the method of treatment. Although a one to one relationship is usual group therapy has been described and can be successful. They must have confidence in their techniques and be able to impart their knowledge with enthusiasm. Second, the patient must have been properly assessed prior to the selection of treatment. Although other types of incontinence will respond to these methods it is the patient who has been found to have troublesome but not severe urinary leakage due to urethral sphincter incompetence and poor function of the peri-urethral muscles who responds best. More scientific quantification has been difficult to produce but Tapp et al. [19] suggested that good results were obtained in premenopausal women who only had a short duration of symptoms and who had a maximum urethral closure pressure of above 9.4 cmH$_2$O. Third, and most importantly, it is the long-term motivation of the patient which produces satisfactory results.

Probably the best management is to combine the modalities of electrical stimulation and pelvic floor re-education. Other workers agree with Kegal that about 30% of parous women do not have the ability to control their perineal muscles. Other than being used for sexual purposes or to stop the flow of urine this muscle group is not used consciously. Trick movements are legion and patients will contract their glutei, their abdominal muscles, their adductors and even hold their breath believing themselves to be using their pelvic floor. Bearing down instead of pulling up is another common mistake. For these women active exercises are without value until such a time as cortical awareness is restored – thus electrical stimulation in the absence of a spontaneous contraction should be used prior to a programme of progressive resisted exercises.

Adjuncts to Pelvic Floor Re-education

The Perineometer

In 1949 Kegel [4] described a pneumatic device for measuring vaginal pressure. He used this both as a method of assessment and to encourage progress during exercises. Since his early description many attempts have been made to produce an effective perineometer. To be effective such a device needs to be cheap, reliable in recording vaginal pressure, robust and acceptable to the patient. Three prototypes were described in 1983 [20] but, despite a proven need, none of these have been marketed. The Bourne Perineometer (Fig.13.1) fills many of the requirements but is expensive. It has the persisting problem that it is not possible to exclude trick movements due to an increase in intra-abdominal pressure. If a cheaper version were available patients could use the device at home in a programme of resisted exercises increasing the strength and duration of the contractions.

Recent advances in the development of a perineometer have included more

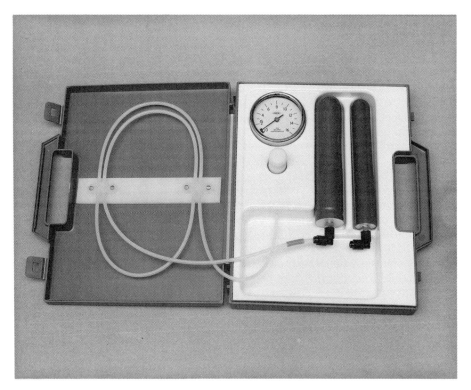

Fig 13.1. The Bourne perineometer: a simple and robust piece of equipment suitable for assessment of pelvic floor function and as a progressive resistance during exercise.

and more lavish equipment. Some incorporate vaginal and abdominal electrodes with a series of flashing lights, some use a vaginal probe with abdominal electrodes. The designs are elaborate and expensive but there is no doubt that they fill a need and help to maintain motivation. However, without proper explanation they are useless and all physiotherapists and continence advisers have experienced the frustrated enthusiast who contacts the department because they are unable to use the equipment effectively on their own.

Vaginal Cones

The most innovative technique in pelvic floor re-education is the use of vaginal cones introduced by Plevnik [21]. Stanton et al. first described their clinical application in 1986 [22] and in 1988 Peattie and Plevnik [23] found an 80% subjective and 60% objective improvement rate. She compared cones with physiotherapy and concluded that fewer patients who had had cone therapy needed subsequent surgery and that the time involved in conventional physiotherapy was three times that required to teach and use cones. Also in 1988 Bridges et al. [24] compared the use of cones to interferential therapy and came to the same conclusion – that they were time-saving and effective.

Current Physiotherapy Practice

Undoubtedly there is a place for the conservative management of genuine stress incontinence. A survey of all the English Health Authorities completed in 1989 [25] gives some idea of the type of treatments currently in practice. A 98.4% response rate showed the interest of the physiotherapists who were involved in returning the questionnaire. The data showed that gynaecologists are six times more likely to send patients to the physiotherapy department than urologists. Urologists rarely refer but it may be that they use their Continence Advisors more readily. When asked to rank the importance of physiotherapy in the management of incontinence the majority saw it as a first line of treatment. Of those physiotherapists involved in treatment 62% had made it their sub-specialty and 57% were of senior grade.

All physiotherapy departments offered pelvic floor exercises and 93% had interferential therapy available. Only 26% used a perineometer but 16% had access to vaginal cones. For a technique which has only been advocated during the past two years this suggests the possibility of wide application in future. Those completing the questionnaire considered pelvic floor re-education to be 72% effective with interferential therapy being rated as 63% effective. Only 18% of responders gave their views on vaginal cones rating them as 59% successful. On the negative side, a poor prognosis was anticipated from patients who were obese, who had had previous surgery, whose symptoms had been long-lasting or who had a prolapse. Lack of motivation was also quoted as a bad sign. Alternatively positive motivation and recent onset of symptoms were considered to herald an optimistic outcome. A similar survey into the practice of the continence advisors needs to be undertaken. Pelvic floor re-education constitutes a large part of their work load. Other professional carers who should be in the forefront of prevention and management are the midwives and health visitors. Their curriculum needs reviewing to ensure that this aspect is addressed properly.

Therapeutic Assessment

There are no specifications for patient selection or for therapeutic practice. Despite considerable attempts to select those women who would respond best it seems that there are no absolute subjective or objective criteria and these will be difficult to achieve. However, pre- and post-treatment assessment is essential to measure the success of treatment. For this purpose a subjective questionnaire, a standardised pad test and a reliable method of assessing pelvic floor contraction are required. For more accurate quantification, measurement of urethral closure pressure or of the position of the bladder neck and proximal urethra within the abdominal cavity would be ideal. The former can only be undertaken by invasive investigation but both the increment in urethral pressure due to pelvic muscle contraction and changes in urethral electric conductance should be considered. Alteration in the position of the bladder neck during pelvic floor contraction can be visualised readily on ultrasound and it may be that this technique can be further developed.

The Need for Standardisation

For methods of treatment to be compared there must be definitions of the types of electrical stimulation and the content of re-education programmes. So many variables exist in management and patient response that standardisation of nomenclature and techniques needs to be addressed urgently. Only then can the results of trials be interpreted usefully and the best techniques applied to each individual. So far the one factor which emerges regardless of patient selection or the type of therapy is motivation. In the long term conservative management will be found to complement and supplement all the other recognized ways of treating genuine stress incontinence.

References

1. Wilson PM. Understanding the pelvic floor. S Afr Med J 1973; 7:1150–67.
2. Green-Armytage VB. The role of physiotherapy in obstetrics and gynaecology. J Obstet Gynaecol Br Emp 1948; 52:21–3.
3. Kegel AH. The physiologic treatment of tone and function of the genital muscles and of urinary incontinence. West J Surg 1949; 57:527–35.
4. Kegel AH. Progressive resistance exercises in functional restoration of the perineal muscles. Am J Obstet Gynecol 1949; 56:238–48.
5. Fairbairn JS. Changes in thought in a half century of obstetrics. Obstetrics 1934; 2:63–77.
6. Scott BD, Green J, Couldrey BM. Pelvic faradism. Investigation of methods. Physiotherapy 1969; 50:302–5.
7. Laycock J, Green RJ. Interferential therapy in the treatment of incontinence. Physiotherapy 1988; 74(4):161–8.
8. Fall M, Ahlstrom K, Carlsson CA, Ek A, Erlandson BE, Frankenberg S, Mattiasson A. Pelvic floor stimulation of female stress incontinence. Urology 1986; 27(3):282–7.
9. Wilson PD, Al Samarral T, Deakin M, Kolbe E, Brown A. The value of physiotherapy in female genuine stress incontinence. Proceedings of the fourteenth annual meeting of the International Continence Society, Innsbruck, Austria, 1984; 156–7.
10. Shepherd AM, Blannin JP, Winder A. The English experience of intravaginal electrical stimulation. Proceedings of the fourteenth annual meeting of the International Continence Society, Innsbruck, Austria, 1984; 224–5.
11. Bent AE, Sand PK, Ostergard DR. Transvaginal electrical stimulation in the treatment of genuine stress incontinence and detrusor instability. Proceedings of the nineteenth annual meeting of the Continence Society, Ljubljana, Yugoslavia. Neurourol Urodynam 1989; 8: 363–4.
12. Perkins J, Shepherd AM. The pelvic floor saga. J Assoc Chartered Physiotherapists Obstet Gynaecol 1987; 61:15–17.
13. Laycock J. Graded exercises for the pelvic floor muscles in the treatment of urinary incontinence. Physiotherapy 1987; 63:371–3.
14. Shepherd AM, Montgomery E. Electrical stimulation and graded pelvic exercises for genuine stress incontinence. Physiotherapy 1983; 69:112.
15. Klarskov P, Belving D, Bischoff N et al. Pelvic floor exercises versus surgery for female urinary stress incontinence. Proceedings of the fourteenth annual meeting of the International Continence Society, Innsbruck, Austria, 1984; 159–61.
16. Klarskov P, Kroyer K, Kromann, Maegaard E. Long term results of pelvic floor training and surgery for female genuine stress incontinence. Proceedings of the nineteenth annual meeting of the International Continence Society, Ljubljana, Yugoslavia. Neurourol Urodynam 1989; 8:357–8.
17. Henella SM, Hutchins CJ, Breeson AJ. Treatment of female genuine stress incontinence with pelvic floor re-education in two different hospitals. Proceedings of the eighteenth annual meeting of the International Continence Society, Oslo, Norway. Neurourol Urodynam 1988; 7:262–3.

18. Tapp AJS, Hills B, Cardozo LD. Randomised study comparing pelvic floor physiotherapy with the Burch colposuspension. Proceedings of the nineteenth annual meeting of the International Continence Society Ljubljana, Yugoslavia. Neurourol Urodynam 1989; 8:356–7.
19. Tapp AJS, Cardozo L, Hills B, Barnick C. Who benefits from physiotherapy? Proceedings of the eighteenth annual meeting of the International Continence Society, Oslo, Norway. Neurourol Urodynam 1988; 7:259–61.
20. Shepherd AM, Montgomery E, Anderson RS. A pilot study of a pelvic floor exerciser in women with stress incontinence. J Obs & Gynae 1983; 3:201–02.
21. Plevnik S. New method for testing and strengthening of pelvic floor muscles. Proceedings of the fifteenth annual meeting of the International Continence Society, London, 1985; 267–8.
22. Stanton S, Plevnik S, Peattie A. Cones: a conservative method of treating genuine stress incontinence. Proceedings of the sixteenth annual meeting of the International Continence Society, Boston, USA, 1986; 227–8.
23. Peattie AB, Plevnik S. Cones versus physiotherapy in conservative management of genuine stress incontinence. Proceedings of the eighteenth annual meeting of the International Continence Society, Oslo, Norway. Neurourol Urodynam 1988; 7:265–6.
24. Bridges N, Denning J, Olah RS, Farrar OJ. A prospective trial comparing interferential therapy and treatment using cones in patients with symptoms of stress incontinence. Proceedings of the eighteenth annual meeting of the International Continence Society, Oslo, Norway. Neurourol Urodynam 1988; 7:267–8.
25. Mantle MJ, Versi E. English physiotherapeutic practice; stress incontinence. Proceedings of the nineteenth annual meeting of the International Continence Society, Ljubljana, Yugoslavia. Neurourol Urodynam 1989; 8:352–3.

Discussion

Stanton: One of the snags about physiotherapy is that while certainly one offers it in patients who want it and do not want surgery, or want to complete their childbearing, or who are physically not fit for surgery, it has to be stated that the physiotherapy has to be continued for life, and that is often forgotten in weighing surgery and physiotherapy in the balance.

Second, I should like comments as to whether there is an upper age limit for physiotherapy and what patients are told in terms of how long the therapy has to continue. I always have in my mind the picture of an athlete who really, if she wants to get into reasonable shape and use muscles which she has not used for a while, has to consider upwards of an hour a day for three months, if not six months, before effect is shown.

Shepherd: I do not think there is any upper age limit. If the woman has the motivation she will learn to use her pelvic floor muscles and will probably get satisfactory results. We know certainly of a number of women in their late 70s and 80s who have had very satisfactory results.

Stanton: If I might respectfully mention, one needs hard data and I have not found any hard data in the literature to support this objectively. That has been my difficulty when I have referred patients for physiotherapy.

Shepherd: There are very few hard data. I am just talking from our experience. Certainly we do not have any upper age limit beyond which we would restrict treatment.

We have always found that perhaps one of the most important things is that this has to be a way of life and it is something that the woman must be aware of for ever. During the retraining programme we recommend that patients do this every hour, but more particularly that they associate it with certain features of their daily living; in other words they should do their pelvic floor exercises whilst they are standing in queues, whilst they are doing their ironing, and particularly whilst they are talking on the telephone. One of the most important aspects of pelvic floor re-education is the trick movements which go along with it, and we find that women are tightening their abdominal muscles, they are tightening their gluteal muscles and abductors, and they are holding their breath. But if they try to do their exercises while they are on the telephone they cannot hold their breath. It is not an exercise; it is a way of life. And this should be perpetuated.

Cardozo: This is a problem because there are no hard data on the elderly and physiotherapy and its actual objective cure rates as well as its subjective cure rates, and no one has addressed the issue of how long physiotherapy needs to be continued – whether duration of individual sessions or duration of management altogether.

One thing that we tried to show, which perhaps did not come over very well, is not that physiotherapy should not be used, but that women should not be led to expect that they will be completely cured by this treatment. It should perhaps be used as an adjunct to other treatments – surgery, drugs, oestrogens, and so on – and not be set up as a method of cure for all in stress incontinence. Women probably need to be counselled appropriately before treatment: this may improve them but they have to continue it long term, and if it does improve them it is unlikely to cure their problem completely.

Versi: There are no hard data and the nearest that we have available is a survey that we carried out where we had almost 100% response and we asked specific questions about prognostic features. In answer to the question about age, a number of physiotherapists did respond that age was important, and specifically they pointed to the menopause. They felt that after the menopause patients were unlikely to accrue so much benefit.

We also asked about pelvic floor exercise regimens and the mean response was that they should carry out a contraction for 5 s, have eight contractions per session, and practise every hour during the retraining period.

The feeling was that if a patient is to have physiotherapy, it is for life. It is a change of habit. It is like dieting. One should not go on a crash diet but should adopt and maintain a different lifestyle.

But the issue that was most prominent was that of motivation. If we are to look for predictor variables in patients who are likely to succeed with physiotherapy, we need to try to assess motivation. We need some objective and reproducible method of assessing it so that we can pick out those who will benefit.

Shepherd: I agree absolutely.

DeLancey: The underlying question that many of us think about with physiotherapy is what does it do to the continence mechanism? That may lead us to be able to say will this individual improve? If, for example, the patient has had a completely denervated muscle there is no way for them to improve. If it is a patient in whom the connection between the muscle and the urethral supportive tissues has been lost, they can improve the strength of the muscle but that will not have an influence on urethral support. It would be then the person who has a weak muscle, in whom there is perhaps some innervation but not perfect innervation and who can improve the performance of that muscle, who would be the one to benefit.

I was intrigued by the suggestion that by putting a speculum into the vagina and stretching the levator ani one can see a change in the resting pressure. It may be that these individuals in whom the connections are there, and who when the levator ani is stretched have a decrease in pressure, would be the people in whom if we could improve their pelvic floor function, that would then translate into better increases in intraurethral pressure during a cough.

I am curious as to whether the cough reflex may be lost in some of these individuals. There is wilful contraction; there is resting tone, that is non-wilful contraction of the pelvic floor; and there is that increase, as I understand it, that happens at the time of a cough that is a contraction in the levator ani muscle and that can be seen on anorectal manometry. Maybe we should separate out those three: what is wilful contraction? what is resting tone? and what is cough reflex? That may be a way of being able to predict who will respond.

Swash: There is a corollary to that, that is whether there is any sensory disturbance. This is something that struck us as being important in anorectal incontinence, although I do not hear much mention of it in stress urinary incontinence. And yet there must be a sensory disturbance if there is some damage to the nerve, which after all is a mixed nerve.

Swash: One of the ways in which physiotherapy might work might be simply to increase sensory awareness of the contiguity of sensory structures by the lining of the vagina and the sensory receptors in the urethra.

Cardozo: This is very possible.

Shepherd: And this is perhaps why using a vaginal electrode may be one of the most satisfactory methods of using electrical stimulation, because it is tactile.

Swash: I do think, if I may say so, that this sort of treatment requires extremely rigorous methods of objective assessment. Otherwise it degenerates into the sort of folklore that appears on "The Saturday Page" in *The Times*, and either one believes in it – people actually say, "I believe in this sort of treatment" – or one does not. We are not interested in belief. We are interested in facts.

Cardozo: We are very much aware of this need for objective assessment.

Swash: What we need now is to devise some appropriate tests, and I should have thought the appropriate test would be some measure of urethral function, such as measuring the pressure generated in bladder–vaginal contraction. And I would have thought sensory threshold was important as well.

Cardozo: There has been a major change in this area in the last five years. Prior to that there were no scientific data on non-surgical intervention for genuine stress incontinence. Within the last five years there have been increasing data with both subjective and objective evidence of cure, improvement and so on. But it still needs to go much further and terminology needs to be sorted out.

Sutherst: One of my questions was about objective measurement and there are methods arising. One of them, I would suggest, is the simple pad test which can be applicable to physiotherapy before and after treatment, which is a fundamental investigation of how wet people are before and afterwards.

Shepherd: But that is an assessment for any sort of treatment.

Sutherst: Yes, but it would be useful in physiotherapy departments that did not have access to urodynamic testing.
   Standardisation was mentioned. There must be a lot of variation between departments on what faradism is and what electrical stimulation is. Is it realistic to talk about standardised treatment in physiotherapy and is it even necessary?

Shepherd: The only reason for it being necessary is if we compare our results. We cannot say how effective things are if there are no basic definitions.

Cardozo: It is like saying, "Does it matter whether your colposuspension is the same as my colposuspension?"

Swash: No it is not. One has to know that the muscles are actually contracting in the way one says that they are contracting.

Cardozo: It is desperately important to know what the physiotherapy is.

Swash: And when they are using different sorts of electrical stimulations, some of them none too well described anyway, one really has to know that the muscles are contracting to a certain degree. The force of the contraction that is occurring has to be measured, the impedance across the tissue, and so on. And there are several objective measurements of the treatment itself that are required as well as knowing the result. It is a very important point.

Sutherst: Are the physiotherapy departments across the country likely to standardise their programmes?

Shepherd: No, not in therapeutic practice. But if they are undertaking research they will need to.

Cardozo: Mr Versi's look into this has shown the differences in practice that arise around the country.

Versi: With interferential therapy, which is offered by over 90% of places in the UK, we had 60 different treatment regimens offered, which is ridiculous. And one-third of the respondents used two electrodes only, not four. I cannot understand how two electrodes can work for interferential therapy because the basic premise is that two currents interact. Two electrodes will not produce two currents that interact, so it makes no sense.

Andersson: What is the current status of pharmacotherapy in treatment of genuine stress incontinence? I am thinking specifically of the α-adrenoceptor agonists as an adjunct to physiotherapy or as a treatment per se.

Cardozo: Is anyone actually using them?

Stanton: I have had a patient or two on them but the Ministry of Health will not now allow us to prescribe phenylpropanolamine (PPA).

Hilton: We used it in conjunction with both vaginal and oral oestrogens, in a group of women with GSI and did not find very convincing objective evidence of urodynamic changes aside from a reduction in urine leakage on pad tests, which was highly significant in those who were treated with vaginal oestrogens plus PPA. In previous studies using midodrine (rather than PPA) alone in women of all ages, we did not find any objective changes at all. But I have used PPA along with oestrogen in some postmenopausal women.

DeLancey: We have been using oestrogen in combination with imipramine, which as an α-like effect. In the postmenopausal woman with atrophy and with good support it seems to work very well. In the younger woman who does not have atrophy and who has a lot of mobility it does not seem to work at all.

We have data on 11 patients but not a big enough series to be conclusive.

Cardozo: It requires further evaluation. But I do not think the majority of people are using the alpha drugs for genuine stress incontinence any more.

Andersson: I know of no long-term studies. How long should treatment be continued and is an initial good response maintained?

Cardozo: If there was any evidence of good results there would be more studies and more long-term studies available. And so the answer to the question is that it is not a very effective form of treatment.

Warrell: Whether physiotherapy will work may well reflect on the integrity of the connections between the pelvic floor and the urethra. When a woman with normal urinary control contracts her pelvic floor we can see the urethral occlusive forces shoot up and this cannot be seen in women who have stress incontinence.

But why should a woman be unable to contract her pelvic floor? Although these women no doubt have nerve-damaged pelvic floors it cannot be nerve damage alone because that would be a completely paralysed muscle. And it is very evident that these are not completely paralysed muscles. Why cannot someone contract her pelvic floor given time, electrical stimulation, and any other relevant stimulus? What is happening neurophysiologically?

Shepherd: This is not very scientific but I would suggest that if any muscle group is not used for a certain length of time, the cortex becomes alienated from that muscle group. If I may draw a parallel with a footballer who has had a meniscectomy: he goes into hospital with a perfectly healthy quadriceps muscle and the next day he simply cannot contract that muscle group because he is afraid of the pain, and there is some sort of inhibition due to the pain factor. It may be that something similar happens at the time of delivery, there is pain from an episiotomy, or a tear, or something that involves stitches, and the woman does not want to contract that muscle group, and if that continues for a long time her cortex becomes alienated from that group, and it is not until cortical awareness is restored by electrical stimulation that she gets a contraction.

Warrell: There are some women who never get that.

Shepherd: Yes.

Cardozo: But it may be even longer term than that. It may be like people who can abduct and adduct their great and little toes. Maybe it is developmentally something that some people are better and some people are less well able to do.

Stanton: Women do not have to contract their pelvic floor. They do not stand and stop and start, except for one group.

I wonder if the fact that Western women do not have to worry about stopping and starting their stream is a factor, whereas men are in a very different category.

Warrell: Can one walk without contracting the pelvic floor?

DeLancey: It is contracted all the time.

Cardozo: But not that extra voluntary contraction. It is resting contraction.

Chapter 14

Which Operation and for Which Patient?

P. Hilton

Introduction

The earliest documented surgical approach to the problem of stress incontinence was that of Baker-Brown [1] in 1864, and since his description of suprapubic cystostomy procedure over 150 different operations have been devised for the treatment of this condition. Views regarding the pathophysiology of genuine stress incontinence have evolved considerably in this time, and much has been said of this in earlier chapters. Nevertheless, the large number of operations available reflects our continuing uncertainties over this condition and the likely mechanism of its cure, and also the inadequacy of any current procedure to deal satisfactorily with all cases.

The aims of incontinence surgery have been variously described as: tightening of the pubocervical fascia; elevation of the bladder neck; restoration of the posterior urethrovesical angle; increasing urethral pressure; increasing functional urethral length; and increasing urethral resistance. There is, however, little information as to the extent to which these aims are achieved by the various operative techniques. Cure rates between 30% [2] and 100% [3] have been reported, but what aspects of the procedures, or of urethral function, determine success or failure are still only poorly understood.

Clearly it would be impossible to deal with all operations within this paper, and rather I would hope to cover the basic philosophies of the selection of patients for surgical treatment, and the selection of the most appropriate operative technique for any individual patient. As regards the first of these questions, the decision as to which patients should undergo surgery, this would seem to depend on a number of secondary considerations: which patients are least likely to respond to other, more conservative treatments? which are most likely to respond to surgery? and which are least likely to develop complications from surgery? The decision as to the most appropriate operative technique for any individual patient is in turn dependent on the clinical and urodynamic status of the patient, and on the impact of individual procedures – not simply in terms of success rate, but also how they achieve continence, and what effect they may have on voiding function.

Which Patients Should Undergo Surgical Treatment?

Which Patients Are Least Likely to Respond to Conservative Treatment?

The most widely accepted form of conservative treatment for genuine stress incontinence (Chapter 13) is that of pelvic floor exercise. Many studies have attested to the success of physiotherapeutic management [4–17] although whilst "cure and improvement" rates of between 42% and 78% have been reported, cures average less than 20%. Patient motivation and continuing reinforcement appear to be vital factors to success. Wilson et al. [8] and Bo et al. [17] both compared the success of pelvic floor exercise carried out by the patient at home after preliminary instruction from a physiotherapist, with an intensive, hospital-based regimen; both found substantially more responders in the latter groups.

Wilson et al. [8] also attempted to identify patient-related factors which were predictive of successful treatment. Age, severity of leakage, and previous unsuccessful incontinence operations were found to be of positive predictive value, younger women, with mild incontinence, and without previous surgery being the most likely to respond. In a similar study reported by Sandri et al. [10] these factors were not found to be predictive, and neither group found parity, weight, or initial perineometry readings to be of any value. In an objective study comparing both clinical and urodynamic factors in patients cured by physiotherapy with those with persisting evidence of incontinence, Tapp et al. [11] found that premenopausal women with a shorter duration of symptoms were most likely to be cured; they also developed a method of selection for physiotherapy based on a visual analogue symptom-score and parameters of the urethral stress profile which allowed the identification of all patients likely to respond to exercise, with the exclusion of many of those who would not be cured from unnecessary and time-consuming therapy. Mayne and Hilton [9], however, were unable to confirm any variable from resting or stress urethral pressure profiles, or from urethral electrical conductance profiles to have any predictive value of either cure or improvement with physiotherapy.

Such data as exists therefore are unconvincing, but it would seem that those parameters that have ever been shown to be of predictive value point simply to the identification of those patients with the least severe symptoms as being those most likely to be cured or improved by pelvic floor exercise; such patients are of course also those most likely to benefit from surgery. Since patient motivation is clearly a vital factor in success from physiotherapy, it would seem appropriate to offer this form of treatment to all patients keen to avoid surgery.

Which Patients Are Most Likely to Respond to Surgery?

Surgery in Detrusor Instability

Since the clinical significance of uninhibited detrusor activity was recognised by Hodgkinson et al. [18] in 1963, it has become accepted wisdom that the identification of detrusor instability in an incontinent woman should contraindicate conventional bladder neck surgery. Stanton et al. [19] reported their results from colposuspension in a group of 60 women with stress incontinence of both "detrusor stable" and "detrusor unstable" types. They found an objective cure rate of only 43% in those with detrusor instability, compared with 85% in those with genuine stress incontinence.

More recently several authors have re-addressed this question [20–25] reporting subjective cure rates of around 80%, and objective cures in approximately 60% of patients with suprapubic procedures, although only 30% from vaginal repair [20]. Meyhoff et al. [21] and Lockhart et al. [22] both reported significantly poorer results in patients showing spontaneous or high pressure detrusor contractions, but obtained subjective results in those with low detrusor pressures or contractions only on provocation which were comparable with those in genuine stress incontinence.

Certainly there is now sufficient evidence that we should review our traditional beliefs, and not consider detrusor instability to be the absolute contraindication to bladder neck surgery that it has previously been held. Those patients with detrusor instability, or combined genuine stress incontinence and instability, for whom the symptom of stress incontinence is a major element of their complaint, and who have failed to respond to conventional treatment by way of pharmacotherapy or behaviour modification techniques, may certainly be offered surgery with a reasonable prospect of success, provided they accept that it is aimed at the relief of incontinence, and that they may have residual frequency and urgency postoperatively.

The Significance of Urethral Pressure

McGuire [26] in 1981, reporting on the urodynamic findings following unsuccessful incontinence surgery found that a "low pressure urethra", by which he meant a maximum urethral closure pressure (MUCP) less than $20\,cmH_2O$, was present in 75% of patients who had undergone multiple failed operations, compared to only 13% of those with primary incontinence. In the same year I presented urethral pressure data from a group of 120 women with genuine stress incontinence [27] and found the MUCP and functional urethral length (FUL) to be inversely related to the number of previous failed procedures (Fig. 14.1). Several studies have now shown that patients suffering unsuccessful surgery by colposuspension [28], suburethral sling [29,30], anterior colporrhaphy [31]; Stamey [30,32] and Marshall–Marchetti–Krantz [33,34] procedures have lower preoperative MUCP and FUL than those treated successfully (Fig. 14.2). However, none of these studies identified any particular value for these variables which made failure inevitable or success assured.

In 1987, Sand et al. [35] described a group of 86 women undergoing colposuspension; patients with a preoperative MUCP less than $20\,cmH_2O$ were three times more likely to have an unsatisfactory outcome (54% compared to 18%). The same group [36], in 1989, reported a study of 21 women with failed colposuspension and 21 matched controls; the results were similar, confirming the poor prognosis associated with low MUCP (80% failures in the low urethral pressure group compared to 23% failures in those with MUCP greater than $20\,cmH_2O$). In response to the paper from Bowen et al. [36] I reviewed our own urethral pressure data in relation to patients undergoing Stamey procedure [32]. Only 30% of failures

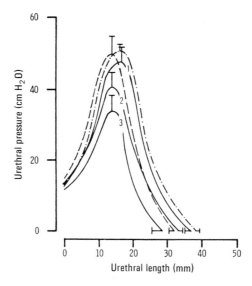

Fig. 14.1. Average resting urethral pressure profiles in a group of 120 stress incontinent women, categorised according to previous surgical history. – · – ·, no pelvic surgery; ——, 1, 2, 3 or more previous operations for continence; – – –, previous pelvic surgery other than for continence. From Hilton and Stanton [149] with permission of the authors and publisher.

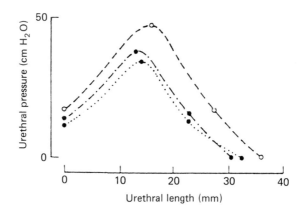

Fig. 14.2. Average preoperative resting urethral pressure profiles in a group of 100 women treated by Stamey procedure, categorised according to outcome. O, cures; ● – · – · – ●, eventual failure; ● · · · · ●, immediate failure. From Hilton and Mayne [32].

had a preoperative MUCP less than 20 cmH$_2$O compared to 22% of those successfully treated; the long-term cure rate in those with a preoperative MUCP less than 20 cmH$_2$O was not significantly different from those with higher values (52% compared to 63%).

Whilst there is good evidence that a low urethral pressure mitigates against successful surgical treatment, I think the case for 20 cmH$_2$O as an absolute cut-off value remains unproven. Whilst the data from the American group in relation to colposuspension is convincing, the position with regard to other procedures is less clear.

Which Patients Are Most Likely to Develop Complications?

Postoperative Voiding Dysfunction

Delay in resumption of spontaneous micturition, and voiding dysfunction in the long term, are known complications of surgery for urinary incontinence [37,38]. Between 12% [39] and 25% [40] of patients treated by colposuspension are reported to suffer delayed voiding, and between 11% [39] and 20% [40] have increased residual volumes and reduced flow rates at three months postoperatively; what is more, there seems to be only limited overlap between these two groups. Whilst there are clearly important surgical influences in this regard which will be considered later, many of these problems can be predicted on the basis of preoperative urodynamic assessment. Schmidt [41] emphasises the pivotal influence of the sphincter muscles on the bladder, and views detrusor function as the natural consequence of neuromuscular reflexes controlling the pelvic floor. An acontractile bladder, therefore, he sees as being almost always due to failure of sphincter relaxation. Infrequent micturition because of prolonged suppression of the urge to void leads to overstretching of the detrusor muscle, and a large thin-walled bladder in middle or old age may result. In this situation the altered dynamics of voiding may not be readily demonstrable, as, typically, such patients void by straining rather than by co-ordinated sphincter relaxation.

Rud et al. [42] investigated the initiation of voiding in normal and stress incontinent women and found a high incidence of abnormal voiding patterns. Whilst all continent women initiated micturition by a reduction in urethral pressure followed by an increase in bladder pressure, 20% of stress incontinent women voided by a reduction in urethral pressure alone, 40% voided by Valsalva manoeuvre, and only 40% appeared to use the normal voiding mechanism. Bhatia and Bergman [43] found a very similar distribution of abnormal voiding patterns among 30 women treated by colposuspension; they also found that in those voiding by Valsalva the duration of postoperative catheterisation was approximately doubled. In a later study [44] the same authors reported that patients with a poor preoperative voiding pressure had an increased likelihood of delayed voiding, and those who in addition had a low flow rate all required catheterisation for more than seven days. Lose et al. [40] confirmed the predictive value of voiding pressure in terms of immediate postoperative voiding difficulty, but found preoperative urethral resistance, calculated as:

$$detrusor\ pressure\ at\ maximum\ flow/maximum\ flow^2$$

to be a more reliable predictor of long-term problems. In 1979, Coolsaet [45] pointed out that many patients voiding with little or no increase in detrusor pressure may in fact have a perfectly adequate detrusor contraction; since the bladder is contracting against relatively little urethral resistance, minimal pressure is generated. As a consequence he advocated the use of the height of the isometric detrusor contraction on interruption of micturition (P_{stop}) as a more reliable predictor of postoperative voiding difficulties, and my own experience would certainly accord with this.

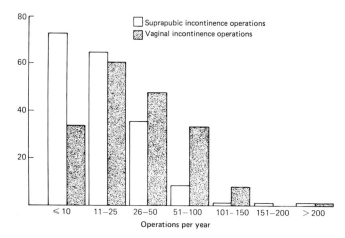

Fig. 14.3. Frequency distribution of workload with respect to suprapubic and vaginal incontinence surgery, among 186 gynaecologists in the British Isles with a special interest in gynaecological urology. From Hilton [46].

In summary, therefore, it would seem that preoperative urodynamic evaluation is important in the prediction of postoperative voiding difficulties. The most reliable predictive parameters remain in debate, although cystometric bladder capacity, maximum voiding pressure (detrusor pressure at maximum flow), maximum flow rate, urethral resistance, and isometric detrusor pressure should all be considered. Perhaps the "diagnostic parameters" P_o and v_{max} described in Chapter 5 may prove of benefit in this respect in future.

Which Operation is Appropriate for a Given Patient?

The traditional gynaecological approach to incontinence surgery has been to perform the operation most suited to the surgeon, rather than that most appropriate for the patient. "Do a vaginal repair first, and if that fails go above" is a philosophy which persists to a considerable extent, in the British Isles at least. In a recent survey of all Members and Fellows of the Royal College of Obstetricians and Gynaecologists [46] responses were obtained from 67% of Consultants and Senior Registrars. Of these, 186 individuals described themselves as having a major special interest in gynaecological urology, and even they estimated that they undertook twice as many vaginal as suprapubic incontinence operations. Most undertook between one and four vaginal procedures, but less than one suprapubic procedure per month (Fig. 14.3). Clearly this philosophy needs re-evaluation.

What Are the Effects of Any Given Operation?

Success Rates

Many studies appear in the literature each year purporting to describe the results of one or more different incontinence operations. Unfortunately the methods used, and the outcome measures applied vary widely. Authors differ in their view as to whether absolute continence, near continence, or simply any improvement in symptoms, constitute satisfactory outcome. Many studies report evaluation on only a proportion of those recruited. Methods of evaluation vary from the assumption of cure in patients who do not return for further treatment, to the use of postal questionnaires, to the use of urodynamic tools which may demonstrate alteration in lower urinary tract function, but do not necessarily distinguish cure or failure (e.g. urethral pressure profilometry), to full urodynamic investigation. The International Continence Society [47] has recommended that all studies should include some objective evaluation and quantification of urine loss preferably by perineal pad testing, before and after treatment.

Anterior colporrhaphy. Many of those studies describing the effects of vaginal incontinence surgery have been lacking in objective assessment; those that have, however, been evaluated in this way report cure rates between 30% and 70% [2,31,48–54]. It is well to point out that these studies as far as one can tell included all patients with stress incontinence. Warrell, in carefully selected cases obtained a three year cure rate of 80% [55]. In the studies by Green [56] only patients with what he describes as type I stress incontinence were treated, with a much improved cure rate of 90%. Similarly, the paper from Walter et al. [57] involving a selected group having the radiological appearance of a posterior suspension defect [58], reported a cure rate of 84%.

Colposuspension. Results reported from suprapubic procedures in general are more often supported by objective evaluation. Cure rates from colposuspension vary from 70% to 100% [28,40,57,59–71]. Results in patients with primary incontinence are significantly better than those with previous unsuccessful surgery; Stanton et al. reported cure rates of 96% and 77% respectively at 12 months [62] and 86% and 67% respectively at five years [63] following surgery.

Marshall–Marchetti–Krantz (MMK) procedure. The MMK procedure [72] was until recently, and perhaps remains in some parts of the world, the most widely used suprapubic incontinence operation. However, in the survey referred to earlier [46], in the UK the colposuspension is currently performed by twice as many gynaecologists as the MMK; among those with a special interest in gynaecological urology five times as many prefer the Burch procedure.

Results with the procedure again lack objectivity in many cases. Subjective results averaging 84% are reported [53,56,72–76], although recent studies with pre- and postoperative urodynamic evaluations [77,78] give cure rates averaging only 57%.

Suburethral Sling Procedures. Sling procedures have been in use since the beginning of this century [79], and in view of their more complicated nature, and greater associated morbidity as compared to other procedures [30], have been largely reserved for the management of recurrent incontinence. Many different materials have been employed, including a variety of autogenic tissues (gracilis, pyramidalis, levator and rectus muscle, round ligament, fascia lata and rectus fascia), allogenic tissues (ox fascia, lyophilised dura, and porcine dermis), and synthetic materials (mersilene, nylon, polypropylene and silastic). Results are not clearly better for any particular material; overall cure rates average around 82% for organic slings [30,80–95] and 88% for synthetic materials [29,96–105].

Needle Suspension Procedures. The first needle suspension procedure was that of Pereyra [106] in 1959. Reported results have been inconsistent with cure rates between 50% and 94% [31,106–109]. Although preliminary results with the Raz modification [110] were encouraging with a 94% cure rate at two years [111], longer follow-up, albeit only on a subjective basis, suggests cure in only 51% [112].

The Stamey bladder neck suspension [113] is a further modification of the Pereyra procedure which has been widely used and evaluated by urologists, but relatively little employed by gynaecologists. In the last ten years at least 20 papers have examined the results of this technique with an average cure of 73% [30,114–129] . The short operating time, minimal dissection and blood loss, low morbidity and ease of performance in the obese or "difficult pelvis" [30] would seem to make it ideally suited to those with multiple previous operations and to the elderly or physically frail. Peattie and Stanton [130], however, reported their experience of the operation in women over 65 years of age and found a cure rate of only 41% at three months. Hilton and Mayne [32], using a modified Stamey, in an actuarial follow-up over four years found better maintenance of cure in older patients (76%) as compared to those under 65 years (53%).

Periurethral Injections. The use of perineal injections of "Teflon" was first proposed by Politano et al [131] in 1974, as a means of treating postprostatectomy incontinence in men; the technique was subsequently extended to women [132]. Subsequent reports suggest cure rates averaging 62% [133–136], although the results of Schulman et al. [133] indicate a 52% cure from a first injection, 40% from a second, and 40% from a third, to give the total figure of 70% in his paper. More recently Appell et al. [137] reported the use of periurethral injections of bovine collagen with an 81% cure rate at six months from a single injection. This material would seem preferable to "Teflon" in being biocompatible; it is also biodegradable, being replaced by host collagen over a period of approximately six months. Long-term results are therefore awaited with interest.

How Operations Achieve Continence

Clearly different operations may achieve continence by different means; I should like to describe some of the studies involving the Burch colposuspension, which has perhaps been more thoroughly investigated than other procedures, and use this as a model to extrapolate to other procedures for further discussion.

Hilton and Stanton [28] reported a clinical and urodynamic evaluation of 25 patients undergoing colposuspension including cystometric and urethral pressure data. An increase in maximum voiding pressure from 28 cmH$_2$O preoperatively to 40 cmH$_2$O postoperatively, and a reduction in urine flow rate from 33 ml s^{-1} preoperatively to 20 ml s^{-1} postoperatively was reported. It seems unlikely, however, that the induction of outflow obstruction is critical to a successful outcome in terms of continence. The three patients whose operations failed showed a similar degree of obstruction, and 13 of the 22 whose operations were successful had normal voiding pressures and flow rates postoperatively.

No change was found in variables of the resting urethral pressure profile, although a highly significant increase in MUCP and FUL on stress was found in successfully treated cases. This resulted from a significant enhancement in pressure transmission ratio (PTR) in the proximal urethra which was not present in those whose operations failed (Figs. 14.4 and 14.5).

The nature of the enhancement in PTR remains in debate. It has previously been held to be due simply to elevation of the bladder neck and proximal urethra thus allowing improved passive transmission to the region [138]. Whilst this may explain PTRs approaching 100%, it clearly cannot account for ratios exceeding 100% which have now been recorded following not only colposuspension [28,31], but also the MMK [31,139,140], Stamey [30,32,141], and both abdominal [29] and abdominovaginal sling procedures [30,139]. It is possible that the bladder neck elevation allows not only improved passive transmission, but also promotes greater efficiency of the pelvic floor reflex, and an accentuation of urethral closure by active means [142]. Against this suggestion, however, is the observation that in healthy continent women the maximum PTR is found in the mid-distal urethra, whereas in those made continent by colposuspension maximum transmission is evident in the proximal urethra (Fig. 14.6). Hilton [27] has thus suggested that the colposuspension induces a novel mechanical urinary sphincter rather than restoring normal physiology. Hertogs and Stanton [143] showed that inserting a vaginal speculum during stress urethral profilometry had the effect of converting the typical postoperative PTR pattern to one approaching the preoperative state; in 27 out of 30 patients who were subjectively and objectively cured by the operation this manoeuvre led to the demonstration of incontinence. These studies suggest that the anatomy of the bladder neck, and its relationship to the symphysis anteriorly and the pelvic viscera posterosuperiorly are crucial to continence following colposuspension. In further radiological studies [144] they found that elevation of the bladder neck alone was not sufficient for a successful outcome, but relocation in proximity to the pubic symphysis was critical to cure. By this repositioning the proximal urethra is exposed to compression against the symphysis by descent of the pelvic viscera during increases in intra-abdominal pressure. It is likely that this mechanism accounts for the enhancement in PTR postoperatively.

The Effect of Surgery on Voiding

The extent of enhancement in PTR is related not only to the success or failure of the procedure, but also to the development of voiding dysfunction. Hilton et al. [145] showed a progression in PTRs from preoperative (genuine stress incontinence) and postoperative (unsuccessful) to postoperative (successful with normal flow) to postoperative (successful with reduced flow) (Fig. 14.7). A similar trend was shown in the radiological studies by Dundas et al. [146] who examined the position of the bladder neck at rest, on straining, and on voiding, from videourodynamic studies before and after colposuspension. Elevation was no greater in successful than failed operations, but was significantly greater in those with reduced flow rates postoperatively than in those with normal flows. Bladder neck mobility was markedly reduced in those with impaired voiding, and thus "super-elevation" and fixation of the bladder neck was held to be responsible for such problems following colposuspension.

The impact of bladder neck surgery on voiding characteristics has been relatively

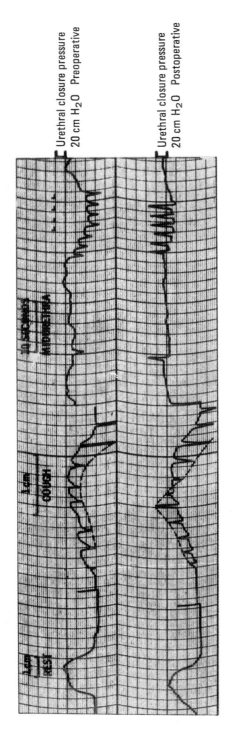

Fig. 14.4. Urethral closure pressure traces before (above) and after (below) successful treatment by colposuspension. From Hilton and Stanton [28] with permission of the authors and publisher.

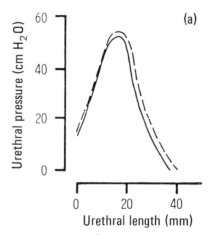

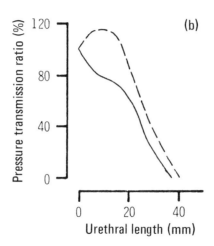

Fig. 14.5. (a) Average resting urethral pressure profiles and (b) pressure transmission profiles in 22 women before (——) and after (– – –) successful treatment by colposuspension. From Hilton [27].

little investigated. Four studies have examined the maximum voiding pressure (MVP) and peak flow rate (PFR) following colposuspension, with very consistent results [28,40,57,62]; all have found a significant increase in MVP and decrease in PFR postoperatively, suggesting that the procedure is markedly obstructive.

With sling procedures [29,30,104] three studies have shown a reduction in PFR, although only one showed any increase in MVP [30]. Whilst most surgeons consider this to be an obstructive procedure, the evidence is less clear, perhaps because of variation between surgeons in operative technique, and in particular in terms of sling tension.

The same may account for the disparities in data relating to the Stamey procedure. Mundy [64] found the operation to be markedly obstructive, but did not

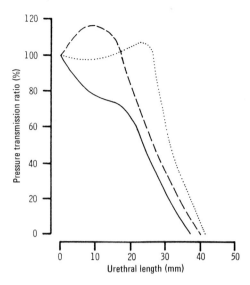

Fig. 14.6. Average pressure transmission profiles in stress incontinent women before (——) and after (– – –) successful colposuspension, compared to a group of 20 symptom-free women (· · · ·). From Hilton and Stanton [28] with permission of the authors and publisher.

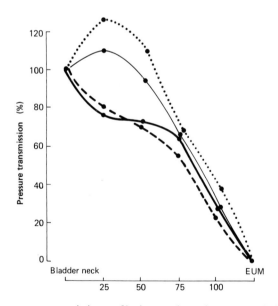

Fig. 14.7. Average pressure transmission profiles in stress incontinent women before colposuspension (– – –), after unsuccessful surgery (——), after successful surgery with normal voiding postoperatively (——) and after successful surgery with reduced flow postoperatively (· · · ·). From Hilton et al. [145].

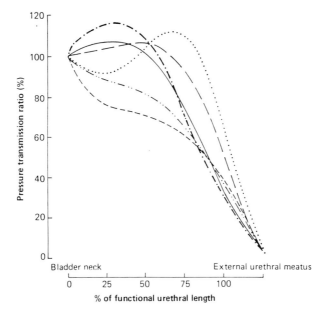

Fig. 14.8. Average pressure transmission profiles in symptom-free women ($\cdots$), stress incontinent women ($---$), and in those undergoing successful treatment by colposuspension ($-\cdot-$), suburethral sling ($———$), Stamey procedure ($——$) and anterior colporraphy ($-\cdot\cdot-\cdot\cdot$). After Hilton [30].

quote MVP or PFR results. My own early results [30] showed a reduction in MVP and increase in PFR, and two other series [32,118] showed no significant alteration in either variable. Clearly it is possible to perform this procedure successfully without inducing obstruction.

Only three reports have assessed voiding parameters following anterior colporrhaphy. Two found no significant change in MVP or PFR [2,51] whereas Walter et al. [57] reported a reduction in MVP and increase in PFR. It is of note that these authors took a selected group of patients with the radiological appearance of a posterior suspension defect; such patients characteristically have a high MVP and low PFR, indicating a degree of obstruction preoperatively which was relieved by colporrhaphy in this series.

Thus we can construct a league table of operations from the most obstructive (colposuspension) to the least obstructive (colporrhaphy). This table roughly parallels the extent of PTR changes (Fig. 14.8), and success rates, by these procedures. For the colposuspension we have shown that the greater the degree of bladder neck elevation and relocation achieved, the greater the enhancement of PTR and the greater the likelihood of cure; but at the same time the greater the likelihood of inducing compression of the urethra, and along with that obstruction. Similarly for bladder neck surgery as a whole, those operations capable of inducing the most marked elevation are most likely to be successful, but carry the greatest risk of obstruction. In patients with compromised voiding on preoperative assessment it is often appropriate to select a procedure with a lower risk of obstruction, accepting that this may carry a slightly poorer prognosis for the cure of incontinence.

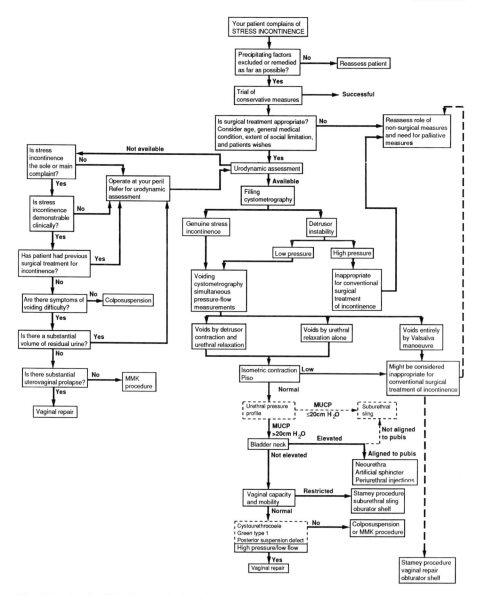

Fig. 14.9.   An algorithm for the selection of operative procedure in the treatment of stress incontinence. Solid lines and boxes indicate the author's current practice; dotted lines indicate other possible approaches based on literature. After Hilton [147].

An Algorithmic Approach to the Choice of Surgery

To collate all these factors into a rational plan for the choice of operation in genuine stress incontinence is not straightforward, but is perhaps best achieved by the use of a clinical algorithm (Fig. 14.9) [147].

In considering surgical treatment for incontinence it is clearly important that stress incontinence should be a major element of the patients' complaints. As noted earlier, predisposing or precipitating factors should be identified and remedied where possible, and in all patients (or at least all who wish to avoid surgery) conservative measures should be employed first. If these measures fail to relieve the incontinence, and surgery is in general terms appropriate, further assessment should be undertaken.

Emphasis has already been placed on the importance of urodynamic assessment in the selection for, and of, incontinence surgery; it is appreciated however that such facilities are not readily available in all departments. If incontinence surgery is to be performed without such information it is the author's view that it should be restricted to those patients whose sole or main complaint is stress incontinence, in whom the physical sign of stress incontinence is clinically demonstrable, who have not had previous incontinence or prolapse surgery, and who have no clinical evidence of voiding dysfunction. Under such circumstances the author's preferred procedure is the Burch colposuspension. Reference has been made to the obstructive effect of this procedure, and therefore in the absence of objective evidence of normal voiding characteristics, it is probably best avoided in those patients with symptoms of voiding difficulty preoperatively. In this latter group a vaginal repair (where there is significant anterior vaginal wall prolapse) or a Stamey or MMK procedure (where there is no prolapse) are less likely to compromise voiding and are therefore advocated. In all other circumstances urodynamic assessment is important and if not available locally should be obtained by secondary referral.

The important questions to be answered from this evaluation are first, "is the urodynamic abnormality likely to be amenable to conventional incontinence surgery?" That is to say, is the diagnosis from the filling phase of the cystometrogram one of genuine stress incontinence or "low pressure" detrusor instability? If the diagnosis is one of "high pressure" instability conventional surgery is inappropriate. Second, "is the voiding pattern normal, and is there adequate detrusor reserve?" From analysis of the voiding phase of the cystometrogram patients may be divided into those voiding by urethral relaxation and detrusor contraction, those voiding by urethral relaxation alone, and those voiding entirely by abdominal straining; in the first two groups further confirmation may be obtained from the isometric contraction on interruption of micturition. Those in whom there is evidence of compromised voiding as evidenced by strain voiding or a poor or absent isometric contraction might, by some, be considered inappropriate for surgical treatment; they should certainly be held to be at increased risk of postoperative voiding problems, and treated where possible by a non-obstructing procedure; my own preference would be for Stamey procedure or anterior colporrhaphy.

A further urodynamic question that could be added into the algorithm at this point (although it is not the author's current practice to do so) might be "is the resting urethral pressure adequate?" As evidenced by Ostergard et al. [35,36] those patients with a resting urethral pressure less than $20\,cmH_2O$ may carry a relatively poor prognosis for cure by colposuspension, and may be better served by sling procedure.

Where voiding characteristics are normal the selection of operation is based on clinical findings, in particular in relation to the degree of elevation of the bladder neck, the capacity and mobility of the vagina, and the presence of associated vaginal wall prolapse. If the bladder neck is already well elevated then most incontinence operations, being elevating procedures, are unlikely to be successful;

a urethral reconstruction using an anterior bladder flap (Tanagho's procedure), an artificial sphincter implantation, or periurethral injections are the only procedures with any real possibility of success. Stanton [148] makes the distinction between the situation where the bladder neck is elevated and aligned with the symphysis, which he manages as above, and that where the bladder neck is elevated but not aligned, in which case he considers a sling to be the operation of choice.

In the remaining patients, and these will be by far the majority, the bladder neck will be inadequately elevated in its resting position, or will descend on coughing or straining. In a proportion of these the vagina will be restricted in capacity or mobility. These are particularly the nulliparous, those with marked atrophic genital changes, and those with previous pelvic irradiation or surgery (including incontinence surgery), and in such cases a colposuspension will not be technically feasible; here a modified Stamey operation or suburethral sling are the author's preferred procedures. On the basis of our more recent work [32], I am inclined to undertake the Stamey procedure in older women and sling in those under 65 years. In the remaining patients, where vaginal capacity is adequate, many would take the view that an anterior colporrhaphy should be performed where there is significant vaginal prolapse, and the MMK where there is not. Others would categorise patients at this stage on the radiological rather than clinical appearance. In the presence of Green's type I stress incontinence [56] or a posterior suspension defect [57,58] anterior colporrhaphy might be preferred; with Green's type II stress, or an anterior suspension defect, a suprapubic procedure would be more appropriate. In the author's opinion, however, the colposuspension is the optimal procedure for the control of stress incontinence whether or not there is co-existent vaginal prolapse, provided that voiding function has been shown to be normal. In the small group of patients recognised as having a high pressure/ low flow voiding pattern, anterior colporrhaphy should certainly be preferred on the evidence of Walter et al. [57].

Any clinical algorithm will inevitably have its flaws, and this is surely no exception. Different surgeons perform the "same" operation in their individual ways, with differing results, and will therefore find varying indications for these, and other, procedures. This chapter simply aims to emphasise that patients considered for surgical treatment of their incontinence, even though they may all have genuine stress incontinence, have widely varying clinical and urodynamic backgrounds, and different operations may modify that in different ways. The philosophy that a single operation is appropriate for the first-line management of all cases can no longer be considered appropriate, and any surgeon with a significant commitment to such patients should have a range of operations in his repertoire.

References

1. Baker-Brown I. On diseases of women remediable by operation. Lancet 1864; i:263–6.
2. Stanton SL, Hilton P, Norton C, Cardozo LD. Clinical and urodynamic effects of anterior colporrhaphy and vaginal hysterectomy for prolapse with and without incontinence. Br J Obstet Gynaecol 1982; 89:459–63.
3. Morgan JE. A sling operation using Marlex polypropylene mesh for treatment of recurrent stress incontinence. Am J Obstet Gynecol 1970; 106:369–77.
4. Kujansuu E. The effect of pelvic floor exercises on urethral function in female stress urinary incontinence: a urodynamic study. Ann Chir Gynaecol 1983; 72:28–32.

5. Fischer W. Physiotherapeutic aspects of urine incontinence. Acta Obstet Gynecol Scand 1983; 63:579–83.

6. Castleden CM, Duffin HM, Mitchell EP. The effect of physiotherapy on stress incontinence. Age Ageing 1984; 13:235–7.

7. Klarskov P, Belving D, Bischoff N et al. Pelvic floor exercise versus surgery for female urinary stress incontinence. Urol Int 1986; 41:129–32.

8. Wilson PD, Al Samarrai T, Deakin M, Kolbe E, Brown ADG. An objective assessment of physiotherapy for female genuine stress incontinence. Br J Obstet Gynaecol 1987; 94:575–82.

9. Mayne CJ, Hilton P. A comparison of urethral electrical conductance and perineometry during a course of pelvic floor exercises for genuine stress incontinence. Proceedings of the eighteenth annual meeting of the International Continence Society, Oslo, Norway. Neurourol Urodynam 1988; 7:264–5.

10. Sandri SD, Biggioggero L, Fanciullacci F, Zanollo A. Are there limitations to pelvic floor rehabilitation in female urinary incontinence? Proceedings of the eighteenth annual meeting of the International Continence Society, Oslo, Norway. Neurourol Urodynam 1988; 7:358–9.

11. Tapp AJS, Cardozo LD, Hills B, Barnick C. Who benefits from physiotherapy? Proceedings of the eighteenth annual meeting of the International Continence Society, Oslo, Norway. Neurourol Urodynam 1988; 7:259–61.

12. Henalla SM, Hutchins CJ, Breeson AJ. Treatment of female genuine stress urinary incontinence with pelvic floor reeducation in two different hospitals. Proceedings of the eighteenth annual meeting of the International Continence Society, Oslo, Norway. Neurourol Urodynam 1988; 7:262–3.

13. Bridges N, Denning J, Olah KS, Farrar DJ. A prospective trial comparing interferential therapy and treatment using cones in patients with symptoms of stress incontinence. Proceedings of the eighteenth annual meeting of the International Continence Society, Oslo, Norway. Neurourol Urodynam 1988; 7:267–8.

14. Peattie AB, Plevnik S. Cones versus physiotherapy as conservative management of genuine stress incontinence. Proceedings of the eighteenth annual meeting of the International Continence Society, Oslo, Norway. Neurourol Urodynam 1988; 7:265–6.

15. Tapp AJS, Hills B, Cardozo LD. Randomised study comparing pelvic floor physiotherapy with the Burch colposuspension. Proceedings of the nineteenth annual meeting of the International Continence Society, Ljubljana, Yugoslavia. Neurourol Urodynam 1989; 8:356–7.

16. Klarskov P. Kroyer K, Kromann B, Maeggaard E. Long-term results of pelvic floor training and surgery for female genuine stress incontinence. Proceedings of the nineteenth annual meeting of the International Continence Society, Ljubljana, Yugoslavia. Neurourol Urodynam 1989; 8:357–9.

17. Bo K, Hagen R, Jorgenssen J, Kvarstein B, Larsen S. The effect of two different pelvic floor muscle exercise programmes in the treatment of urinary stress incontinence in women. Proceedings of the nineteenth annual meeting of the International Continence Society, Ljubljana, Yugoslavia. Neurourol Urodynam 1989; 8:355–6.

18. Hodgkinson CP, Ayers MA, Drukker BH. Dyssynergic detrusor dysfunction in the apparently normal female. Am J Obstet Gynecol 1963; 87:717–30.

19. Stanton SL, Cardozo LD, Williams JE, Ritchie D, Allan V. Clinical and urodynamic features of failed incontinence surgery in the female. Obstet Gynecol 1978; 51:515–20.

20. Jorgensen L, Lose G, Mølsted-Pedersen L. Vaginal repair in female motor urge incontinence. Eur Urol 1987; 13:382–5.

21. Meyhoff HH, Walter S, Gerstenberg T, Olesen KP, Nordling J, Pedersen PH, Hald T. Incontinence surgery in females with motor urge incontinence. Proceedings of the tenth annual meeting of the International Continence Society, Los Angeles, USA, 1980; 109–12.

22. Lockhart JL, Vortsman B, Politano VA. Anti-incontinence surgery in females with detrusor instability. Proceedings of the thirteenth annual meeting of the International Continence Society, Aachen, FRG, 1983; 280–1.

23. Koonings P, Bergman A, Ballard CA. Combined detrusor instability and stress urinary incontinence: where is the primary pathology? Gynecol Obstet Invest 1988; 26:250–6.

24. Langer R, Ron-El R, Newman M, Herman A, Caspi E. Detrusor instability following colposuspension for urinary stress incontinence. Br J Obstet Gynaecol 1988; 95:607–10.

25. Karram MM, Bhatia NN. Management of co-existent stress and urge urinary incontinence. Obstet Gynecol 1989; 73:4–7.

26. McGuire EJ. Urodynamic findings in patients after failure of stress incontinence operations. Prog Clin Biol Res 1981; 78:351–60.

27. Hilton P. Urethral pressure measurement by microtransducer: observations on the methodology,

the pathophysiology of genuine stress incontinence and the effects of its treatment in the female. MD Thesis, University of Newcastle-upon-Tyne, 1981.

28. Hilton P, Stanton SL. A clinical and urodynamic evaluation of the Burch colposuspension for genuine stress incontinence. Br J Obstet Gynaecol 1983; 90:934–9.

29. Hilton P, Stanton SL. A clinical and urodynamic evaluation of the polypropylene ("Marlex") sling for genuine stress incontinence. Neurourol Urodynam 1983; 2:145–53.

30. Hilton P. A clinical and urodynamic study comparing the Stamey bladder neck suspension and suburethral sling procedures in the treatment of genuine stress incontinence. Br J Obstet Gynaecol 1989; 96:213–20.

31. Weil A, Reyes H, Bischoff P, Rottenberg RD, Krauer F. Modifications of the urethral rest and stress profiles after different types of surgery for urinary stress incontinence. Br J Obstet Gynaecol 1984; 91:46–55.

32. Hilton P, Mayne CJ. The Stamey endoscopic bladder neck suspension: a clinical and urodynamic evaluation including actuarial follow-up over four years. Proceedings of the nineteenth annual meeting of the International Continence Society, Ljubljana, Yugoslavia. Neurourol Urodynam 1989; 8:336–7.

33. Behr J, Winkler L, Schwiersch U. Urodynamic observations on the Marshall–Marchetti–Krantz operation. Geburtshilfe Frauenheilkd 1986; 46:649–53.

34. Francis LN, Sand PK, Hamrang K, Ostergard DR. A urodynamic appraisal of success and failure after retropubic urethropexy. J Reprod Med 1987; 32:693–6.

35. Sand PK, Bowen LW, Panganiban R, Ostergard DR. The low pressure urethra as a factor in failed retropubic urethropexy. Obstet Gynecol 1987; 69:399–402.

36. Bowen LW, Sand PK, Ostergard DR, Franti CE. Unsuccessful Burch retropubic urethropexy: a case controlled urodynamic study. Am J Obstet Gynecol 1989; 160:452–8.

37. Delaere KPJ, Moonen WA, Debruyne FMJ, Michiels HGE, Renders GAM. Anterior vaginal repair, cause of troublesome voiding disorders? Eur Urol 1979; 5:190–4.

38. Stanton SL, Cardozo LD, Kerr-Wilson R. Treatment of delayed onset of spontaneous voiding after surgery for incontinence. Urology 1979; XIII:494–6.

39. Stanton SL, Cardozo LD, Chaudhury N. Spontaneous voiding after surgery for urinary incontinence. Br J Obstet Gynaecol 1978; 85:149–52.

40. Lose G, Jorgensen L, Mortensen SO, Mølsted-Pedersen L, Kristensen JK. Voiding difficulties after colposuspension. Obstet Gynecol 1987; 69:33–8.

41. Schmidt RA. Post-operative voiding dysfunction. In: Stanton SL, Tanagho EA, eds. Surgery for female incontinence, 2nd ed. Berlin: Springer-Verlag, 1986; 259–66.

42. Rud T, Ulmsten U, Anderssen K-E. Initiation of voiding in healthy women and those with stress incontinence. Acta Obstet Gynecol Scand 1978; 57:457–62.

43. Bhatia NN, Bergman A. Urodynamic predictability of voiding following incontinence surgery. Obstet Gynecol 1984; 63:85–91.

44. Bhatia NN, Bergman A. Use of pre-operative uroflowmetry and simultaneous urethrocystometry for predicting risk of prolonged post-operative bladder drainage. Urology 1986; XXVIII:440–5.

45. Coolsaet BLRA. Stop-test. A pre-operative determination of bladder contractility. Proceedings of the ninth annual meeting of the International Continence Society, Rome, Italy, 1979; 253–4.

46. Hilton P. Bladder drainage: a survey of practices among gynaecologists in the British Isles. Br J Obstet Gynaecol 1988; 95:1178–89 (with unpublished observations regarding surgical practices).

47. Abrams P, Blaivas JG, Stanton SL, Andersen JT. Standardisation of terminology of lower urinary tract function. Neurourol Urodynam 1988; 7:403–27.

48. Bailey KV. A clinical investigation into uterine prolapse with stress incontinence. Treatment by modified Manchester colporrhaphy. J Obstet Gynaecol Br Emp 1954; 61:291–8.

49. Jeffcoate TNA. Principles governing treatment of stress incontinence of urine in females. Br J Urol 1965; 37:633–43.

50. Ross RA, Shingleton HM. Vaginal prolapse and stress urinary incontinence. West Va Med J 1969; 65:70–9.

51. Stanton SL, Cardozo LD. A comparison of vaginal and suprapubic surgery in the correction of incontinence due to urethral sphincter incompetence. Br J Urol 1979; 51:497–9.

52. Stanton SL, Chamberlain GVP, Holmes DM. Randomised study of the anterior repair and colposuspension operation for the control of genuine stress incontinence. Proceedings of the fifteenth annual meeting of the International Continence Society, London, 1985; 236–7.

53. Park GS, Miller EJ. Surgical treatment of stress urinary incontinence: comparison of the Kelly plication, Marshall–Marchetti–Krantz and Pereyra procedures. Obstet Gynecol 1988; 71:575–9.

54. Bergman A, Koonings P, Ballard CA. Primary stress urinary incontinence and pelvic relaxation:

a prospective randomised comparison of three different operations. Am J Obstet Gynecol 1989; 161:97–101.

55. Warrell D. Anterior repair. In: Stanton EL, Tanagho EA, eds. Surgery for female incontinence, 2nd ed. Berlin: Springer-Verlag, 1986; 77–86.

56. Green TH. Urinary stress incontinence: differential diagnosis, pathophysiology and management. Am J Obstet Gynecol 1975; 122:368–400.

57. Walter S, Olesen KP, Hald T, Jensen HK, Pederesen PH. Urodynamic evaluation after vaginal repair and colposuspension. Br J Urol 1982; 54:377–80.

58. Olesen KP, Walter S. Posterior bladder suspension defects in the female. Acta Obstet Gynecol Scand 1980; 59:543–8.

59. Burch JC. Urethrovaginal fixation to Coopers ligament for correction of stress incontinence, cystocele and prolapse. Am J Obstet Gynecol 1961; 81:281–90.

60. Burch JC. Coopers ligament urethrovesical suspension for stress incontinence. Am J Obstet Gynecol 1968; 100:764–72.

61. Stanton SL, Williams JE, Ritchie D. The colposuspension operation for urinary incontinence. Br J Obstet Gynaecol 1976; 83:890–5.

62. Stanton SL, Cardozo LD. Results of colposuspension for incontinence and prolapse. Br J Obstet Gynaecol 1979; 86:693–7.

63. Stanton SL, Hertogs K, Cox C, Hilton P, Cardozo LD. Colposuspension operation for genuine stress incontinence: a five year study. Proceedings of the twelfth annual meeting of the International Continence Society, Leiden, Netherlands, 1982; 94–6.

64. Mundy AR. A trial comparing the Stamey bladder neck suspension procedure with colposuspension for the treatment of stress incontinence. Br J Urol 1983; 55:687–90.

65. Gillon G, Stanton SL. Long-term follow-up of surgery for urinary incontinence in elderly women. Br J Urol 1984; 56:478–81.

66. Bhatia NN, Bergman A. Modified Burch versus Pereyra retropubic urethropexy for stress urinary incontinence. Obstet Gynecol 1985; 66:255–61.

67. Galloway NT, Davies N, Stephenson TP. The complications of colposuspension. Br J Urol 1987; 60:122–4.

68. Pigne A, Keskes J, Maghioracos P, Boyer F, Marpeau L, Barrat T. Clinical and urodynamic results of the Burch colposuspension operation in the treatment of female urinary stress incontinence. A study a propos of 370 cases. J Gynecol Obstet Biol Reprod 1988; 17:922–30.

69. Borstad E, Rud T, Skrede M. Mechanisms for success or failure after colposuspension for urinary stress incontinence. Proceedings of the annual meeting of the International Urogynecological Association, Riva-del-Garda, Italy, 1989; 42.

70. Meschia M, Barbacini P, Carena Maini M, Marri R, Mele A. Unsuccessful Burch colposuspension: an analysis of risk factors. Proceedings of the annual meeting of the International Urogynecological Association, Riva-del-Garda, Italy, 1989; 45.

71. Bergman A, Koonings P, Ballard CA. Ball-Burch for the treatment of low urethral pressure type of stress urinary incontinence. Proceedings of the annual meeting of the International Urogynecological Association, Riva-del-Garda, Italy, 1989; 3.

72. Marshall VF, Marchetti AA, Krantz KE. The correction of stress incontinence by simple vesicourethral suspension. Surge Gynecol Obstet 1949; 88:509–18.

73. Giesen JE. Stress incontinence: a review of 60 Marshall–Marchetti operations. J Obstet Gynaecol Br Commonw 1962; 69:397–402.

74. Lee RA, Symmonds RE, Goldstein RA. Surgical complications and results of modified Marshall–Marchetti–Krantz procedure for urinary incontinence. Obstet Gynecol 1979; 53:447–50.

75. Parnell JP, Marshall VF, Vaughan ED. Primary management of urinary stress incontinence by the Marshall–Marchetti–Krantz vesicourethropexy. J Urol 1982; 127:679–82.

76. Lee RA. The surgical treatment of recurrent stress incontinence. Proceedings of the annual meeting of the International Urogynecological Association, Riva-del-Garda, Italy, 1989; 40.

77. Behr J, Winkler M, Schwiersch U. Urodynamic observations on the Marshall–Marchetti–Krantz operation. Geburtshilfe Frauenheilkd 1986; 46:649–53.

78. Briel RC. Follow-up of a new modification of the Marshall–Marchetti–Krantz procedure. Arch Gynecol 1986; 239:1–9.

79. Hohenfellner R, Petri E. Sling procedures. In: Stanton SL, Tanagho EA, eds. Surgery for female incontinence, 2nd ed. Berlin: Springer-Verlag, 1986; 105–13.

80. Jeffcoate TNA. Results of Aldridge sling operation for stress incontinence. J Obstet Gynaecol Br Emp 1956; 63:36–9.

81. Wharton I, Te Linde RW. Evaluation of fascial sling operation for urinary incontinence in female patients. J Urol 1959; 82:776–9.

82. Kennedy C. Stress incontinence of urine: a survey of 34 cases treated by the Millin 1 sling operation. Br Med J 1960; 2:263–7.

83. McLaren HC. Late results of sling operations. J Obstet Gynaecol Br Commonw 1968; 75:10–13.

84. Beck RP, Lai AR. Results of treating 88 cases of stress incontinence with the Oxford fascia lata sling procedure. Am J Obstet Gynecol 1982; 142:649–51.

85. Heidenreich J, Faber P, Beck L. Suspension mit Lyoduraband. In: Verh Dtsch Ges Urol 27. Berlin: Springer-Verlag, 1976; 221–2.

86. Gaudenz R. Die Bedeutung einer Zusatzoperation bei der primaren operativen Behandlung einer Urethralinsuffizienz. Geburtshilfe Frauenheilkd 1976; 39:393–401.

87. Altmann P, Georgiades E, Rudelstorfer B. Zur Technik der Inguinovaginal Schlingenoperation (Modifikation nach Narik-Palmrich) und ihre Spätergebnisse. In: Verh Dtsch Ges Urol 27. Berlin: Springer-Verlag, 1976; 213–15.

88. McGuire EJ, Lytton B. Pubovaginal sling procedure for stress incontinence. J Urol 1978; 119:82–4.

89. Parker RT, Addison WA, Wilson CJ. Fascia lata urethrovesical suspension for recurrent stress urinary incontinence. Am J Obstet Gynecol 1979; 135:843–52.

90. Hagele D, Fruhwirth O, Kriesche H, Nol C, Berg D. Ergebnisse nach Schlingenoperation mit Tutoplast-Dura. Geburtshilfe Frauenheilkd 1983; 43:762–5.

91. Petri E, Beckhaus I, Frohneberg D, Thuroff JW. Inguinovaginal fascial sling according to Narik and Palmrich – indications, problems, long-term results. Aktuel Urol 1983; 14:286–90.

92. Jarvis GJ, Fowlie A. Clinical and urodynamic assessment of the porcine dermis bladder sling in the treatment of genuine stress incontinence. Br J Obstet Gynaecol 1985; 92:1189–91.

93. Rottenberg RD, Weil A, Brioschi BA, Bischoff P, Krauer F. Urodynamic and clinical assessment of the Lyodura sling operation for urinary stress incontinence. Br J Obstet Gynaecol 1985; 92:829–34.

94. McIndoe GA, Jones RW, Grieve BW. The Aldridge sling procedure in the treatment of urinary stress incontinence. Aust NZ J Obstet Gynaecol 1987; 27:238–9.

95. Enzelsberger H, Sagl R, Heytmanek G, Schatten C, Wagner G. Comparison of urodynamic findings before and after loop operations for recurrent incontinence. Geburtshilfe Frauenheilkd 1988; 48:264–7.

96. Moir JC. The gauze-hammock operation. J Obstet Gynaecol Br Commonw 1968; 75:1–9.

97. Zoedler D. Die operative Behandlung der weiblichen Harnikontinenz mit dem Kunststoff-Netzband. Aktuel Urol 1970; 1:28–34.

98. Morgan JE. A sling operation, using Marlex polypropylene mesh for recurrent stress incontinence. Am J Obstet Gynecol 1970; 106:369–77.

99. Spencer T, Jaquier A, Kersey H. The gauze-hammock operation in the treatment of persistent stress incontinence. J Obstet Gynaecol Br Commonw 1972; 79:666–9.

100. Nicholas DH. The Mersilene mesh gauze-hammock for severe urinary incontinence. Obstet Gynecol 1973; 41:88–93.

101. Fiaanu S, Soderberg G. Absorbable polyglactin mesh for retropubic sling operations in female urinary stress incontinence. Gynecol Obstet Invest 1983; 16:45–50.

102. Weinhower R, Merten M, Zoedler D. Ergebnisse urologischer Rezidiv-Inkontinenz-Operationen. In: Verh Dtsch Ges Urol 27. Berlin: Springer-Verlag, 1976; 222–4.

103. Morgan JE, Farrow GA. Recurrent stress urinary incontinence in the female. Br J Urol 1977; 49:37–42.

104. Stanton SL, Brindley GS, Holmes DM. Silastic sling for urethral sphincter incompetence in women. Br J Obstet Gynaecol 1985; 92:747–50.

105. Korda A, Peat B, Hunter P. Silastic slings for female incontinence. Int Urogyn J 1989; 1:5–7.

106. Pereyra AJ. A simplified surgical procedure for the correction of stress incontinence in women. West J Surg 1959; 67:223–6.

107. Pereyra AJ, Lebhertz TB. Combined urethro-vesical suspension and vagino-urethroplasty for correction of urinary stress incontinence. Obstet Gynecol 1967; 30:537–46.

108. Kursch E, Wainstein N, Persky L. Pereyra procedure and urinary stress incontinence. J Urol 1972; 108:591–3.

109. Backer MH, Probst RE. The Pereyra procedure. Am J Obstet Gynecol 1977; 125:346–52.

110. Raz S. Modified Pereyra bladder neck suspension for female stress incontinence. Urology 1981; XVII:82.

111. Leach GE. Raz S. Modified Pereyra bladder neck suspension after previously failed anti-incontinence surgery. Surgical technique and results with long-term follow-up. Urology 1984; XXIII:359–62.

112. Leach GE, Kelly MJ, Roskamp DA, Knielsen K, Bruskewitz R. Long-term follow-up of the

modified Pereyra bladder neck suspension. Proceedings of the nineteenth annual meeting of the International Continence Society, Ljubljana, Yugoslavia. Neurourol Urodynam 1989; 8:257.

113. Stamey TA. Endoscopic suspension of the vesical neck for urinary incontinence. Surg Gynecol Obstet 1973; 136:547–54.

114. Vordemark JS, Brannen GE, Wettlaufer JN, Modarelli RO. Suprapubic endoscopic bladder neck suspension. J Urol 1979; 122:165–7.

115. Stamey TA. Endoscopic suspension of vesical neck for urinary incontinence in females: a report of 203 consecutive patients. Ann Surg 1980; 192:465–71.

116. Diaz DL, Fox BM, Walzak MP, Nieh PT. Endoscopic vesico-urethropexy: experience and complications. Urology 1984; XXIV:321–3.

117. Gaum L, Ricciotti NA, Fair WR. Endoscopic bladder neck suspension for stress urinary incontinence. J Urol 1984; 132:1119–21.

118. Ashken MH, Abrams PH, Lawrence WT. Stamey endoscopic bladder neck suspension for stress incontinence. Br J Urol 1984; 56: 629–34.

119. Fleischer AN, Vinsor RK, Jumper B. Endoscopic vesico-urethropexy for stress urinary incontinence. Urology 1984; XXIV:577–9.

120. Huland H, Butcher H. Endoscopic bladder neck suspension (Stamey–Pereyra) in female urinary stress incontinence: long-term follow-up of 66 patients. Eur Urol 1984; 10:328–41.

121. Fowler JE. Experience with suprapubic vesico-urethral suspension of the vesical neck for stress incontinence in females. Surg Gynecol Obstet 1986; 162:437–41.

122. Spencer JR, O'Connor VJ, Schaeffer AJ. A comparison of endoscopic suspension of the vesical neck with suprapubic vesico-urethropexy for the treatment of stress urinary incontinence. J Urol 1987; 137:411–15.

123. Lawrence WT, Thomas DJ. The Stamey bladder neck suspension operation for stress incontinence and neurovesical dysfunction. Br J Urol 1987; 59:305–10.

124. Kirby RS, Whiteway JE. Assessment of the results of Stamey bladder neck suspension. Br J Urol 1989; 63:21–3.

125. Wujanto R, O'Reilly PH. Stamey needle suspension for stress urinary incontinence: a prospective study of 40 patients. Br J Urol 1989; 63:162–4.

126. Jones DJ, Shah JR, Worth PHL. Modified Stamey procedure for bladder neck suspension. Br J Urol 1989; 63:153–61.

127. Theodorou C, Metropoulos D, Alivizatos G, Dimopoulos C. Urodynamic parameters related to the final outcome after the Stamey procedure for correction of stress urinary incontinence. Proceedings of the nineteenth annual meeting of the International Continence Society, Ljubljana, Yugoslavia. Neurourol Urodynam 1989; 8:272–3.

128. Shah PJR, Holder P. A comparison of the modified Stamey and Pereyra–Raz endoscopic bladder neck suspension. Proceedings of the nineteenth annual meeting of the International Continence Society, Ljubljana, Yugoslavia. Neurourol Urodynam 1989; 8:264–5.

129. Kirby RS, Eardley R, Parkhouse H. Analysis of the reasons for failure of the Stamey endoscopic bladder neck suspension and early results of a modified procedure. Proceedings of the nineteenth annual meeting of the International Continence Society, Ljubljana, Yugoslavia. Neurourol Urodynam 1989; 8:249–50.

130. Peattie AB, Stanton SL. The Stamey operation for correction of genuine stress incontinence in elderly women. Br J Obstet Gynaecol 1989; 96:983–6.

131. Politano VA, Small MP, Harper JM, Lynne CM. Periurethral Teflon injection for urinary incontinence. J Urol 1974; 111:180–3.

132. Politano VA. Periurethral polytetrafluorethylene injection for urinary incontinence. J Urol 1982; 127:439–42.

133. Schulman CC, Simon J, Vespes E, Germeau F. Endoscopic injections of Teflon to treat urinary incontinence in women. Br Med J 1984; 288:192.

134. Vicente J, Arano P. Endoscopic injection of Teflon in urinary incontinence in women. J Urol (Paris) 1984; 90:35–8.

135. Fischer W, Hegenscheid F, Jende W, Vogler H, Abet L. Is Teflon treatment of female urinary incontinence still justified? Zentralbl Gynakol 1986; 108:833–40.

136. Vesey SG, Rivett A, O'Boyle PJ. Teflon injection in female stress incontinence. Effect on urethral pressure profile and flow rate. Br J Urol 1988; 62:39–41.

137. Appell RA, Goodman JR, McGuire EJ, Wang SC, Bennett AH, DeRidder PA, Webster GD. Multi-centre study periurethral and transurethral GAX-collagen injection for urinary incontinence. Proceedings of the nineteenth annual meeting of the International Continence Society, Ljubljana, Yugoslavia. Neurourol Urodynam 1989; 8:339–40.

138. Enhorning GE. A concept of urinary continence. Urol Int 1976; 31:3–5.

139. Henriksson L, Ulmsten U. A urodynamic evaluation of the effects of abdominal urethrocystopexy and vaginal sling urethroplasty in women with stress incontinence. Am J Obstet Gynecol 1978; 113:78–82.

140. Raz S, Maggio AJ, Kaufman JJ. Why Marshall–Marchetti operation works – or does not. Urology 1979; XIV:154–9.

141. Constantinou CE, Faysal MH, Rother L, Govan DE. The impact of bladder neck suspension on the mode of distribution of abdominal pressure along the female urethra. In: Zinner NR, Sterlin AM, eds. Female incontinence. Progress in Clinical and Biological Research, Volume 78. New York: AR Liss, 1981, 121–32.

142. Heidler H, Wolk H, Jonas U. Urethral closure mechanism under stress conditions. Eur Urol 1979; 5:110–12.

143. Hertogs K, Stanton SL. Mechanism of urinary continence after colposuspension: barrier studies. Br J Obstet Gynaecol 1985; 92:1184–8.

144. Hertogs K, Stanton SL. Lateral bead-chain urethrocystography after successful and unsuccessful colposuspension. Br J Obstet Gynaecol 1985; 92:1179–83.

145. Hilton P, Langer R, Hertogs K, Stanton SL. Urethral pressure measurement before and after Burch colposuspension – results in patients with cured and recurrent stress incontinence and with voiding difficulties. Proceedings of the twelfth annual meeting of the International Continence Society, Leiden, Netherlands, 1982, 130–1.

146. Dundas D, Hilton P, Williams JE, Stanton SL. Aetiology of voiding difficulty following colposuspension. Proceedings of the twelfth annual meeting of the International Continence Society, Leiden, Netherlands, 1982;132.

147. Hilton P. Clinical algorithms: urinary incontinence in women. Br Med J 1987; 295: 425–32.

148. Stanton SL. The choice of surgery. In: Stanton SL, Tanagho EA, eds. Surgery for female incontinence. 2nd ed. Berlin: Springer-Verlag, 1986; 275–82.

149. Hilton P, Stanton SL. Urethral pressure measurement by microtransducer: results in symptom-free women and in those with genuine stress incontinence. Br J Obstet Gynaecol 1983; 90:919–34.

Chapter 15

Why Operations Fail

S. L. Stanton

The reasons for incontinence following continence surgery are varied: literature reviews are often unsatisfactory because despite the growing use of pre- and post-operative urodynamic investigations, many papers exist where only clinical data are presented and therefore, in terms of failure, only conjectures rather than objective answers are available.

Aim of Surgery for Genuine Stress Incontinence (Urethral Sphincter Incompetence)

Continence surgery aims to correct either the descent of the bladder neck, whereby intra-abdominal pressure fails to be transmitted to the proximal urethra as it is to the bladder, or to increase urethral resistance or pressure when it is below that of the intravesical pressure at rest (a negative closure pressure), e.g. found in epispadias and following repeated bladder neck surgery.

Definition of Failure

Failure has to be defined and may represent recurrence of the symptom of stress incontinence or occurrence of another type of incontinence.

1. Stress incontinence secondary to genuine stress incontinence, may be

Table 15.1. Results of colposuspension for mixed detrusor instability and genuine stress incontinence [6]

Preoperative	Postoperative	Result
Systolic DI-9	8 Systolic instability	6 Wet, 2 Dry
	1 Stable	1 Wet
Low compliant DI-4	3 Low compliant instability	Dry
	1 Stable	Dry

failure to correct the original anatomical lesion or is stress incontinence due to worsening of preoperative detrusor instability or occurrence de novo, of postoperative instability.

2. Presence of urge incontinence may represent deterioration of the preoperative symptom or its occurrence de novo. It is often strongly linked to detrusor instability.

3. Precipitation of voiding disorders leading to retention may cause symptoms of overflow incontinence (i.e. incontinence all the time) or stress incontinence.

4. Surgical trauma may cause a urinary fistula with incontinence all the time.

Failure can be considered according to whether it arises before, during or after surgery.

Preoperative Causes

The following are incriminated.

Previous Bladder Neck Surgery

Bladder neck surgery either to correct incontinence or anterior vaginal wall prolapse is a commonly cited cause of recurrence. Stanton et al. [1], Galloway et al. [2] and Hilton [3] have all shown that previous surgery is associated with a higher failure rate.

Detrusor Instability

Either low compliant or phasic (systolic) instability is likely to reduce the success rate of continence surgery [1,4]. Lockhart et al. [5] were the first to note that if a cut off of 25 cmH$_2$O detrusor pressure was taken, patients whose systolic contractions were below that had a lower chance of failure than those above. Wilkie et al. [6] studied 13 patients, nine with instability and four with low compliance instability (Table 15.1). Six patients with systolic instability remained wet and all the low compliant patients were dry.

Table 15.2. Results of three operations on patients with stable and unstable bladders [7]

Procedure	Urodynamic diagnosis	Cure (%)	Number of patients with high pressure instability
Burch	17 Stable	94	0
	6 Unstable	67	4
Stamey	19 Stable	74	0
	6 Unstable	17	0
Pereyra	22 Stable	91	0
	12 Unstable	66	2

A further study on 98 women by Pow-Sang et al. [7] confirmed the differences in cure rates between stable and unstable bladders and again noted the presence of "high pressure" instability amongst the failures (Table 15.2).

By contrast McGuire [8] and Blaivas and Olesen [9] felt that detrusor instability had no bearing on outcome provided that stress incontinence was objectively demonstrated. However, in neither of these papers are these statements confirmed by postoperative urodynamic studies.

Frozen/Drain-Pipe Urethra

This condition is frequently alluded to as a cause of failure and usually follows repeated bladder neck surgery for continence [9,10]. Little objective data are available as to its exact cause or nature. Usually more than one bladder neck operation has been performed. Radiologically, the urethra is fixed and immobile, sometimes visualised to be completely open. At operation, the urethra is surrounded by fibrous tissue and adherent to the back of the symphysis pubis. There is lack of hermetic closure and of urethral contractility.

Incorrect Diagnosis

Failure to correctly diagnose genuine stress incontinence as the cause of stress incontinence may lead to continence surgery being used to treat a variety of causes of the symptom of stress incontinence, e.g. detrusor instability, overflow retention, epispadias and urethral diverticulum. Having correctly diagnosed genuine stress incontinence, it is important to determine whether the bladder neck needs elevation or urethral resistance needs to be increased or both need to be attended to.

Age

Increasing age is a deleterious factor [1–3,10], because tissues are atrophic, do not heal properly and the hermetic closure of the urethra is ineffective. Patients are also less able physically and mentally to cope with major surgery.

Lowered Maximum Urethral Closure Pressure

It is a common clinical observation, that some patients with stable bladders and a well elevated bladder neck, are still not continent following surgery. It is assumed that the urethral resistance (pressure) is lower than normal. Sand et al. [11] using dynamic urethral profilometry, found a 54% failure rate in patients with a urethral closure pressure below 20 cmH$_2$O. This was a significant risk factor for patients under 50 years of age. Hilton [3] reviewed 10 patients treated by sling and 10 by Stamey operation, and found (like many others) that the maximum urethral closure pressure was unchanged and that although three patients who had failed surgery (two Stamey, one sling) all had preoperative closure pressures less than 20 cmH$_2$O, so had five patients who were successfully treated. Urethral pressure profilometry is consistently unreliable in the measurement of urethral resistance which may explain the disparity of findings here.

The other preoperative deleterious factors include chronic obstructive pulmonary disease, asthma and dosage with maintenance steroids. Obesity is not regarded as prejudicial to the cure rate although it may make surgery more difficult to perform and may increase postoperative morbidity.

Operative Causes

Incorrectly Chosen Operation

Choice of the wrong procedure is likely to lead to failure. The current argument for vaginal versus suprapubic procedures is now leaning in favour of the latter. Stanton et al. (unpublished observations) compared the anterior repair and colposuspension in a prospective study with randomisation of patients to either operation and to either of two surgeons: 54% of patients after anterior repair and 92% of patients after colposuspension were objectively cured at 2 years. Iosif [12] reported similar results although he only performed preoperative urodynamic studies and the postoperative results were subjective. Nevertheless, some clinicians are expert in the selection of patients and in their technique of anterior colporrhaphy and obtain better results [13]. The other controversy concerns performing a bladder neck elevating procedure when an increase in urethral resistance per se is required; as referred to earlier, the difficulty here lies in being able accurately to determine urethral resistance, which at present we are unable to do consistently.

Failure to Elevate the Bladder Neck

Bladder neck elevation is a fundamental goal of continence surgery. This is achieved either by "pushing" the bladder neck up using the vaginal route or "pulling" it up from above, as in the suprapubic and needle suspension operations. The "pulling up" and supporting the bladder neck in its new position seems more readily (and permanently) accomplished by a suprapubic operation. Hertogs and Stanton [14] using lateral bead-chain urethrocystography, showed that bladder neck elevation was directly related to the successful outcome of colposuspension surgery, whilst failure was related to inadequate elevation.

Table 15.3. Surgical causes of failure

Colposuspension	DI
Anterior repair	Poor elevation
Sling	Wrongly placed
	Erosion
	Voiding difficulty
Artificial urinary sphincter	Mechanical
	Erosion
Raz/Stamey	Suture breakage
Stamey	Migration of buffer

Suture Material

A variety of sutures have been used to secure bladder neck elevation. Catgut has been popular, only to be superseded now either by longer-lasting absorbable sutures such as the polyglycolic acid suture (Vicryl, Dexon) or permanent sutures (Tevdek, Nylon or Ethibond), as clinicians have become increasingly aware of the rapid loss of tensile strength of some absorbable sutures [15–17].

Patient's Tissues

The poorer success rate associated with surgery in the elderly, is partly due to atrophic change in their tissues, which cannot always be reversed by preoperative administration of oestrogen [18]. Some tissues are less able to resist stress and "wear and tear" as evidenced by the appearance of stress incontinence on exercise in nulliparous patients in their teens. Impaired collagen formation is one mechanism which is proposed.

The causes of failure relating to a specific operation are summarised in Table 15.3.

Postoperative Causes

Suture Breakage or Pulling Through

Breakage of a suture is more of a problem with needle suspension operations, where success depends on a single suture either side of the bladder neck, than the suprapubic operations where two to four sutures either side of the bladder neck are employed. The common history is a successful operation followed by a fall in the convalescent period with a tearing sensation and the development again of incontinence; hence the preference by many surgeons, for a non-absorbable suture.

Similarly, a bout of postoperative coughing or a fall can lead to a suture pulling through; this is more common in the elderly.

Detrusor Instability

The appearance of postoperative detrusor instability is unfortunately not to be foretold. It occurs either because it is not detected prior to operation, perhaps

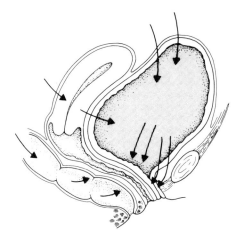

Fig. 15.1. Sagittal section of pelvis, to show direction of forces during intra-abdominal pressure rise acting on the bladder and proximal urethra.

owing to a lack of urethral resistance leading to incontinence occurring before instability can be encountered in the cystometrogram, or it is produced de novo by the surgery. Certainly the preoperative presence of urge incontinence associated with seeing running water is significant and often associated with instability. Postoperative instability is not due to obstruction in the female (although this is a common cause in the male), but likely to occur following repeated continence procedures [19]. Its appearance is bad news as 50% will continue to have symptoms of urge incontinence and frequency and will be resistant to treatment [20].

Loss of Compression by High Cystocele or Rectocele

Correction of a high cystocele and sometimes a rectocele, may lead to recurrence of stress incontinence as either the cystocele or rectocele now fails to exert pressure/force on the proximal urethra during a cough or on exertion (Fig.15.1). These are anecdotal clinical events not necessarily evaluated by scientific measurement.

Conclusion

Failure following surgery is likely to be due to one or more of the above factors. Some are observed clinical phenomena, others have been confirmed by objective measurement. The following questions need to be answered: what are the goals of continence surgery? how does one assess urethral function? can one be more effective in selecting the right operation for each patient? and can one foretell failure?

References

1. Stanton SL, Cardozo L, Williams J, Ritchie D, Allan V. Clinical and urodynamic features of failed incontinence surgery in the female. Obstet Gynecol 1978; 51:515–20.

2. Galloway N, Davies N, Stephenson T. Complications of colposuspension. Br J Urol 1987; 60:122–4.
3. Hilton P. A clinical and urodynamic study comparing the Stamey bladder neck suspension and sub-urethral sling procedures in the treatment of genuine stress incontinence. Br J Obstet Gynaecol 1989; 96:213–20.
4. Bates CP, Loose H, Stanton SL. The objective study of incontinence after repair operations. Surg Gynecol Obstet 1973; 136:17–22.
5. Lockhart J, Vorstman B, Politano V. Anti-incontinence surgery in females with detrusor instability. Neurourol Urodynam 1984; 3:201–7.
6. Wilkie D, Barzilai M, Stanton SL. Combined urethral sphincter incompetence and detrusor instability: does colposuspension help? Proceedings of the sixteenth annual meeting of the International Continence Society, Boston, 1986; 618–20.
7. Pow-Sang J, Lockhart J, Suarez A, Lansman H, Politano V. Female urinary incontinence: pre-operative selection, surgical complications and results. J Urol 1986; 136:831–3.
8. McGuire E. Abdominal procedures for stress incontinence. Urol Clin North Am 1985; 12:285–90.
9. Blaivas J, Olesen C. Stress incontinence: classification and surgical approach. J Urol 1988; 139:727–31.
10. Maggio A, Raz S. Why vesicourethral suspensions work or fail. In: Raz S, ed. Female urology. Philadelphia:WB Saunders, 1983; 299–307.
11. Sand P, Bowen L, Panganiba R, Ostergard D. The low pressure urethra as a factor in failed retropubic urethropexy. Obstet Gynecol 1987; 69:399–402.
12. Iosif C. Results of various operations for urinary stress incontinence. Arch Gynecol 1983; 233:93.
13. Walter S, Olesen K, Hald T, Jensen H, Pedersen P. Urodynamic evaluation after a vaginal repair and colposuspension. Br J Urol 1982; 54:377–80.
14. Hertogs K, Stanton SL. Lateral bead chain urethrocystography after successful and unsuccessful colposuspension. Br J Obstet Gynaecol 1985; 92:1179–83.
15. Lee R, Symmonds R, Goldstein R. Surgical complications and results of modified Marshall – Marchetti–Krantz for urinary incontinence. Obstet Gynecol 1979; 53:447–50.
16. Karran M, Bhatia N. Transvaginal needle bladder neck suspension procedures for stress urinary incontinence: a comprehensive review. Obstet Gynecol 1989; 73:906–14.
17. Stanton SL. Colposuspension. In: Stanton SL, Tanagho EA, eds. Surgery of female incontinence. Heidelberg: Springer-Verlag, 1986; 95–103.
18. Versi E, Cardozo L, Brincat M, Cooper D, Montgomery J, Studd J. Correlation of urethral physiology and skin collagen in post-menopausal women. Br J Obstet Gynaecol 1988; 95:147–52.
19. Cardozo L, Stanton SL, Williams JE. Detrusor instability following surgery for genuine stress incontinence. Br J Urol 1979; 51:204–7.
20. Steel S, Cox C, Stanton SL. Long term follow up of detrusor instability following colposuspension. Br J Urol 1985; 58:138–42.

Discussion

Swash: I do not understand detrusor instability and its relationship to these surgical procedures. As I understand it, detrusor instability is not necessarily present prior to the operation but can be there afterwards. Is that not important in relation to considering why operations do not work? If a patient is likely to be incontinent because of detrusor instability, that is surely of importance.

Stanton: The only factor that seems to be relevant is the number of previous operations. Patients with previous continence operations were more likely to develop instability than those without. We do not think it is obstructive because when we looked back at the figures the amount of obstruction was equal in the failed and the successful groups. It certainly did not stand out as a cause for instability.

These patients did not have any neuropathy and it still remains a mystery as to why this occurred.

Cardozo: One could raise hypotheses. It is possible that the detrusor instability was not identified preoperatively although it already existed. There is an impression – although this is not statistically proven – that more women who did develop postoperative detrusor instability have urgency and urge incontinence prior to the surgical procedure than those who do not. It would require a very large series to detect whether or not this was so.

In men with outflow obstruction, when the outflow obstruction is relieved the detrusor instability may go, and most of these operations, particularly colposuspension, are obstructive to some extent.

Because of previous surgery, a further operation might be disrupting the nerve supply so much as to cause detrusor instability de novo.

Quinn: In our small series, where the surgery has been inaccurate, or for one reason or another the supporting shelf underruns the trigone rather than the bladder neck and the indentation of the trigone by the supporting shelf can be clearly seen, detrusor instability can be produced de novo under those circumstances. We have objectively demonstrated this in only a very few patients, but it certainly was new in one patient and was persistently problematical in another, who had pre-existent detrusor instability.

Versi: Does the postoperative detrusor instability go away with time?

Cardozo: No. In fact the initial patients that I reviewed from Mr Stanton's colposuspensions were re-reviewed some five years later: they were still symptomatic in 56% of cases and the number that were available for review still showed detrusor instability.

Sutherst: And it did not go away when we undid the colposuspension.

Stanton: How long afterwards was it undone?

Sutherst: About 6 months.

Warrell: Detrusor instability would seem to be very much related to the technique of operation. The two things that characterise the sort of surgery that seems ideal from my point of view – either slings or colposuspension – is not to overdo them. The philosophy of the sort of surgery that I carry out is just to take the tension out of the anterior vaginal wall and to take out the slackness; and for a sling, again just to take the slackness out of the sling so that the degree of elevation is minimal.

Ever since Ms Cardozo wrote about postoperative testing in 1979 we have carried out postoperative provocative cystometry on slings, vaginal surgery and colposuspensions, and although a number of patients have developed the symptom of urgency, only one out of several hundred who have had slings or colposuspensions has developed detrusor instability that did not have it beforehand.

The other thing which would characterise my surgery but would appal many of my colleagues is the minimum of dissection for a colposuspension and the minimum of dissection for a sling. I would suspect that what I am not doing is upsetting the nerve supply.

The point that I am making is that detrusor instability as a postoperative phenomenon for the first time need not arise, certainly from the evidence I have from the 6 months follow-up.

Cardozo: Obviously surgical technique needs to be compared. The patients that I studied were operated on mainly by Mr Stanton, who does, or did, carry out, quite an extensive dissection.

In my own practice there are patients who have developed detrusor instability de novo following colposuspension, and also following a Stamey, which does not have dissection. So it cannot be related to just the one thing and may be multifactorial.

Hilton: I would agree with Mr Warrell that surgical technique and the extent of dissection are important features. I am not sure I would agree that disruption of nerve supply is likely to be of great relevance. I find it difficult to see how dissecting as peripherally as we do can produce a lesion like detrusor instability.

The other important issue is that of misdiagnosis before operation. I do not mean patients who have not been investigated preoperatively but patients in whom we have failed to demonstrate unstable contractions, either because we have got them on a good day, or more likely because these are patients who prior to their surgery have a very low urethral resistance. We know that patients with low urethral resistance can contract their bladder without any measured pressure rise. If they then have an operation that increases their urethral resistance, the detrusor contractions – which have been happening all along – become manifest as an increase in pressure. The way to detect this is to do the preoperative assessment using a Foley catheter rather than a standard Nelaton catheter, get them to cough and strain at bladder capacity and then pull the catheter down against the bladder neck so that they are obstructed. We have quite a few patients in whom we have demonstrated detrusor contractions by that means which were not present on a conventional cystometric analysis.

Stanton: That is fairly unphysiological. I would not like a catheter pulled on my bladder neck if I was conscious.

Hilton: I am sure Mr Stanton is right, but I am equally sure that we are missing the diagnosis of instability in a number of patients.

Stanton: How many of us stand the patient erect and then repeat cystometry routinely? I mean fill them and see nothing happening, then empty them, tip them erect and fill them again in the erect position.

Cardozo: Not routinely, but we do in some cases.

Stanton: I am led to believe this is the best method of picking up instability that is not detected in horizontal cystometry.

Cardozo: To do a second test picks up more. To do a complete second test will identify more detrusor instabilities than just to repeat the filling, because only 50% of patients manifest their detrusor instability on filling. This can be increased to 70% by erect filling but it can be increased even more by doing a completely separate test of filling and voiding.

DeLancey: How do we prove that someone does not have instability? If somebody has one episode of instability every couple of days, it would seem that only ambulatory monitoring for a week or so would really tell us that they do not have instability. I wonder if some of what we are picking up is just what Ms Cardozo is saying: the more times we sample them, the longer an observation period we have. This is why Mr McGuire has such very different data. If a woman says she is standing and feels the urge to urinate and a gush of water runs down her leg, he accepts that as detrusor instability even if the cystometrogram is normal. It may be the sampling error of what we use as the definition that gives rise to the different figures, but disproving detrusor instability without ambulatory monitoring is something we cannot do.

Cardozo: The problem is that she may be standing, give a cough and feel urine leak down her leg, and Mr McGuire would not have differentiated one from the other. That is why if we look back at some of the data that Mr Hilton showed, the American results of surgery for a woman with detrusor instability are uniformly higher than the cure rates in any other part of the world, because the diagnosis of detrusor instability is different in those centres where the surgery is performed and the follow-up is not the same either. This makes it difficult to compare data on both sides of the Atlantic.

Sutherst: I find this discussion about whether we are missing detrusor instability worrying. Recently we were doing two sets of tests. One involved filling patients up naturally and then on a different occasion doing cystometry. In some women who had quite marked detrusor instability during cystometry we found on a separate occasion they had quite stable bladders and could control huge amounts of urine. I suppose this is the nature of instability; sometimes it is there and sometimes it is not.

Cardozo: I think that is right, but there was a study some years ago doing repeat cystometrograms of symptomatic women and far fewer manifested detrusor instability on one occasion and not another than one would have expected. Cystometry may not be the perfect test but it is still a reasonable option to use at the moment.

Warrell: Can I change the focus of discussion and ask about the place of pelvic floor reconstruction or posterior repair in this problem of stress incontinence. How do surgeons assess the pelvic floor and how do they decide whether or not to repair it?

Stanton: I initially go on what the patient complains of. If she says that she has a prolapse feeling and that when she tries to empty her bowels it is incomplete and she can reduce it digitally, and if I see a rectocele or an enterocele I will repair those. I will also ascertain whether the patient is having an active sex life because this colours the degree to which one repairs them.

I am conscious of not wanting to do too many posterior repairs because of the dyspareunia that it can produce. Not all rectoceles produce problems; neither do all enteroceles. I am also influenced by whether I intend doing a Burch colposuspension, an operation that can lead to an increase in enteroceles, and therefore I may well prophylactically do something at the same time.

I also note that a repair to an enterocele or a rectocele, with nothing at all being done to the anterior vaginal wall or to the bladder neck, has been known to precipitate stress incontinence. I make my decision with the balance of all these things taken into account.

I am a little puzzled as to why incontinence can be produced, except on the theory that reducing the rectocele may then prevent transmission of the force coming forward.

Hilton: There seem to be two separate issues here. The first issue is: does the patient have any posterior wall prolapse, enterocele or rectocele prior to their stress incontinence surgery, and is any operation likely to make it worse – or make it arise de novo in a patient who did not have it before? Therefore should one undertake a repair, either of an existing prolapse or prophylactically?

The second issue is: does posterior repair have any role in terms of the restoration of urinary continence? Those are two completely separate questions.

With regard to the first, I tend to take the same stand as Mr Stanton. If the patient has a symptomatic rectocele or evident enterocele, that should certainly be dealt with in association with any colposuspension.

Cardozo: Before or after?

Hilton: Personally I would do it after, because I suspect it would be technically very difficult to do a colposuspension after doing an effective posterior repair. But I have no hard data on that.

As for the question of whether posterior repair has any place in the maintenance of continence, again I have no evidence to that effect. It is not something that I do as a matter of routine, either at the time of suprapubic surgery or for that matter at the time of anterior vaginal wall surgery.

Warrell: Two or three comments. First, if the fascial tissues of the patient with prolapse are genuinely different from the fascial tissues of the patient without prolapse, then clearly for that sort of patient one should use non-absorbable sutures with a suprapubic kind of approach.

If the bladder neck is under greater stress because the vagina is nearer vertical than horizontal, it would seem rational to me to try and reconvert the vagina to lie more parallel with the floor. This would minimise the strain on the anterior vaginal wall, and would minimise the chance of enterocele occurring.

My other point is that pregnancy damage, parity damage, is broad brush damage. It is never just bladder, or just rectum. As a philosophical approach there is a lot to be said for considering the pelvic structure as an interdependent set of units, and rather than saying, "I shall fix the urethra", one should say, "I shall do my best to restore this dynamic collection of structures back to as near normal as possible".

Stanton: There used to be a point of view among the older clinicians that they got a good cure of incontinence by doing a posterior repair together with the anterior repair because they tightened the levator ani muscle.

Warrell: Can I add something on the subject of painful intercourse following a posterior repair. Again this is technique dependent. If no skin is removed, dyspareunia never results.

Cardozo: It is the "registrar's ring", is it not, that causes the dyspareunia?

Warrell: I think it is the scar on the skin. Either one repairs the Denonvilliers' fascia or one sutures the levator muscles together, and these always move a bit and never cause it.

Cardozo: My patients have been inherited from one of the older school of surgeons who believed that he could cure incontinence by a pelvic floor repair and who always did a posterior repair when doing any incontinence procedure because he felt that it supported the anterior vaginal wall. The patients come back and they report that as being so, and so although I have no data on it I am led to believe that probably posterior wall support is relevant to the bladder neck.

Sutherst: Can I put in a good word for slings? As part of a prospective study on intraoperative ultrasound measurement, we compared slings with colposuspensions and our results were very much the same provided the anatomical result at the end of the operation was what we set out to achieve. We did not have all the complications which people have talked about in the past couple of days. But again it is a question of technique. I have no experience with "Silastic" slings and I do not know how they compare. Usually I use ox fascia.

Cardozo: The advantage of ox fascia is that it does not erode into the bladder in the same way as synthetic material.

Warrell: Why not use the patient's own tissue?

Stanton: It is never very good. It is why she is incontinent in the first place.

Warrell: It is muscle and endopelvic fascia, and there is nothing wrong with the abdominal wall fascia.

Cardozo: But if her skin collagen content is less than the equivalent woman who is not incontinent, then perhaps ox fascia, which contains more collagen, might be better.

Sutherst: I agree with Mr Stanton. I would not take out clumps of fascia from a woman with that sort of tissue deficit to start with. She is really in bad shape and she gets hernias.

Warrell: Not true. I do a lot of slings and have followed them up for as many as ten years, and their cure rate is as good as or better than any other abdominal procedure. The point is that ox fascia is replaced by the patient's own tissue, and so that is not a rational argument.

Cardozo: In my experience, slings have the highest complication rate of any operation for stress incontinence and therefore I try to avoid them.

Stanton: We need to qualify that by saying that they are the more complicated patients.

Warrell: I use it as a secondary and a primary procedure and we have done more than 400 without a fistula. The long-term voiding problem is of the order of 5% and is less now than it used to be. They do not produce detrusor instability; we have had two hernias, and really they are a trouble-free collection of patients.

Cardozo: Perhaps the difference is that I reserve slings for patients who have had previous surgery and who are likely to have complications and I also use inorganic material. Organic material does not seem to have the same complication rate and maybe we should be more interested in it.

Warrell: Patients' own abdominal wall fascia lasts certainly for 10 years plus, which is as long as I have followed them up, and does not leave them with an unacceptable incidence of abdominal wall hernias.

Cardozo: While we are talking about different types of operation it is important to mention urethrocleisis, which is not much used but which may be relevant in women who require narrowing of the urethra, particularly those who have a "drainpipe", fixed or frozen urethra. I wonder whether anyone has experience of this?

Stanton: Mr Mundy did mention this in an earlier discussion. He has not at the moment evaluated it so I think the question must remain open.

Cardozo: There is a need for some sort of reduction sphincteroplasty for women who have a urethra that will not be helped by support or elevation.

Warrell: I have experience of operating on more than 60 patients who, for want of a better term, have a fibrosed damaged urethra stuck by a lot of previous surgery. The operation which I have practised for 20-plus years I heard described by Turner Warwick as a reduction urethroplasty, which is to cut away completely the floor of the urethra vaginally and clear away what fibrous tissue one can from above and below and then bring in the patient's fat to try and prevent the adhesions forming again. Whether it works or not depends on what is left in the urethral muscle, in other words whether the reconstructed tube is reasonable muscle or very poor quality tissue. In this very difficult set of patients the 6-month cure rate was two out of three, so it was not very good.

Sutherst: Do you ever couple that with any bladder operation like making the first part of the urethra out of trigone or bladder flap?

Warrell: No. I have only a handful of these.

Stanton: I have done seven such urethroplasties involving bladder tube. They were characterised by blood loss and I might have got 60% improvement/cure. But I gave them up when the artificial sphincter became available because this seemed a much more consistent and certain procedure.

Cardozo: But artificial sphincters are now falling out of favour for women, particularly those with recurrent surgery, because they are the most difficult in whom to implant them and the most likely for them to erode.

Sutherst: Yet from Dr Scott's original reports on artificial sphincters, of all the groups he operated on the results were best in those very women.

Cardozo: It may be that in the early days he operated on women with less severe problems who are now being operated on by other methods.

Warrell: A woman with a lot of fibrous tissue and a matted urethra is probably incurable and our emphasis should be on preventing that sequence of events from happening.

Cardozo: Mr Stanton is still putting in sphincters.

Stanton: Yes. We have put in 22 or 23 so far and most of them are of the "knackered urethra" variety. They certainly are beset by problems of erosion and mechanical failure, but some are cured and they are very grateful. I shall continue to put them in until someone indicates that there is a better alternative.

Shah: Do urologists and gynaecologists see this problem from a different perspective? We have discussed problems with voiding and now we are discussing incontinence and it is always very interesting. Yet our clinical practices might be quite different. For instance, I never do a sling and neither does Mr Mundy. I wonder whether either we see things from a different perspective and treat the patients differently, or we see a different group of patients who require different treatment. That is something that perhaps we should consider, and look specifically at cases that we would perhaps approach in a different way.

Stanton: Is that answered by the comment that there are several ways to skin a cat, and we cannot say that the only way to manage this patient is by such and such operation. There is still a wide diversity of opinion.

The main difference that I see is that perhaps urologists are not so aware of the relevance of treating prolapse at the same time as they might manage sphincter incompetence.

The urologists are very jaundiced about slings (as are some gynaecologists); I notice more enthusiasm for Stameys, whereas some gynaecologists have great reservations about needle suspensions for certain categories of patients.

Shah: Patients with pipe-stem urethras and incontinence who have descent do well with cleisis and Pereyra procedures. I only do Pereyras; I do not do Stameys at all. If a patient has previously had a Stamey procedure that has failed and the tissue has welded, by mobilising as in a Pereyra Raz one can get very good elevation.

Cardozo: What difference does it make doing a Pereyra Raz or doing a Stamey?

Shah: It makes a significant difference to technique. With a Stamey one does not mobilise whereas with a Pereyra all the tissues adjacent to the urethra are mobilised, and the urethra can be elevated as far as one wants. It can be lifted as high as any colposuspension would ever achieve.

Stanton: I would agree. One should also make the point that what Mr Hilton is doing is not a pure Stamey but a much more effective procedure that is actually incorporating part of the anterior vaginal wall. Probably it should be re-named.

Hilton: We call them needle suspensions.

Everybody's approach to any of these operations is different, and to name them eponymously is a great mistake. We should be looking at needle suspensions as a whole.

Raz himself is now less enthusiastic for his modified Pereyra procedure than he was. In his earlier results he quoted 90% but he is now talking about 50% cures.

Cardozo: Needle suspensions fail because the stitches pull through the fascia. Having done Stameys and modified Pereyras I cannot see much difference in why they should fail. If the patient has inherently poor fascia then under certain circumstances they will pull through, and if not, they will not.

Shah: That argument does not apply to using fascia as a basis for the suspension. The fascia is used in a Stamey but it is not used in a Pereyra. In a Pereyra the para-bladder neck tissue and subvaginal tissue are used, and that is a much better basis for sutures than the endopelvic fascia, which is very thin in some elderly patients.

The other point is that there is not the same mobilisation. If the Stamey is expected to lift just by pulling on the endopelvic fascia, it will break, whereas with the Pereyra the formal mobilisation will lift it up. The Pereyra is the more logical operation but the results do not seem to be much better than the Stameys.

Stanton: The point about dissection is not so much the elevation but that it will prepare the ground for more fibrosis, so that when the suture eventually breaks then hopefully it will not all come down because there is fibrosis either side. Which I am sure is also part of the effect of the colposuspension.

Cardozo: But the fibrosis is not being produced where it is needed. The operation still only provides a narrow tract from the bottom to the top.

Stanton: I also bring into question how much elevation one is really trying to achieve. I do not elevate at all with the slings and I do elevate with the colposuspension. With the Raz or the modified Pereyra I elevate much less than I would do with the colposuspension. The bladder neck suspensions are one of the few operations, apart from the sling, where the surgeon has a certain amount of choice as to what the end point is. With the colposuspension it is pulled up and that is that. With any of the needle suspensions, either one does as some urologists do – they look down the cystoscope and when the bladder neck is closed then that is it – or one pushes up one's fingers and ties when it feels tight, or one does empirical bladder neck urethral closure and works it out on a process of clamping. We are trying to evaluate those.

Plevnik: What is important is to have some idea of how much it is elevated regardless of the control that is used. There should be some measure, perhaps in millimetres, irrespective of what method is used, of how much elevation is achieved. We have no real idea. One surgeon claims he is elevating very little and another that he elevates a lot. But by how much? Is it 2 mm, 1 mm, 5 mm?

Warrell: We are discussing why some operations succeed and why some operations fail. If cystometry and urethrometry are carried out postoperatively the one thing that does not change is the urethral occlusive forces, and one would expect not to change them because they are probably dependent more on striated muscle in the urethra than anything else. If this has been denervated, no surgery will change it. The one thing that can be changed is cough transmission and I would go along entirely with the concept, advanced some years ago, that an entirely different urinary control mechanism has been created. But what I do not know is whether in postoperative cough transmission it is possible to pick out the failures and say their postoperative cough transmission is poorer. Is it because the urethra is extremely feeble and the cough transmission does not compensate? Or is it because the urethra is fibrosed and cough transmission does not squash the urethra? Do we have any data on those three things? The only positive factor that anyone has come up with in success of operations as to why they work is the changed cough transmission.

Hilton: In the colposuspensions that fail, that enhancement in pressure transmission has not been achieved and the postoperative transmission profiles are exactly the same as the preoperative transmission profiles. Much the same applies to our results in relation to slings. In those that do not work, we do not get the enhancement in transmission. But with the slings in addition the resting profile is markedly eroded; that is to say that after an unsuccessful sling the urethra is a lot less than it was before an unsuccessful sling. Whether that is a result of fibrosis and pipe stemming we do not have the data to say.

Warrell: This must be very individual because in the many that we have done it did not make any measurable difference either way.

Hilton: The other data we have are in relation to the Stamey, where with success one gets marked enhancement on transmission even with what I would call relatively little tension on the sutures and relatively little elevation. But in the ones that fail immediately, that is to say they come back at three months wet and have never been dry, their transmission profiles are as they were preoperatively.

Warrell: Why?

Hilton: I do not know that I can answer that in terms of what happens at operation or whether there are lesser degrees of elevation. The ones that we can say something about are those who fail later, where our evidence is that those who are cured initially and subsequently relapse are also a group with lower preoperative pressures. They seem to be doomed from the outset. They are also a group in whom the initial transmission is somewhere in between the failures and the ones that maintain cure.

Quinn: I agree with Mr Stanton about support of the bladder neck in that many of the operations that we carry out do elevate the bladder neck by virtue of the technique that is employed. The bladder neck can be elevated with one side of a needle suspension procedure but that will not cure the patient's stress incontinence; it has to be supported in its new position. The support of a mobile urethra is as important as elevation itself.

Cardozo: That is not strictly true. Mr Worth showed that in certain patients one could cure with just one side of a needle suspension not with two, showing that elevation rather than support may be important.

Quinn: There are occasional patients. They will be very tightly elevated. Some women may be lucky in that when one side of a suspension breaks down they remain dry. Depending on the time course with which that happens fibrosis may be significant. But in patients with a mobile urethra, on the observations that I have made with the ultrasound, simply supporting them is often all that needs to be done.

General Discussion on Genuine Stress Incontinence

Cardozo: When Ms Shepherd discussed conservative measures she spoke about physiotherapy and about electrical stimulation but she did not discuss devices. It would be relevant, especially with certain new sponges on the market, to see if the group finds any real need for prophylactic devices against the occasional incontinence episode, such as tampons or any other obstructive device which is placed in the vagina, or perhaps even the urethral plug which the Americans are trying to investigate at the moment.

Does anyone have any views on this type of device for the occasional stress incontinence episode? Sponge tampons to go in the vagina are being sold very heavily. Should we be encouraging the idea, that three days of wearing and washing and then replacing is an appropriate treatment for genuine stress incontinence?

Sutherst: We have used them for 20 years in the occasional patient.

DeLancey: The one problem where it might be useful is the patient who has exercise incontinence, where it is a specific situation over a limited period of time and their continence is good at other times. If there were something that people could use during that period of time, that might be a role for it.

Cardozo: We have been using Lillets Super-plus for many years or advising patients to use them. I am not sure that the sponge tampons are any better and I certainly have not seen any data on them from experimental studies.

Shepherd: I understood that they caused less vaginal dryness. Cottonwool absorbs all vaginal secretion and may be associated with ulceration.

Warrell: Our experience is to echo Ms Shepherd. It is patient motivation. I have never had a patient who stuck to it long term. They all resented the change in their vaginal flora and the associated discharge.

Cardozo: What do we advocate then, for young women who have not yet completed their families? Should we operate on them and risk the recurrence of their incontinence? Do we advocate physiotherapy, which is a long-term training? Or should we ask them to wait for treatment until they have completed their families?

The use of oestrogens is another aspect that we have not fully discussed. It is important. I recently reviewed the literature for the Consensus Conference at the NIH and found that although many people advocate the use of oestrogens for women with genuine stress incontinence, there is no study which shows that oestrogens have actually cured genuine stress incontinence; that is, no controlled properly randomised study that has done. Do we use them? Are they good adjuncts for physiotherapy or for surgery? Or should the use of oestrogens not be advocated when the diagnosis is genuine stress incontinence?

Hilton: I think they do have a role. My own preference is to use oestrogens with a-stimulants, but there is no reason why they cannot be used as an adjunct with physiotherapy or with surgery for that matter, where it is only partially effective.

I would agree that they do not produce cure but I am not entirely sure that absolute cure is the only outcome measure we should be aiming for. Many patients are happy with symptomatic improvement and would use that as an argument to support their use.

Cardozo: Could the reason that oestrogens help perhaps be that they improve patients' general wellbeing and make them feel better, and they can then cope with their incontinence? Or is it that oestrogens raise the sensory threshold of the bladder, so that the women have fewer symptoms of nocturia, urgency and frequency, thereby improving their incontinence?

Hilton: It may be both of those things and it may be modification in urethral function as well. The evidence for a change in transmission is not very sound. Whether it is a change in vascularity and hermetic closure, which theoretically it ought to be but again nobody has been able to show, I am not sure. I suspect it is a combination of all of these things. These women feel generally better and are perhaps more inclined to put up with substantially more in the way of leakage. But as I said before, we have shown that these women do get a reduction in terms of perineal pad weight and so on.

Andersson: Could oestrogens improve tissue quality?

Cardozo: That is one of the hypotheses that we made when we studied skin collagen in incontinent women.

Warrell: All of these are questions, but we have no data on them.

Cardozo: That is why it is important to raise them. There are quite a lot of data on surgery now and why operations do not work, but there are few data on other methods of treatment and I think it is important because not all women are suitable for surgery.

Kulseng-Hanssen: We did a double-blind study with vaginal oestriol. We evaluated the patients with the pad test over 48 hours and visual analogue scales and found no differences between placebo and the oestriol.

Cardozo: Oestriol is a very weak oestrogen, and if it does not increase serum oestradiol or oestrone levels then it is quite possible that it does not have significant effect on the lower urinary tract.

Sutherst: The point was made that occlusive forces are the best method we have of measuring success. But whilst I agree entirely with the concept of pressure transmission, at the end of the day what one is trying to detect is fluid going down the urethra. We have a urodynamic test in which we can see change pre- and postoperatively by the extent of descent of urine down the urethra, which seems to be far more logical and sensible than invoking inferences from pressure transmissions or from occlusive forces.

Plevnik: There have been a number of references to pressure transmission as the objective means to assess the effects of surgery. I would completely disagree that it is objective. I think it is a complete artefact. It has been shown on many occasions, especially in the static UPPs and in the dynamic situation, that these artefacts can multiply, whether on second or third potency we do not really know. I would suggest that one should be very careful when talking about transmission. I believe that we are talking about the artefacts, and unless we really know what sort of artefact this is we cannot draw any conclusions.

Cardozo: On that note I shall sum up.
     I started by saying the importance of genuine stress incontinence is that we all have to deal with a lot of it and therefore it is appropriate that we should consider it in detail.
     Mr Warrell (Chapter 12) discussed the pathophysiology of genuine stress incontinence and explained two studies carried out at Manchester, saying that stress incontinence generally occurs in multiparous women with bladder prolapse.
     He also described studies on fascial damage in genuine stress incontinence and the possibility of weakness of collagen. (A more detailed summary of this contribution is given on p. 203.) The discussion which followed provoked many new ideas for further work in this field.
     Ms Shepherd (Chapter 13) discussed conservative treatment of genuine stress incontinence. She divided the treatment into pelvic floor exercises and electrical stimulation, and suggested a five-part programme of re-education involving education, demonstration, stimulation, facilitation and quantification, and suggested that if patients were unable to produce any pelvic floor contraction, they need to have electrical help before pelvic floor exercises would be useful to them. She also mentioned cones, which have become popular since 1985, and talked about the study of physiotherapeutic practices in England and Wales [1] showing that we need to have more standardisation of definitions and types of treatment in this conservative area of management of genuine stress incontinence.
     Mr Hilton (Chapter 14) discussed "Which operation for which patient?" He first tried to identify which patients should undergo surgery as being those least likely to respond to other forms of treatment, those most likely to respond to

surgery and those least likely to develop complications from surgery. He looked at which operations were appropriate in terms of clinical and urodynamic status and suggested that it is important to know how the operation works. He made the very important comment that many of us operate for the preference of the operator rather than necessarily looking at which patients need which operations. He then went on to discuss the relevance of low urethral closure pressures and the prediction of postoperative voiding difficulties from the preoperative investigations. He felt that colposuspensions were likely to be the most obstructive operations, followed by slings, then Stameys, and then repairs, and felt that it was important, therefore, to teach patients clean intermittent self-catheterisation prior to surgery if they were likely to develop postoperative voiding difficulties.

Mr Stanton (Chapter 15) looked at the difference between a recurrence of genuine stress incontinence and failure due to the coexistence of detrusor instability either before or after surgery. Mr Stanton stressed the need to avoid producing urge incontinence in those that had preoperative stress incontinence and to avoid the occurrence of voiding difficulties following surgery. He looked at failures in terms of preoperative complications, operative complications and postoperative problems, and his final summary was that low urethral pressure is a factor in the genesis of failure of surgery and we need to look at it further. Failure to elevate the bladder neck is important and postoperative detrusor instability is to be avoided and needs to be looked into further.

We discussed at some length the different types of operation which are used for genuine stress incontinence. There is no consensus as yet and this needs further work. The overall view of the session was that there are many different views on the management of this difficult problem and that we have not yet identified which types of treatment are suitable for which types of patient.

References

1. Mantle MJ, Versi E. English physiotherapeutic practice: stress incontinence. Neurourol Urodynam 1989: 8:352–3.

Section V
Detrusor Instability

Chapter 16

The Aetiology of Detrusor Instability

A. R. Mundy

Introduction

Detrusor instability is the term applied to the occurrence of involuntary detrusor contractions in an individual who has no evidence of neurological disease. Because these contractions commonly occur when the bladder is only partly full, they usually give rise to symptoms of frequency; because they create the sensation that the bladder is about to empty (which it is) they usually give rise to the sensation of urgency; and if the urethral sphincter mechanism is unable to resist the detrusor contractions, or if the individual has no sensory awareness of their occurrence, they give rise to urge incontinence. On urodynamic investigation the diagnosis is usually made by observing the presence of a detrusor contraction during bladder filling at a time when the patient is not attempting to initiate voiding. Such a contraction may occur spontaneously or on provocation, usually on coughing or changing from a lying to a standing position.

The aetiology of detrusor instability has not been fully elucidated. Involuntary detrusor contractions have been recognised for a long time as being associated with neurological disease and in such circumstances the term detrusor hyperreflexia is more correct. In the neurologically normal individual the only factor known to be associated with detrusor instability is bladder outflow obstruction in males [1]. The same association does not seem to occur in females, among whom bladder outflow obstruction causing a high detrusor pressure and a low urinary flow rate is rare. Thus although some cases of detrusor instability in males are secondary to bladder outflow obstruction, many, if not most instances in males and all instances of detrusor instability in females are idiopathic.

Neonates and toddlers do not void voluntarily in the generally accepted sense of the word. Most will learn to control their bladders during the first few years of life but some will never achieve this goal. For this reason and because many patients with frequency, urgency and urge incontinence have disorders of affect [2], many investigators have felt that detrusor instability is due to a loss of "central control" of the bladder.

Thus in general terms, the theories of causation of detrusor instability can be divided into two main categories: first, disorders of "central control" of the bladder and second, peripheral disorders as exemplified by bladder outflow obstruction in males.

The Physiology of Detrusor Contraction

This is not the place to discuss this issue in detail but there are several points of relevance to a discussion of the aetiology of detrusor instability.

It is clear from pharmacological studies that the excitatory stimulus to detrusor contraction is mediated by the pelvic parasympathetic nerves and that the excitatory neurotransmitter at the neuromuscular junctions within the bladder wall is acetylcholine [3]. In other animal species, other excitatory neurotransmitters have been proposed and there are grounds for believing, whatever the neurotransmitters may be, that an alternative neurotransmitter does exist [4]. In humans this is not the case.

Another fairly well established fact is that although there may be some co-ordinating activity in relation to detrusor behaviour in the sacral segments of the spinal cord, the main co-ordinating centre for initiating and maintaining detrusor contractions is in the rostral pons [5]. A normal detrusor contraction, therefore, is initiated in the rostral pons from which efferent pathways descend to emerge from the sacral spinal cord in the pelvic parasympathetic nerves which run forwards to the bladder where they lead to a release of acetylcholine at the neuromuscular endings within the detrusor layer of the bladder wall. It is not clear what stimulates the rostral pons to initiate a single and sustained co-ordinated detrusor contraction or why the bladder contracts in a co-ordinated fashion rather than fibrillating. It is also not clear whether or not there are inhibitory pathways that affect detrusor function. Nevertheless this seems to be the case and neuropeptides seem to be involved in mediating this inhibitory or modulatory effect [6].

If we return to our original postulate, stated at the end of the last section, that detrusor instability may be due to "central" or "peripheral" factors, then there may in theory be either excessive suprapontine excitation or reduced suprapontine inhibition (involving neurological pathways and neurotransmitters that are, as yet, only poorly understood). Alternatively, there may be excessive peripheral cholinergic excitation or reduced peripheral neuropeptide-ergic inhibition.

Histological and Histochemical Studies of Bladder Innervation

There have been various studies at a microscopic level of the innervation of the normal and unstable human bladder [7] and the normal and unstable bladder in various animal models, notably in the obstructed pig model devised in Oxford [8]. From these studies there is neither evidence of any increased excitatory parasympathetic neurological component in the bladder wall, nor indeed evidence of the presence of any alternative excitatory neurological mechanism [9]. Neither is there any evidence of increased afferent nerve endings which may be responsible for an increased peripheral excitatory stimulus to detrusor contraction. Thus it seems more likely that detrusor instability is due either to a central or to a peripheral reduction in inhibitory innervation or neuromodulation rather than to an altered excitatory component [10].

Indeed histochemical studies of the detrusor in obstructive instability in the pig model have shown that there is in fact a reduced number of cholinergic excitatory nerves and nerve endings [11], and in human studies of female patients with idiopathic detrusor instability there is a relative paucity of nerve endings containing vasoactive intestinal polypeptide (VIP) which is the main candidate for an inhibitory neurotransmitter involved in the control of detrusor contractile activity [10].

Physiopharmacological Studies of the Normal and Unstable Detrusor

The same groups that have studied idiopathic detrusor instability in humans and obstructive detrusor instability in the pig, have reported the results of physiopharmacological studies in these models as compared with normal. The conclusions in the various species vary only in detail.

In the human studies, detrusor muscle strips in vitro from patients with idiopathic detrusor instability show an increased response to direct electrical stimulation, a slight but definite increase in sensitivity to stimulation with acetylcholine and an increased sensitivity to low frequencies of electrical stimulation when compared with muscle from normal subjects [9].

In the obstructed pig model the response to electrical stimulation was less marked than in the human model and near normal, whereas the increased response to stimulation with acetylcholine was more marked than in the human study [12]. The Oxford group who studied the pharmacological aspects of the pig model concluded that their findings represented postjunctional supersensitivity due to partial denervation of the detrusor, which correlated very well with the findings of their colleagues in Manchester of a reduced number of cholinergic nerves in the obstructed unstable detrusor [11]. This finding of a relative cholinergic denervation has also been found in obstructed male humans [13,14].

The Guy's Hospital group that studied human idiopathic detrusor instability in women had one other interesting finding which was an increase in the incidence of spontaneous detrusor contractile activity when compared with normal (as distinct from that induced by electrical or pharmacological stimulation). Furthermore this spontaneous detrusor contractile activity, when it did occur in vitro, was of a greater amplitude and higher frequency than that seen in muscle strips taken from normal individuals [9].

In essence then, the unstable detrusor is supersensitive. Indeed the detrusor smooth muscle cell membranes could be said to be "unstable", possibly due to hypopolarisation when compared with normal, leading to enhanced spread of electrical activity from cell to cell [15]. It is thus more likely to respond to lower levels of stimulation, either electrical or pharmacological. In vivo this would correspond to a sensitivity to a lower level of neurological efferent activity or a lower level of acetylcholine release than would initiate detrusor contraction in a normal individual.

It is not, however, clear whether this "instability" or supersensitivity of the detrusor smooth muscle cell membrane is due to a relative cholinergic denervation or to a reduced inhibitory or modulatory neurological activity, possibly mediated by VIP. Given the proposal that acetylcholine and VIP may be released from the same nerve endings as "contransmitters" [16] the coincidental finding of a reduction in both elements, albeit in two different models, may well be significant.

The Cause of Instability or Supersensitivity of the Detrusor Smooth Muscle Cell Membrane

Unfortunately, although these histological, histochemical, physiological and pharmacological studies tell us what has happened to the final common pathway in detrusor instability, they tell us nothing of how these changes have developed. There is however, evidence to suggest that when detrusor instability is resolved by whatever means, the histological, physiological and pharmacological studies return towards normal, if not entirely to normal [6]. (Gosling, personal communication).

It is easier to hypothesise on the basis of the obstructed pig model. One might propose that bladder outflow obstruction leads to a reduction in the number of smooth muscle fibres and a corresponding increase in the collagen content of the detrusor as described by Gosling et al. [13]. It is not unreasonable to suggest that as a result of this reduction in the number of muscle fibres, there might be a corresponding reduction in the number of cholinergic and VIP-containing nerves, and that as a result of the inevitably uneven distribution of these changes, a partial denervation might occur which would lead in turn to denervation supersensitivity of the remaining muscle fibres.

Relief of bladder outflow obstruction might cause a reduction of the increased collagen content and an associated regeneration of smooth muscle fibres followed by a corresponding return towards normal of the neurological component. The physiological mechanism or mechanisms by which such a cycle of events might occur is unknown but presumably could occur at an entirely peripheral level. There are thus good reasons for invoking a peripheral aetiology for detrusor instability.

The grounds for proposing a central aetiology for detrusor instability are less satisfactory. There are three grounds for invoking a possible disorder of central control:

1. The facts that normal bladder control is a learned phenomenon and that some individuals never acquire it.
2. The association between increased bladder activity and anxiety, recognised in normal individuals by a desire to void under stress conditions.

3. The fact that some patients with detrusor instability can be cured of their symptoms, or at least improved, by programmes of bladder retraining [17].

Against these three facts it has to be said that anxiety makes a normal individual more aware of his or her bladder, but does not actually make it unstable, and that the other two factors simply confirm that the bladder is subject to voluntary control, both excitatory and inhibitory, which is well known. We are therefore no nearer a conclusion.

Conclusions

We do not know the aetiology of detrusor instability. We know that in detrusor instability the detrusor smooth muscle cell membrane is supersensitive and therefore more responsive to lower levels of stimulation than the levels that would induce a detrusor contraction in normal individuals. Why this should be the case is not clear but of the two postulated mechanisms, central and peripheral, the evidence seems stronger for a peripheral mechanism. On the other hand the two proposed mechanisms are not necessarily mutually exclusive and it is perfectly possible that several different mechanisms may be involved in different subgroups of patients.

References

1. Murray KH, Mundy AR. Obstruction and detrusor instability. In: Freeman RM, Malvern J. eds. The unstable bladder. London: Wright, 1989; 30–7.
2. Frewen WK. The significance of the psychosomatic factor in urge incontinence. Br J Urol 1984; 56:330.
3. Kinder RB, Mundy AR. Atropine blockade of nerve-mediated stimulation of the human detrusor. Br J Urol 1985; 57:418–21.
4. Burnstock G, Dumsday B, Smythe A. Atropine resistant excitation of the urinary bladder: the possibility of transmission via nerves releasing purine nucleotide. Br J Pharmacol 1972; 44:451–61.
5. Mundy AR. Clinical physiology of the bladder, urethra and pelvic floor. In: Mundy AR, Stephenson TP, Wein AJ, eds. Urodynamics: principles, practice and application. Edinburgh: Churchill Livingstone, 1984; 14–25.
6. Mundy AR. Neuropeptides in lower urinary tract function. World J Urol 1984; 2:211–15.
7. Gilpin SA, Gosling JA, Barnard RJ. Morphological and morphometric studies of the human obstructed, trabeculated urinary bladder. Br J Urol 1985; 57:525–9.
8. Sibley GNA. An experimental model of detrusor instability in the obstructed pig. Br J Urol 1985; 57:292–8.
9. Kinder RB, Mundy AR. Pathophysiology of idiopathic detrusor instability and detrusor hyperreflexia. An in vitro study of human detrusor muscle. Br J Urol 1987; 60:509–15.
10. Gu J, Restorick JM, Blank MA, Huang WM, Polak JM, Bloom SR, Mundy AR. Vasoactive intestinal polypeptide in the normal and unstable bladder. Br J Urol 1983; 55:645–7.
11. Speakman MJ, Brading AF, Gilpin CJ, Dixon JS, Gilpin SA, Gosling JA. Bladder outflow obstruction – a cause of denervation supersensitivity. J Urol 1987; 138; 1461–6.
12. Sibley GNA. The physiological response of the detrusor muscle to experimental bladder outflow obstruction in the pig. Br J Urol 1987; 60:332–6.
13. Gosling JA, Gilpin SA, Dixon JS, Gilpin CJ. Decrease in the autonomic innervation of human detrusor muscle in outflow obstruction. J Urol 1986; 136:501–4.
14. Harrison SCW, Hunnam GR, Farnman P, Ferguson DR, Doyle PT. Bladder instability and denervation in patients with bladder outflow obstruction. Br J Urol 1987; 60:519–22.

15. Foster CD, Speakman MJ, Fujii K, Brading AF. The effects of cromakalim on the detrusor muscle of human and pig urinary bladder. Br J Urol 1989; 63:284–94.
16. Hokfelt T, Everett B, Meister B, et al. Neurons with multiple messengers with special reference to neuroendocrine systems. Recent Prog Hor Res 1986; 42:1–70.
17. Frewen WK. A reassessment of bladder training in detrusor dysfunction in the female. Br J Urol 1982; 54:372–3.

Discussion

Andersson: At least in bladder overactivity associated with outflow obstructed we have some evidence for depolarisation. We have very good evidence for what was said about an increased sensitivity to release transmitter, although I do not know that we have it to the same degree in hyperreflexia and idiopathic detrusor instability.

If there is depolarisation, not only could we expect the various potassium channel openers to influence reversion of spontaneous activity – we know that this is effective in isolated muscle – but also we could expect that this should also be clinically effective.

Is there any clinical experience with this? That would very much support the hypothesis of depolarisation as the primary cause of the supersensitivity.

Mundy: First, the sensitivity to pharmacological stimulation comparing unstable with hyperreflexic bladders. The response, or rather the sensitivity to pharmacological stimulation, is much greater in the hyperreflexic bladder than in the unstable bladder.

Andersson: Yes. But were the unstable bladders associated with obstruction?

Mundy: No.

Andersson: They were idiopathic?

Mundy: Yes.

Andersson: But my question was related to a comparison between overactive bladders associated with obstruction and the other types.

Mundy: Comparing obstructed with non-obstructed?

Andersson: Yes.

Mundy: There are differences between the two. I did not want to go into that because the differences are really only differences of degree. They are enough to suggest that there is a difference between the unstable bladder that is obstructed and one that is not obstructed but we are not in a position to say that, because we do not have age-matched controls and the observations that we have presented here are only the observations made in women.

Andersson: I think it does. When we electrically stimulate rat bladders that have been obstructed, we have a decreased response to nerve stimulation. That is also because they have a decreased nerve function secondary to the obstruction.

If there is some pure nerve-stimulated response, then either the postjunctional supersensitivity would compensate for the decreased neuronal activity, or there would be nothing at all to be seen, or a decreased response. We see it in hypertrophic rat bladder muscle, which is why I wonder whether there is a difference in the results in the human bladder.

Mundy: There seems to be a difference in as much as the obstructed male bladder behaves more like the obstructed pig bladder than like idiopathic instability in females. In other words, with a dyssynergic bladder neck obstruction or benign prostatic hyperplasia in males, the results would be closer to the results we have seen in the pig model than what we have seen in idiopathic instability in females. The histological similarities would also be closer. Histologically these female bladders show no increased collagen deposition, no increased profile area of smooth muscle bundles, and no alteration in the smooth muscle to connective tissue relation.

We originally concentrated on idiopathic instability in females because it was the only way of being sure that there was no obstructive element, and therefore getting a group for study. But there are problems with studying obstructed men.

As to the cromecalin study – the drug that I mentioned that acts by opening potassium channels – this drug was studied a couple of years ago in the UK and in Scandinavia, but I believe nowhere else. The drug went as far as a Phase III study but was then withdrawn because of toxicological studies in baboons which at high doses got patchy myocarditis. The drug was never released and the company, and I am sure other companies, are now working on analogues. VRL34915 is a mixture of two drugs, one of which they think was the active one, and possibly the other was the one responsible for the myocarditis.

Before it was withdrawn, we did a study which was not a control study. We gave the drug to 20 patients who were waiting to have a clam ileocystoplasty for detrusor instability and who had failed to respond to oxybutynin, terodiline, and in some instances phenol injections as well, and they may in addition have had probanthine, cetiprin, indomethacin, and other drugs. They had all failed to respond to the only two drugs with any effect, namely terodiline and oxybutynin. Three patients withdrew because they got headaches with the drug, which was an established side effect of treatment. Of the remaining 17 patients, half showed a response and continued the drug after the study period until the time when it was withdrawn. Of the remaining eight patients, two stopped taking it when the study period was up and said they were better with voiding diaries that were improved but no urodynamic evidence of improvement, and the remainder showed no response.

So, crudely put, we could say that 50% of patients who had failed to respond to standard anticholinergic therapy showed a significant objective and subjective response.

Andersson: That is very promising.

We have performed with phenacetin a controlled double-blind crossover study in 10 patients with obstructive detrusor instability. We treated them for two weeks and we gave them a dosage which was the highest possible dosage usually recommended in hypertension; we could not go higher. We found absolutely no effect on cystometric variables or subjective symptom scores, but there are differences between drugs. We were very frustrated because the drug was very effective in our rat model; both drugs were equally effective.

I think it is too early to discard the principle, which is an interesting one. We hope that when new analogues appear new trials will be performed in all types of overactivity because there might be differences between the different types in response to a specific drug.

Sutherst: I agree entirely with the comments on the central pathways or central problems. But quite a lot of work has been done on abnormal psychological traits associated with detrusor instability, some of them seemingly showing that there is a cause and effect relationship with some types of psychological abnormality.

Is there any comment on those studies? Are they to be wiped out or is there some aetiological factor there also?

Mundy: Until we know why the bladder contracts as a single sustained contraction rather than fibrillates, why it relates so closely in most instances to specific intravesical volume, and what the mechanisms are by which activity gets down there, the only thing one can do is to start at the final common pathway and work upwards. The point I have made here, I hope, is that there is no need to go higher in studying the aetiology of instability, which is not to say that we cannot get it from there but we do not have to go up there to get a fairly good idea of how it is working. One can, as we all know, say that the bladder is under cortical control and if the cortex is deranged, it is not unreasonable that the bladder should be deranged. Most people who have psychiatric problems, or normal people who get anxious, do have increased frequency and urgency, but I know of no evidence that there is an increased association of instability. If an unselected group of 1000 anxiety-affective disorders or depressive disorders were to be compared with 1000 unselected controls, I do not know that there is any evidence that the incidence of instability is any different.

Sutherst: It has not been done that way round.

Warrell: Has any similar work been done in the adult enuretic, who I suppose is the prime example of failure to inhibit in the absence of gross neurological disease, and who by daytime will have demonstrable failure to inhibit in a cystometric study?

Mundy: Does that mean bedwetters with no urodynamic abnormality?

Warrell: If adult enuretics are tested with provocative cystometry we can demonstrate a failure to inhibit in over 90%.

Mundy: That is a fairly controversial statement.

Warrell: I do not think that it is.

Mundy: Does enuretics mean bedwetters?

Warrell: Yes.

Mundy: Without daytime symptoms?

Warrell: Some of these will have daytime symptoms.

Mundy: If they have daytime symptoms I would agree. Indeed it may be higher than 90%. If they have bedwetting but no daytime symptoms, then I would say that 90% of them would probably be normal. But that is not to answer the question, and I do not think that anybody can answer the question.

To the best of my knowledge there have been odd reports that have looked at one or two, but usually only one individual parameter was being studied: for example, there was a study of the effect of naloxone on adrenergic receptors, and there have been one or two others. But the only two studies that I know of that have looked sequentially at a number of factors were the two I mentioned; on idiopathic instability in humans and obstructive instability in pigs.

Warrell: And the second question, why should there be partial denervation in a patient who is neurologically normal?

Mundy: I do not know the answer to that. I had thought that as a result of the increased work the bladder had to do and partial decompensation, there would be fibrous replacement of the detrusor and that denervation would follow pari passu with the loss of the smooth muscle cells. Smooth muscle cells are quite capable of manufacturing collagen and indeed of turning histologically into fibroblasts. The only snag with that theory is that there is recent evidence to show that they get denervation first and then a change in the smooth muscle thereafter.

We know that if we obstruct a pig, then within three months the first histological or electron microscopic change we get is a 50% reduction in the number of nerve terminals and of cholinergic neurons in the bladder.

Warrell: Is the fact that there is partial denervation a bit of a nudge towards looking higher up in bladder control?

Mundy: Not necessarily. Professor Andersson would probably be better able to comment, but I think that a change in afferent activity within the bladder could probably be provoked from tension receptors in the detrusor layer, having a direct effect locally first of all, and then maybe a secondary effect from up above. But "up above" may be at ganglionic level outside the bladder, or at sacral segment level, before getting up to the pons and higher. Indeed perhaps it goes in stepwise fashion.

But I am just theorising.

Chapter 17

Medical and Surgical Treatment

L. D. Cardozo

Introduction

Treatment of detrusor instability remains unsatisfactory. Many different types have been tried and although few women are ever completely cured, many may have their symptoms improved by one or other of these therapies. The most troublesome symptoms of detrusor instability vary from patient to patient and from time to time. Not all patients will require treatment and some will only need to use simple measures when their symptoms are worst. Many women with detrusor instability benefit from an explanation of their condition and are then able to control their own symptoms by behaviour modification such as drinking less fluid and avoiding tea, coffee and alcohol. For more severe symptoms the following methods of treatment are available: (a) drugs, (b) bladder retraining, (c) phenol injections, (d) augmentation cystoplasty.

In the past other forms of treatment which have been tried but which have not stood the test of time include vaginal denervation [1–3], selective sacral neurectomy [4], cystodistention [5–7] and bladder transection [8]. They all give some short-term benefit in carefully selected cases but may produce significant morbidity and are rarely used nowadays.

Drugs

Mode of Action

Neurotransmitters and drugs combine with cell receptors to initiate a series of biochemical and physiological changes. The neurotransmitters present in the detrusor (in different proportions at different points) are acetylcholine at the preganglionic sympathetic, postganglionic parasympathetic and somatic nerve endings; and noradrenaline at the postganglionic sympathetic neurons.

Stimulation of the parasympathetic pelvic nerves causes a sustained detrusor contraction. Atropine, which is a muscarinic blocking agent, only partially blocks this bladder response. The reason for the relative "atropine resistance" is not properly understood, but may be due to the presence of a non-cholinergic, non-adrenergic neurotransmitter. Two possibilities have been suggested: these are purinergic nerves with adenosine triphosphate (ATP) as the neurotransmitter [9] and peptidergic nerves with vasoactive intestinal polypeptide (VIP) as the neurotransmitter [10]. This obscure neurotransmitter may account for the fact that muscarinic blockers given to patients with detrusor instability are sometimes relatively ineffective.

Evaluation of Drug Therapy

The assessment of drugs used in the management of detrusor instability is problematic. The experimental effect of drugs in vitro may be different from the effect in vivo and animals used to test a preparation may be more or less sensitive than humans. In addition drugs can act at more than one site and have different short- and long-term effects. If a drug has multiple effects they may occur at different times; and the rate of absorption and efficacy depend on the route of administration and the state of the tissues. Unfortunately many drug trials fail to take into account the weight of the patient, the rate of absorption, and the blood levels following administration.

Patients with detrusor instability vary considerably in the severity of their symptoms, expectation, compliance and tolerance to side effects. It is difficult to compare the results of treatment with a specific drug in different locations as the method of assessment may differ. In addition there is known to be a high placebo response rate amongst patients with detrusor instability. Using subjective assessment at least 35% of patients respond to a placebo [11]. In a study by Meyhoff et al. [12] comparing emepronium bromide, flavoxate hydrochloride and placebo, 47% of women actually prefer placebo. And the incidence of side effects among patients taking placebo for urge incontinence is also high with 27% reporting adverse events, mostly anticholinergic in nature [13]. The major categories of drugs used to treat detrusor instability are:

1. Drugs which inhibit bladder contractility
   a) Anticholinergic agents
   b) Musculotropic relaxants
   c) Tricyclic antidepressants
   d) Calcium channel blockers
   e) Beta-adrenergic agonists
   f) Alpha-adrenergic antagonists
   g) Prostaglandin inhibitors
2. Drugs which increase outlet resistance
   a) Alpha-adrenergic stimulators
   b) Beta-adrenergic blockers

3. Drugs which decrease urine production
    Antidiuretic hormone analogues
4. Drugs which improve the state of the tissues
    Oestrogens

In clinical use not all of these categories of drugs are helpful. Those which increase outlet resistance are rarely effective on their own as the main symptoms of detrusor instability (urgency and urge incontinence) are due to detrusor contraction rather than urethral weakness. However, they may be helpful in conjunction with oestrogens especially when detrusor instability and urethral sphincter weakness coexist.

Anticholinergic Agents

Atropine, propantheline (probanthine) and emepronium (cetiprin) produce competitive blockade of acetylcholine receptors at postganglionic parasympathetic receptor sites. They have the typical side effects of dry mouth, blurred vision, tachycardia, drowsiness and constipation. Nearly all the drugs which are truly beneficial in the management of detrusor instability produce these unfortunate, unwanted side effects to a lesser or greater extent. This makes double-blind trials difficult. In addition the severe side effects produced by atropine make it unusable for this indication in clinical practice.

Propantheline bromide is relatively inexpensive and in in vitro studies has a direct antimuscarinic binding potential similar to atropine [14]. The recommended adult dose is 15–30 mg four times daily, but in practice this may be inadequate and it is possible to prescribe up to 90 mg four times daily providing the drug is introduced slowly to minimise side effects. Absorption from the gastrointestinal tract is improved if the drug is given before meals [15]. Parenteral drug studies have shown that propantheline does suppress detrusor contractions in some patients and these will usually respond well to oral therapy [16]. Unfortunately there are no good recent clinical trials of this drug. In general it is tolerated by patients but unfortunately it is also often ineffective. It is most helpful for those patients whose main problem is frequency of micturition.

Emepronium bromide was widely used for many years. However, it has now been withdrawn from the market in the United Kingdom. Emepronium carrageenate is available in some European countries and is still quite a useful drug [17].

Musculotropic Relaxants

Oxybutynin chloride (cystrin, ditropan), dicyclomine hydrochloride (merbentyl) and flavoxate hydrochloride (urispas) are direct-acting smooth muscle relaxants which predominantly act on the bladder. Their side effects are anticholinergic.

Oxybutynin

This is probably the most effective drug currently available for the treatment of detrusor instability. Unfortunately as yet it can only be prescribed in the United

Kingdom on a "named patient" basis. When given in the maximum recommended dose of 5 mg three times daily many women find the side effects less tolerable than the symptoms of detrusor instability. The worst problem is a very dry mouth and throat with a lingering bad taste. Some women manage to achieve symptomatic relief on lower doses with fewer side effects.

In the original placebo-controlled study [18], 30 unselected patients with detrusor instability underwent treatment. Symptomatic improvement was achieved in 69% of those receiving oxybutynin and only 8% receiving placebo. There was also urodynamic improvement in half the patients on oxybutynin. Seventeen of the patients suffered side effects while taking oxybutynin, five so severe that they had to discontinue therapy. However, it is impossible to perform a truly double-blind trial of oxybutynin as patients can always tell when they are taking it because of the unpleasant side effects.

In a double-blind crossover placebo-controlled trial of oxybutynin in the management of postmenopausal women with detrusor instability we have found a significant improvement in the symptom of urgency, but at the expense of an increase in residual urine volume and a very high incidence of intolerable side effects [19]. Recently Baigrie et al. [20] reviewed 192 consecutive patients for whom oxybutynin was prescribed in a district general hospital. They found that 57% derived benefit while 76% noted side effects, none of which was dangerous or irreversible. Holmes et al. [21] compared oxybutynin with propantheline in a crossover variable-dose trial. They found that only oxybutynin improved symptoms and cystometry but the number of patients in the study was small and the dose of propantheline low (90 mg day^{-1}).

Despite its problems oxybutynin is useful in the day-to-day management of patients with detrusor instability. It is particularly good for those patients with severe urgency and urge incontinence. Unpleasant side effects can be minimised by starting on a low dose and increasing it gradually. There is a noticeable difference between young and older women in their response to oxybutynin. Those over the age of 75 years may only require 3 mg a day as effective treatment for symptoms of urgency and frequency of micturition.

Dicyclomine Hydrochloride

This has been proposed as an alternative to oxybutynin when the side effects of the latter are intolerable. Dicyclomine is usually used to treat gastrointestinal disorders and has very few side effects but it is also considerably less effective than oxybutynin in the management of detrusor instability. Awad et al. [22] showed that 24 of 27 patients improved symptomatically when given dicyclomine 20 mg three times daily and that parenteral administration of 20 mg intramuscularly caused an increase in bladder capacity. However, this drug has never gained real popularity, maybe because the doses prescribed are inadequate [23].

Flavoxate Hydrochloride

This has been used for many years but its popularity is really unfounded. Briggs et al. [24] reported that flavoxate was of no proven benefit in the management of detrusor instability. There is no good evidence that it is effective either orally or intravenously [25].

Tricyclic Antidepressants

Imipramine Hydrochloride (Tofranil)

These preparations have a complex pharmacological action. Imipramine has anticholinergic, antihistamine and local anaesthetic properties. It may also cause increased outlet resistance due to peripheral blockage of noradrenaline uptake, and acts as a sedative. The side effects are anticholinergic with tremor and fatigue.

Imipramine has been used for nocturnal enuresis in children for a long time but is also effective in adults. Castleden et al. [26] showed that six of ten incontinent elderly women became dry with imipramine and they recommended that doses of up to 150 mg at night could be used, although the usual dose is 50 mg twice daily. Raezer et al. [27] found that imipramine was more effective when used in conjunction with an anticholinergic agent such as propantheline. Imipramine is the most effective treatment of nocturia and nocturnal enuresis. It is also helpful in the management of incontinence which occurs at orgasm which may be a difficult symptom to treat.

Calcium Channel Blockers

Terodiline (micturin), flunarizine and nifedipine limit the availability of calcium ions which are required for the contractile process. These drugs also have some anticholinergic action. The side effects are not usually severe but include hypotension, headache, dizziness, constipation, nausea and palpitations. The use of calcium channel blockers in the management of detrusor instability is relatively new.

Terodiline

This is currently the most popular drug in the United Kingdom for the management of urge incontinence. The preliminary work was carried out in Scandinavia. Ulmsten et al. [28] showed that ten out of twelve women studied in a double-blind placebo-controlled crossover trial improved symptomatically and urodynamically while taking terodiline. In a longer-term study they found that all 12 women reported subjective improvement. The dose is 25–50 mg per day in divided doses. Side effects are less severe than those caused by oxybutynin but some patients do complain of a dry mouth on the higher doses.

Among 70 patients who completed a variable-dose multicentre trial of terodiline [29], there were significant improvements in frequency, incontinence episodes and volumes voided in the terodiline group as compared to the placebo group. Significantly more patients (62%) in the treated group considered themselves improved than in the control group (42%). The incidence of anticholinergic side effects was greater in the terodiline group. However, there was no difference in urodynamic parameters following treatment.

Other Drugs Which Inhibit Bladder Contractility

Beta-adrenergic agonists such as clenbuterol and terbutaline stimulate the beta-adrenergic receptors in the bladder and have been shown in animal studies to increase bladder capacity. Their role in the management of detrusor instability is uncertain although there has been one favourable study reporting subjective and objective improvement with clenbuterol [30].

Although both alpha-adrenergic antagonists and prostaglandin synthetase inhibitors have been tried in the management of detrusor instability and have been shown to reduce bladder contraction in animal studies, neither of these groups of drugs is currently used in the management of this condition.

Drugs Which Increase Outlet Resistance

The smooth muscle of the bladder neck contains many alpha-receptor sites which if stimulated increase outlet resistance. Ephedrine, pseudoephedrine (sudafed) and phenylpropanolamine (ornade) are more likely to be helpful in cases of genuine stress incontinence than in detrusor instability. They cause unpleasant side effects such as hypertension, anxiety and insomnia if given in large doses and tachyphylaxis develops so these preparations are not helpful in the long term. Beta-adrenergic antagonists such as propranolol are thought to potentiate the alpha-adrenergic effect thus increasing outlet resistance but there is no good evidence to show that these drugs are useful in any type of urinary incontinence.

Drugs Which Decrease Urine Production

DDAVP (synthetic vasopressin) can be given at a dose of 20–40 µg intranasally as spray or snuff at bedtime. This dose has been shown to decrease urine production by up to 50%. It can be used for children or adults with nocturia or nocturnal enuresis, but obviously it cannot be used to control diurnal frequency as well. Ramsden et al. [31] showed that DDAVP was superior to placebo in reducing the number of wet beds in a series of 21 severe enuretics; and Hilton and Stanton [32] found that the number of night-time voids in 25 women with nocturia could be reduced by both placebo and DDAVP but that the latter was significantly more effective. DDAVP is definitely helpful for a small group of patients with troublesome nocturnal symptoms but is contraindicated in those who have hypertension, ischaemic heart disease or congestive cardiac failure. It has recently been shown that it is safe to use DDAVP in the long-term treatment of nocturnal enuresis [33].

Drugs Which Improve the Tissues

Although there are abundant oestrogen receptors in the urethra they are sparse in the bladder itself. Many authors have shown that oestrogen deprivation following the menopause causes changes in all functional layers of the urethra [34]; but no studies have actually proved that oestrogen therapy is helpful in the management of urinary incontinence due to detrusor instability. However, sensory urgency which may be due to atrophic changes does respond to oestrogen replacement therapy.

Which Drug, Which Patient?

It is difficult to know how to select the most appropriate drug for each patient. Patients respond differently to the various preparations available and it is always

Table 17.1. Possible order of preference of commonly used drugs in detrusor instability

	Prop	Oxy	Imip	Terod	DDAVP
Frequency	1	2		3	
Nocturia		3	1		2
Urgency		1		2	
Urge incontinence		1		2	
Nocturnal enuresis		3	1		2
Coital incontinence		2	1		

Abbreviations: Prop, propantheline; Oxy, oxybutynin; Imip, imipramine; Terod, terodiline.
1, 1st choice; 2, 2nd choice; 3, 3rd choice.

worth remembering that if a drug does not work as well as one would expect it to then the dose may need to be increased or it may be helpful to combine it with another preparation. Table 17.1 shows a possible order of preference for the most commonly used drugs in this condition.

Bladder Retraining

Continence is a learned phenomenon. Most individuals become dry during infancy when they are "potty trained" and remain that way for the rest of their lives. However, it is reasonable to suppose that if continence can be learned during infancy it could also be learned or relearned during adult life. Various different forms of bladder re-education have been tried, including (a) bladder drill; (b) biofeedback and (c) hypnotherapy.

Bladder discipline was first described as a method of treating urgency incontinence by Jeffcoate and Francis [35] in the belief that this type of incontinence was exacerbated or even caused by underlying psychological factors. Since then Frewen [36,37] has shown that many women with detrusor instability "are able to correlate the onset of their symptoms to some untoward event" which can be identified by taking a careful history. He has shown that both inpatient and outpatient bladder drill are effective forms of treatment for many such women.

The technique for performing bladder drill has been established by Jarvis [38] and is shown below:

1. Exclude pathology and admit to hospital
2. Explain rationale to patient
3. Instruct to void every one and a half hours during the day (either she waits or is incontinent)
4. When one and a half hours is achieved increase by half an hour and continue with two hourly voiding etc.
5. Normal fluid intake
6. Fluid balance chart kept by patient
7. Meter success
8. Encouragement from patient, nurses and doctors

Jarvis and Millar [39] performed a controlled trial of bladder drill in 60 consecutive incontinent women with idiopathic detrusor instability. They showed the following inpatient treatment results: 90% of the bladder drill group were continent and 83.3% remained symptom free after six months. In the control group 23.2% were continent and symptom free due to the placebo effect. Despite the excellent early results it has been shown that up to 40% of patients relapse within three years [40].

When bladder drill is successful subjective improvement may precede objective conversion to stability by up to three months. Those patients who have stable cystometrograms following treatment are no less likely to relapse than those who do not. When patients do relapse drugs are more likely to be successful than repeat bladder drill.

Biofeedback

Biofeedback is a form of learning or re-education in which the subject is placed in a closed feedback loop where information about a normally unconscious physiological process is made available to her in the form of an auditory, visual or tactile signal. The objective effects of biofeedback in the treatment of detrusor instability can be recorded on a polygraph trace but the subjective changes may be difficult to separate from the placebo effect. This technique was described by Cardozo et al. [41]. Of a group of 30 women with idiopathic detrusor instability 80% were initially cured or improved, but after five years the relapse rate was high [42]. Biofeedback helps by giving the patient a better understanding of bladder function and of her particular bladder problem. It does not require hospital admission although trained enthusiastic personnel are required to perform the training.

Millard and Oldenberg [43] used bladder training and/or biofeedback to treat 59 women with detrusor instability or sensory urgency. They also employed supportive psychotherapy or drugs. They stated that biofeedback was undoubtedly the most useful of the techniques. Combined behavioural treatment with biofeedback has been used in the management of elderly outpatients with improvement in at least 80% [44]. More recently the successful use of bladder neck electric conductance with biofeedback has been reported in a small series of women with idiopathic detrusor instability [45].

Hypnotherapy

Freeman and Baxby [46] treated 61 women with idiopathic detrusor instability using 12 sessions of hypnosis over a period of one month. The initial results were promising but at two-year follow-up few patients were symptom free. This high relapse rate is in keeping with other forms of behavioural intervention.

Non-Surgical Non-Pharmacological Intervention

Various newer techniques have been tried in the treatment of detrusor instability but they cannot be recommended for routine clinical practice until they have been further evaluated. Anal or vaginal electrical stimulation may inhibit spontaneous detrusor contractions and represents a therapeutic alternative for the management of this condition [47]. The neurophysiological basis for the resulting prolonged bladder inhibition remains unclear. However, this technique is safe and inexpensive and can be performed by specialist nurses. A success rate (cure or improvement) of 77% on objective follow-up at one year after an average initial treatment regimen of seven sessions has recently been reported [48].

Acupuncture has also been tried in the management of detrusor instability and sensory urgency. In a recent study Philp et al. [49] reported that 69% of 16 patients with idiopathic detrusor instability were cured or improved after treatment but only one converted to a stable bladder.

All these forms of "bladder training" are advantageous because there are few unpleasant side effects and no patient is ever made worse. Mild to moderate detrusor instability can be cured or significantly improved by re-educating the bladder. However, the relapse rate is very high and although this type of treatment avoids the mortality and morbidity associated with surgery and the side effects of drug therapy it requires skilled personnel and is time consuming for both the patient and the operator.

Transvesical Phenol

This treatment was originally described for patients with detrusor hyperreflexia [50], but has since been used for women with idiopathic detrusor instability also. Through a 30 degree cystoscope a 35 cm semi-rigid needle is inserted under the bladder epithelium midway between the ureteric orifice and the bladder neck and 10 ml of 6% aqueous phenol is injected on each side. The largest published series [51] reported an improvement for at least one year in 88 of the 116 women treated. The response to treatment was best in those women over the age of 55. A number of side effects and complications were reported, of which transient postoperative haematuria was the most common, but there was no significant morbidity. In a recent study Cameron-Strange and Millard [52] reported a 63% response to transvesical phenol in a mixed group of 40 patients with refractory detrusor instability of whom 35 were followed up for more than 18 months. The only complication they reported was one vesicovaginal fistula following radiotherapy.

Other workers in the field are less enthusiastic about the long-term results of transvesical phenol and more concerned regarding the incidence of significant complications [53]. Wall and Stanton [54] have treated 28 women with refractory urge incontinence. After the first injection, eight (29%) responded, all of whom relapsed during follow-up, and after a second injection only three out of eleven responded and one developed a vesicovaginal fistula. With these recent diametrically opposed views it is difficult to know whether transvesical phenol will continue to be used in the treatment of detrusor instability. Subtrigonal 50% ethanol has also been injected extravesically in a small series of 10 women with severe detrusor instability [55]. This treatment apparently cured or improved seven of the patients at two years but three vesicovaginal fistulas developed and one required urinary diversion.

Surgery

Different surgical techniques have been described for the treatment of detrusor instability but currently the most popular operation is the "clam" cystoplasty [56]. The bladder is bisected almost completely and a patch of gut (usually ileum) equal in length to the circumference of the bisected bladder (about 25 cm) is sewn in place. This operation often cures the symptoms of detrusor instability but inefficient voiding may result. Patients have to learn to strain to void and some have to resort to clean intermittent self-catheterisation, sometimes permanently. There are problems associated with the use of gut as a urinary reservoir. Mucus in the urine can cause outflow obstruction but it has recently been shown that cranberry juice reduces the amount of mucus [57]. Disordered acid–base balance, in the form of a metabolic acidosis, may result and there is an increased risk of cancer developing in the gut segment because of the exposure of the gut mucosa to nitrosamines [58].

For those women with severe detrusor instability or hyperreflexia for whom all other methods of treatment fail, it may be worth considering urinary diversion via an ileal conduit as a last resort. This is particularly helpful in young disabled women, for example those with multiple sclerosis, as it is often easier for them or their carers to empty a bag rather than change wet underclothes or incontinence pads.

Mixed Incontinence

The appropriate management for women with mixed stress and urge incontinence remains a contentious issue. In a series of 603 women treated surgically for stress incontinence 30% also had detrusor instability (172 preoperatively and 23 postoperatively) [59]. Eight weeks postoperatively 4% (14% of those with detrusor instability) were still incontinent. Unfortunately the results of this study are somewhat difficult to interpret as five different operations were employed, an unconventional definition of detrusor instability was used and assessment was subjective only. But the results would imply that routine bladder neck surgery is helpful in the management of women with mixed stress and urge incontinence.

On the other hand Karram and Bhatia [60] treated 52 women with coexistent genuine stress incontinence and detrusor instability. Of these, 27 underwent a colposuspension and 25 were given oxybutynin together with imipramine and/or oestrogen. Of those who were surgically treated 59% were cured and 22% improved whereas of those who were given medical treatment 32% were cured and 28% improved. They suggested that medical management reduces the need for surgical intervention.

As the results of conventional bladder neck surgery are generally considered to be poor in women with detrusor instability then it would seem appropriate to try medical treatment first in the hope that this will avoid the need for surgery and only to resort to surgery with the understanding that any symptoms of urgency and frequency which the patient experiences are less likely to be cured.

General Management

All women who are incontinent benefit from advice regarding simple "self-help" measures which they can take to alleviate their symptoms. Many women drink far more than they need and they should be advised to limit their fluid intake to one litre per day and to avoid tea, coffee and alcohol if these exacerbate their symptoms. The use of drugs which affect bladder function, such as diuretics, should be reviewed and if possible these should be stopped. If there is coexistent genuine stress incontinence then pelvic floor exercises with or without electrical treatment such as faradism may be helpful.

For younger women who leak only when exercising, a tampon in the vagina during sports may be helpful. Peri- or postmenopausal women often benefit from hormone replacement therapy which is unlikely to cure the problem but may increase the sensory threshold of the bladder and make the urinary symptoms easier for the patient to deal with. The most degrading aspect of urinary incontinence for many women is the odour and staining of their clothes and this can be helped by sensible advice regarding incontinence pads and garments.

Conclusion

Detrusor instability is a common condition which adversely affects the quality of life of people of all ages. It is characterised by multiple symptoms which are embarrassing and may cause an increasingly restricted lifestyle. Our lack of understanding of the underlying pathology of detrusor instability is reflected in the numerous methods of treatment which are currently employed, none of which is thoroughly satisfactory. As conventional bladder neck surgery is not usually helpful for women with detrusor instability unless there is concomitant genuine stress incontinence it is important to make an accurate diagnosis before treatment is commenced.

The majority of patients are treated with drug therapy initially and they may need to take this indefinitely as symptoms usually return once tablets are discontinued. Behavioural intervention requires reasonably intelligent well-motivated patients but can produce a cure in some patients without significant morbidity or side effects. Surgical procedures are usually reserved for those women with severe symptoms in whom other forms of treatment have been tried and failed. Although it is rare to completely cure a patient indefinitely with any form of treatment, the majority can have their symptoms significantly reduced so it is important to elicit the patients' main complaints and aim treatment accordingly. As the pathophysiology of detrusor instability becomes clearer it is hoped that there will be significant advances in the management of this unfortunate condition.

References

1. Warrell DW. Vaginal denervation and bladder nerve supply. Urol Int 1977; 32:114–16.
2. Hodgkinson CP, Drucker BH. Intravesical nerve resection for detrusor dyssynergia. Acta Obstet Gynecol Scand 1977; 38:401–8.

3. Ingleman-Sundberg A. Partial bladder denervation for detrusor dyssynergia. Clin Obstet Gynaecol 1978; 21:797–805.

4. Torrens MJ, Griffith HB. The control of the uninhibited bladder by selective sacral neurectomy. Br J Urol 1974; 46:639–44.

5. Ramsden PD, Hindmarsh JR, Price DA et al. DDAVP for adult enuresis – a preliminary report. Br J Urol 1982; 54:256–8.

6. Higson RH, Smith JC, Whelan P. Bladder rupture: an acceptable complication of distension therapy? Br J Urol 1978; 50:529–34.

7. Pengelly AW, Stephenson TP, Milroy GJG, Whiteside CG, Turner Warwick R. Results of prolonged bladder distension on treatment for detrusor instability. Br J Urol 1978; 50:243–5.

8. Mundy AR. The long term results of bladder transection for urinary incontinence. Br J Urol 1983; 55:642–4.

9. Burnstock G, Dumsday B, Smythe A. Atropine resistant excitation of the urinary bladder: the possibility of transmission via nerve releasing a purine nucleotide. Br J Pharmacol 1972; 44:451–61.

10. Gu J, Restovick JM, Blank M et al. Vasoactive intestinal polypeptide in the normal and unstable bladder. Br J Urol 1983; 54:252–5.

11. Benson H, Epstein MD. The placebo effect. J Am Med Assoc 1975; 232:1225–6.

12. Meyhoff HH, Gerstenberg TC, Brendler CB. The urodynamic and subjective results of treatment for detrusor instability with oxybutynin chloride. Br J Urol 1980; 52:474–5.

13. Karlmark B, Jensfett B, Magnusson O. Adverse events with placebo in 458 patients treated for urinary urge and urge incontinence. Neurourol Urodynam 1989; 8:410–11.

14. Levin RM, Staskin D, Wein AJ. The muscarinic cholinergic binding kinetics of the human urinary bladder. Neurourol Urodynam 1982; 1:221–5.

15. Gibaldi M, Grundhofer G. Biopharmaceutic influences on the anticholinergic effect of propantheline. Clin Pharmacol Ther 1975; 18:457–61.

16. Blaivas JG, Labib KB, Michalik SJ, Zayed AAH. Cystometric response to propantheline in detrusor hyperreflexia: therapeutic implications. J Urol 1980; 124:259–62.

17. Massey JA, Abrams PH. Dose-titrated emepronium carrageenate for detrusor instability. In: Proceedings of the fourteenth annual meeting of the International Continence Society, Innsbruck, 1984; 109–10.

18. Moisey CU, Stephenson TP, Brendler CB. The urodynamic and subjective results of treatment of detrusor instability with oxybutynin chloride. Br J Urol 1980; 52:472–5.

19. Cardozo LD, Cooper D, Versi E. Oxybutynin chloride in the management of idiopathic detrusor instability. Br Med J 1987; 280:281–2.

20. Baigrie RJ, Kelleher JP, Fawcett DP, Pengelly AW. Oxybutynin: is it safe? Br J Urol 1988; 62:319–22.

21. Holmes DM, Montz FJ, Stanton SL. Oxybutynin versus propantheline in the treatment of detrusor instability in the female: a patient regulated variable dose trial. In: Proceedings of the fifteenth annual meeting of the International Continence Society, London, 1985; 63–4.

22. Awad SA, Bryniak S, Downie JW, Bruce, AW. The treatment of the uninhibited bladder with dicyclomine. J Urol 1977; 117:161–3.

23. Wein AJ. Pharmacological treatment of non-neurogenic voiding dysfunction. In: Caine M, ed. The pharmacology of the urinary tract. Berlin: Springer-Verlag: 1984; 100–34.

24. Briggs RS, Castleden CM, Asher MJ. The effect of flavoxate on uninhibited detrusor contractions and urinary incontinence in the elderly. J Urol 1980; 123:665–6.

25. Cardozo LD, Stanton SL. An objective comparison of the effects of parenterally administered drugs in patients suffering from detrusor instability. J Urol 1979; 123:399–401.

26. Castleden CM, George CF, Renwick AG, Asher MJ. Imipramine – a possible alternative to current therapy for urinary incontinence in the elderly. J Urol 1981; 125:318–20.

27. Raezer DM, Benson GS, Wein AJ, Duckett JW. The functional approach to the management of the pediatric neuropathic bladder. A clinical study. J Urol 1977; 117:649–54.

28. Ulmsten U, Ekman G, Andersson KE. The effect of terodiline treatment in women with motor urge incontinence. Am J Obstet Gynecol 1985; 193:619–22.

29. Tapp AJS, Fall M, Norgaard J et al. A dose titrated multicentre study of terodiline in the treatment of detrusor instability. In: Proceedings of the seventeenth annual meeting of the International Continence Society, Bristol, 1987.

30. Gruneberger A. Treatment of motor urge incontinence with clenbutarol and flavoxate hydrochloride. Br J Obstet Gynaecol 1984; 91: 275–8.

31. Ramsden PD, Hindmarsh JR, Price DA et al. DDAVP for adult enuresis – a preliminary report. Br J Urol 1982; 54: 256–8.

32. Hilton P, Stanton SL. The use of desmopressin (DDAVP) in nocturnal urinary frequency in the female. Br J Urol 1982; 54:252–5.
33. Knusden UB, Rittig S, Pederen JB, Norgaard JP, Djaarhus JC. Long term treatment of nocturnal enuresis with desmopressin – influence on urinary output and haematological parameters. Neurourol Urodynam 1989; 8:348–9.
34. Tapp AJS, Cardozo LD. The postmenopausal bladder. Br J Hosp Med 1986; 35:20–3.
35. Jeffcoate TNA, Francis WJA. Urgency incontinence in the female. Am J Obstet Gynecol 1966; 94:604–18.
36. Frewen WK. Urge and stress incontinence: fact and fiction. J Obstet Gynaecol Br Commonw 1970; 77:932–4.
37. Frewen WK. An objective assessment of the unstable bladder of psychological origin. Br J Urol 1978; 50:246–9.
38. Jarvis GT. Bladder drill. In: Freeman R, McLaren J, eds. The unstable bladder. London: Wright, 1989; 55–60.
39. Jarvis GT, Millar DR. Controlled trial of bladder drill for detrusor instability. Br Med J 1980; 281:1322–3.
40. Holmes DM, Stone AR, Barry PR, Richards CJ, Stephenson TP. Bladder training – three years on. Br J Urol 1983; 55:660–4.
41. Cardozo LD, Abrams PH, Stanton SL, Feneley RCL. Idiopathic detrusor instability treated by biofeedback. Br J Urol 1978; 50:521–3.
42. Cardozo LD, Stanton SL. Genuine stress incontinence and detrusor instability: a review of 200 cases. Br J Obstet Gynaecol 1980; 87:184–90.
43. Millard RJ, Oldenberg BF. The symptomatic, urodynamic and psychodynamic results of bladder re-education programmes. J Urol 1983; 130:717–19.
44. Burgio KL, Robinson JC, Engel BT. The role of biofeedback in Kogel exercise training for stress urinary incontinence. Am J Obstet Gynecol 1986; 154:64–88.
45. Holmes D, Plevnik S, Stanton SL. Bladder neck electric conductivity in female urinary urgency and urge incontinence. Br J Obstet Gynaecol 1989; 96:816–20.
46. Freeman RM, Baxby K. Hypnotherapy for incontinence caused by the unstable bladder. Br Med J 1982; 284:1831–4.
47. Plevnik S, Janez J, Vrtacnik P, Trsinar B, Vodusek DB. Short term electrical stimulation: home treatment for urinary incontinence. World J Urol 1986; 4:24–6.
48. Eriksen BC, Bergman S, Eik-Nes SH. Maximal electrostimulation of the pelvic floor in female idiopathic detrusor instability and urge incontinence. Neurourol Urodynam 1989; 8:219–30.
49. Philp T, Shah PJR, Worth PHL. Acupuncture in the treatment of bladder instability. Br J Urol 1988; 61:490–3.
50. Ewing R, Bultitude ME, Shuttleworth KGD. Subtrigonal phenol injection for urge incontinence secondary to detrusor instability in females. Br J Urol 1982; 54:689–92.
51. Blackford W, Murray K, Stephenson TP, Mundy AR. Results of transvesical infiltration of the pelvis with phenol in 116 patients. Br J Urol 1984; 56:647–9.
52. Cameron-Strange A, Millard RJ. Management of refractory detrusor instability by transvesical phenol injection. Br J Urol 1988; 62:323–5.
53. Rosenbaum TP, Shah PJR, Worth PHL. Transtrigonal phenol – the end of an era? Neurourol Urodynam 1988; 7:294–5.
54. Wall LL, Stanton SL. Transvesical phenol injection of pelvic nerve plexuses in females with refractory urge incontinence. Br J Urol 1989; 63:465–8.
55. Harris RG, Constantinou CE, Stamey TA. Extravesical subtrigonal injection of 50 per cent ethanol for detrusor instability. J Urol 1988; 140:111–16.
56. Mundy AR, Stephenson TP. Clam idiocystoplasty for the treatment of refractory urge incontinence. Br J Urol 1985; 57:647–51.
57. Rosenbaum JP, Shah PJR, Rose GA, Lloyd Davies RW. Cranberry juice helps the problem of mucus production in enterouroplastics. Neurourol Urodynam 1989; 8:344–5.
58. Nurse DE, Mundy AR. Cystoplasty infection and cancer. Neurourol Urodynam 1989; 8:343–4.
59. McGuire EJ, Savastano JA. Stress incontinence and detrusor instability/urge incontinence. Neurourol Urodynam 1985; 4:313–16.
60. Karram MM, Bhatia NW. Management of coexistent stress and urge urinary incontinence. Obstet Gynecol 1989; 73:4–7.

Discussion

Shah: We might start by discussing behavioural therapy, seeing what people's views are and whether or not they use it. We can then go on to talk about drug treatment.

Andersson: Would combining behavioural therapy and drug therapy improve the results?

Cardozo: I think it would. The problem is that we are then not looking at the same thing. If we give patients drugs usually we do it in the outpatient clinic and we send them away to look after themselves at home. If we teach them bladder drill, then usually we bring them into hospital and we are giving them a high amount of input and encouragement. If drugs are then added, the response rate is increased but it is difficult to know which is doing the best, the drugs or the bladder drill.

Stanton: I am totally unable to tie up Miss Cardozo's lecture with Mr Mundy's lecture. They are both excellent but it does underline a kind of dichotomy in our understanding at the moment with Mr Mundy's view that the genesis of the problem with the unstable bladder is likely to be a peripheral problem and with Miss Cardozo's statement that this is really a central problem.

Cardozo: No. I just looked at behavioural intervention as one method of treatment that was used in the management of detrusor instability. I do not know how many in this group do use behavioural intervention but we certainly have very good results with a certain proportion of patients.

Stanton: That is what I mean. The results are very good but how do we tie this up?

Cardozo: Surely it is like any other autonomic phenomenon, like blood pressure.

Stanton: We do not know.

Cardozo: I mean one can have a certain amount of control over it for oneself.

Shah: Does Miss Cardozo actually use behavioural modification?

Cardozo: Yes.

Shah: Patients are admitted to hospital?

Cardozo: Yes.

Shah: I would imagine that most urologists do not. I could not quite understand why drug therapy and behavioural modification would not be combined.

Cardozo: We do combine them. We give drugs first on an outpatient basis. If the drugs are not effective we then admit the patient for bladder drill and give more drugs on top of that, because then we can see whether they are taking the drugs and whether the drugs are being effective or not. So we do combine them.

Shah: Why not just do the two at the same time?

Cardozo: With every patient? Because if we did that we would be occupying beds and we would be wasting a lot of time that we do not have to waste. Why do urologists not admit patients for bladder drill?

Shah: Because we have other patients we want to admit for more important treatment.

Cardozo: Well, exactly.

Shah: Behavioural modification can be given on an outpatient basis. Is that not so? To combine the two treatments together would save the time of the patient and of the clinician.

Warrell: Can I ask about the place of cystoscopy in the assessment of the patient with idiopathic detrusor instability? There are many patients who have some innate impairment in the capacity to inhibit the micturition reflex and frequently this is brought into focus by something in their bladder like an inflammatory trigger, an atrophic urethritis, or a stone, and I wonder how important people feel it is to have normal endoscopy before making this diagnosis and instituting the sort of drug and behaviour treatment we are discussing.

Cardozo: I do not do a cystoscopy in patients in whom I have shown detrusor instability because I have found a cause for their symptoms. I do carry out cystoscopy in patients who have those symptoms in whom I do not demonstrate detrusor instability.

Mundy: If they do not have sensory symptoms and their bladders are of reasonable capacity urodynamically I would not bother. Most of the urodynamics study results in our patients with instability show lots of instability of course, but the bladder capacity is not grossly reduced. If the bladder capacity was grossly reduced, or if the patient had associated sensory symptoms, then I would tend to cystoscope. The crucial factor is sensory symptoms that cannot be explained by tea, coffee, alcohol or Coca-Cola, and a reduced capacity, and particularly if surgery is under consideration.

Andersson: I do not see the dichotomy between the two presentations. It is necessary to have some nervous activity to induce bladder contraction. The micturition reflex is centrally controlled and even if the end organ has increased sensitivity, nerves are still required to initiate a contraction. That is why I think it is possible to look at therapeutic interventions acting at the central level and at the peripheral level, and they could both be effective.

I also think that it is important to stress the possible role of afferent stimulation and supersensitivity at the afferent side of the micturition arc as a possible cause of bladder instability. If that is correct, we could try to establish increased sensitivity in these patients, which is important information when we are discussing therapeutic approaches.

Mundy: It might be a nice idea as an active surgeon to say something on phenol and surgery, and also on the problem of mixed sensory and urge incontinence. There may be an impression that someone need only walk the streets of Bermondsey to get a segment of bowel slapped into the bladder, which is not the case, and obviously the first line of treatment must be self-help supplemented with drugs. But there are many patients who do not get better with self-help and drugs and something has to be done for them. The suggestion has been made that we should leave them alone. If I were to suggest that a woman with stress incontinence who failed to respond to oestrogens or phenylpropanolamine should be left incontinent for the rest of her life I would probably be laughed out of the room, and I do not see the difference between stress incontinence and the unstable bladder. Something has to be done.

A paper Miss Cardozo quoted made the point that the average response rate in the average patient with detrusor instability is 15%. We said then, and I would still maintain, that this is not a good response rate, but in those people who fail to respond to treatment phenol injection is a day case treatment with minimum morbidity and no mortality to date. It is no worse than cystoscopy. We also said that it should not be used in patients who had had radiotherapy or who had interstitial cystitis or any other evidence of active chronic inflammatory process, and that it should not be injected under the trigone but under the ureteric orifices on each side. With these in mind, it is not possible to develop vesicovaginal fistula, slough the bladder wall or get any other significant complications.

I would still say that phenol does not carry much of a response rate, but it is a trivial procedure and as the alternative is for the patients to tolerate urinary incontinence for the rest of their lives or to have a major abdominal operation, it has a place.

As far as cystoplasty is concerned, I can guarantee a cure for detrusor instability with cystoplasty beyond any question in the groups that have had the most experience of this technique, namely ourselves, with 167 patients to date, the Cardiff group and Mr Shah and Mr Worth's group at the Institute. There have been no failures to control the symptoms of detrusor instability, and in the absence of neurological disease the requirement for self-catheterisation in our experience is two patients in 167. This is a common requirement in patients who have detrusor hyperreflexia due to multiple sclerosis, spinal cord injury or spina bifida. There is thus no complication of significant voiding difficulty (and indeed in patients with mixed incontinence) and those are the patients who are most refractory to drug treatment and self-help treatment. The presence of a small amount of stress incontinence is an actual advantage for a cystoplasty because we can then be sure that, first, the stress incontinence will go away almost invariably, as it usually does if the unstable bladder can be treated, and second, that they will have no voiding difficulty at all. There are two questions hanging over it: of metabolic acidosis and its potential significance in the long term, and also the association with urinary nitrosamines and a possible malignant risk in the long term. The chances are that neither of these is a significant problem but we have drawn attention to them principally to make sure that these patients are followed up.

It is easy to be negative about an operation if one has no experience of it, and it is in fact an extremely useful procedure when all else fails.

Sutherst: I wanted to make the same sort of statement but about a transection. Is that now completely dead as far as those people are concerned? I find myself doing a fair number of those and again it is a fairly simple operation which is useful prior to moving on to cystoplasty.

Mundy: We have found that the response rate to bladder transection in terms of objective response was not sufficient to justify its use. Although there was an objective response, the objective and subjective responses did not match up sufficiently well for us to think we were having anything other than a placebo effect in the long term, and that is with two-year follow-up. I still have patients 10 years out who had a satisfactory result, but I do not think that we can be so sure with that operation as we can with a clam.

Sutherst: I did not say that the two were comparable. I was thinking about it in different terms, perhaps something more akin to phenol.

Mundy: An endoscopic transection?

Sutherst: Yes. Certainly the results from the Liverpool group are quite good.

Mundy: It is interesting that they have not done a follow-up.

Sutherst: But again it is an operation with very little morbidity and mortality, so it can be a useful step on the way to something bigger.

Cardozo: For a technique to be useful, it has to be able to be used by not necessarily everybody but at least the majority of those who treat patients with this condition. Although one practitioner may have very good experience with phenol, others do not have such good experience.

Mundy: I said I had a 15% response rate. That is not a very good experience.

Cardozo: But there were no serious side effects.

Mundy: There are no significant side effects.

Cardozo: But that is obviously not the experience of other people who have reported this type of treatment.

Shah: We reported it and we did not have any side effects either, out of 96 injections. And we used identical techniques.

Cardozo: And there were no side effects?

Shah: No. No complications of the type described by the Middlesex group, which were vesicovaginal fistulae, sloughed ureters and sciatic nerve palsies. We did not have any of those.

Mundy: But the fact is – and I stress this – it has to be injected in the right place and not under the trigone. It is a misnomer to call it subtrigonal phenol as a lot of people do. To do that is to run the risk of fistulae. To treat radiotherapy, interstitial cystitis or any chronic inflammatory process is to invite problems. But Blackford et al. [1] specifically state that it should not be subtrigonal and it should not be used when there is any histological abnormality or chronic inflammation.

Cardozo: In fact the report in which there was a vesicovaginal fistula following radiotherapy is protagonistic towards this type of treatment. But because one group's experiences are on the whole good does not mean that everybody's are, and the people who are embarking on this type of treatment should at least be aware that others have found problems with it.

Mundy: I stressed that the results are not good, but they are better than doing nothing at all.

References

1. Blackford W, Murray K, Stephenson TP, Mundy AR. Results of transvesical infiltration of the pelvis with phenol in 116 patients. Br J Urol 1984; 56:647–9.

Chapter 18

The Management of the Neuropathic Bladder

A. R. Mundy

Introduction

There are three main considerations in the management of a patient with neuropathic lower urinary tract dysfunction.

1. Multiple urodynamic pathology is the general rule.
2. Lower urinary tract dysfunction may lead to secondary upper urinary tract problems and ultimately to renal failure.
3. The lower urinary tract cannot be considered in isolation from other neurological and related problems affecting particularly the bowel, sexual function, the spine and the lower limbs.

   Until comparatively recently most patients with congenital neuropathic dysfunction (i.e. "open" spina bifida) died shortly after birth or in early childhood, usually as a result of overwhelming neurological infection or severe hydrocephalus. Advances in treatment reduced this mortality and it was then found that in the survivors, renal failure and urologically related problems, mainly secondary to bladder outflow obstruction, were a major cause of death in later childhood and early adult life [1]. This was also the experience in the long-term follow-up of many male patients after spinal cord injury [1]. This experience led to the widespread use of ileal conduit urinary diversion as a means of averting renal failure (and also of treating the incontinence) in these patients until the "urodynamic era" led to a better understanding of the urodynamic problems associated with neuropathic bladder dysfunction and consequently to better application of existing treatments and the development of new treatment methods.

   Other neurological diseases, notably multiple sclerosis, Parkinson's disease, diabetes mellitus and cerebrovascular disease, can cause significant problems as far as continence is concerned but rarely if ever cause serious secondary problems in the upper urinary tract. Moreover, with the notable exception of multiple sclerosis, the bladder problems are commonly overshadowed by other effects of these various diseases. On the other hand, in multiple sclerosis and related paraplegias, incontinence is the commonest cause of admission to hospital [2] and probably also the major cause of social disability out of hospital.

Assessment

Although the main purpose of this chapter is to discuss management, this cannot be considered without a few words on assessment. Assessment must include the patient as a whole, with particular reference to overall neurological disability, the stability of the neurological lesion, the likelihood of progression and the effects of the neurological disease on sexual function, on the bowel and on the lower limbs. Reference must also be made to any associated problems affecting the central nervous system above the sacral segments concerned with lower urinary tract function. In this way an assessment can be made of the patient's mobility, manipulative skills, intelligence and motivation, and thus of their ability to appreciate their problem and to co-operate physically and emotionally with their treatment.

Remembering that certain types of neurological lesion, particularly spina bifida in either sex and spinal cord injury in males, may lead to secondary upper tract problems, attention is next directed towards determining whether the patient has any degree of upper tract impairment or is at risk of developing it. This can be assessed either by a good quality ultrasound study or an intravenous urogram (IVU). If either the ultrasound or IVU is abnormal, the serum creatinine should be measured and any appropriate investigations such as dimercaptosuccinic acid or diethylene triamine penta-acetic acid renal scanning should be arranged as appropriate. If there is impairment of renal function, urodynamic investigation should be arranged with a view to treatment. If there is no evidence of impairment of renal function, the only problem is likely to be related to continence and it is reasonable on the basis of clinical assessment and other non-invasive methods of assessment to attempt empirical treatment without recourse to urodynamic assessment. If this fails, or if empirical treatment is not helpful, urodynamic assessment is required.

There are various ways of classifying the urodynamic disturbances seen in neuropathy. The one outlined briefly here is the one the author uses routinely and finds useful and is based on the fact that lower urinary tract dysfunction in neuropathy falls into one of three groups [3–6].

Contractile Dysfunction

In contractile dysfunction (Fig 18.1), contractility of the bladder and urethra is preserved. Detrusor contractions are discrete and are capable by virtue of their amplitude and duration of giving a useful degree of bladder emptying, assuming

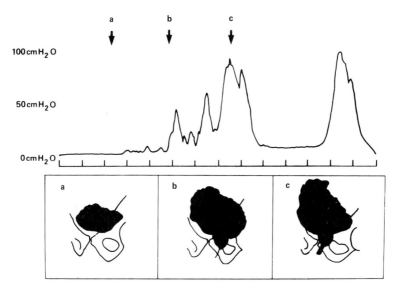

Fig. 18.1. Contractile dysfunction – videourodynamic features. (In this and in Figs 18.2 and 18.3, only the detrusor pressure trace is shown.) The detrusor pressure trace shows high amplitude swings in detrusor pressure (detrusor hyperreflexia). Synchronous video micturating cystourethrogram (MCUG) shows initial bladder neck competence and trabeculation (a); opening of the bladder neck with a detrusor contraction (b); but failure of opening of the distal sphincter mechanism (c) due to detrusor sphincter dyssynergia. From [5].

that any associated bladder outflow obstruction (which is often present, see below) is eliminated. Between contractions, detrusor pressure returns to normal so that baseline pressure during filling is within the normal range. In other words, there is normal bladder compliance. These detrusor contractions may be involuntary, in which case they are called hyperreflexic, but the individual may be capable of initiating a voiding contraction voluntarily. The bladder neck is competent in about 50% of patients and there is no incompetence of the urethral sphincter mechanism.

In patients who have lesions between the sacral parasympathetic outflow and the pons (where detrusor contractile activity, urethral relaxation and the co-ordination between the two are organised) there may be contraction of the urethral sphincter mechanism during a detrusor contraction, rather than the relaxation of the urethral sphincter mechanism that occurs under normal circumstances. This is known as detrusor-sphincter dyssynergia and may be a potent cause of bladder outflow obstruction.

In patients with partial lesions, urethral and bladder sensation may be preserved and there may also be control of the periurethral pelvic floor musculature, so the individual may have sensory awareness of what is happening in the lower urinary tract and some residual ability to resist incontinence during an involuntary bladder contraction.

In patients with lesions above the pons, detrusor hyperreflexia is not associated with detrusor sphincter dyssynergia because the lesion is above the level where detrusor contraction is co-ordinated with reflex urethral relaxation. Typical causes of suprapontine lesions are cerebrovascular disease, Parkinson's disease and some

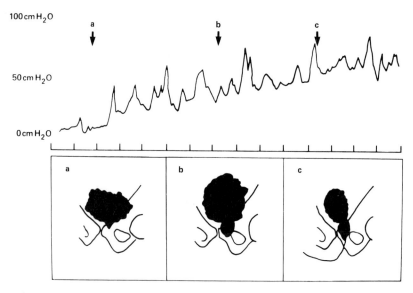

Fig. 18.2. Intermediate dysfunction. The detrusor pressure trace shows a steady rise in baseline pressure (low compliance) and constant detrusor activity of varying amplitude. However, as distinct from Fig. 18.1 this activity is poorly sustained and therefore ineffective – it is sufficient to restrict filling but insufficient to produce voiding. Synchronous video-MCUG shows bladder neck incompetence (a), which gets progressively worse (b) with sphincteric obstruction allowing filling of the urethra only when intravesical pressure exceeds urethral resistance (c). From [5].

cases of multiple sclerosis; typical causes of suprasacral cord lesions are spinal cord injury, spina bifida and multiple sclerosis.

Intermediate Dysfunction

In the intermediate group (Fig 18.2), bladder and urethral contractile activity are also preserved but such contractile activity is not discrete: instead it takes the form of high frequency, low amplitude, short duration contractile activity, which gives no degree of useful bladder emptying but simply serves to restrict bladder filling. Between contractions base line pressures do not return to normal; in other words there is poor compliance. Similar contractile activity in the urethra causes sphincteric obstruction unless intravesical pressure exceeds the level of urethral resistance, in which case incontinence may occur, giving the seemingly paradoxical combination of sphincteric obstruction and sphincteric incompetence. The combination of high intravesical pressures due to poor compliance and sphincteric obstruction is a particularly potent cause of secondary upper tract problems, particularly when combined with recurrent urinary tract infections and vesicoureteric reflux. The bladder neck sphincter mechanism is always incompetent at usual bladder volumes in this group of patients.

Intermediate type of dysfunction is almost always due to spinal cord injury and spina bifida, particularly extensive and complete thoracolumbar or low sacral lesions.

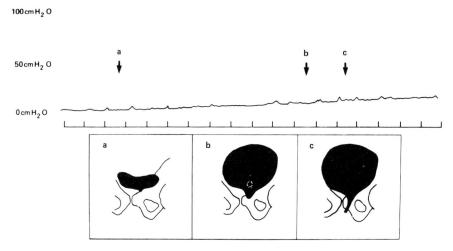

Fig. 18.3.   Acontractile dysfunction. The detrusor pressure trace shows no evidence of detrusor contractility. Synchronous video-MCUG shows bladder neck incompetence with early "beaking" of the bladder neck (a), which becomes marked with filling (b). On coughing or attempted voiding by straining, sphincter weakness incontinence occurs (c) but the urethra in the region of the distal sphincter mechanism fails to open adequately because of static distal sphincter obstruction. From [5].

Acontractile Dysfunction

In the acontractile group (Fig.18.3) there is no contractile activity at all. Bladder compliance is normal and the bladder fills until it reaches a point at which intravesical pressure exceeds urethral resistance and overflow incontinence then develops. Although the urethra is not contractile it exerts a fixed resistance although this may be very low. As in the intermediate group, the bladder neck is always incompetent at usual bladder volumes. If urethral resistance is fairly high there may be a considerable volume of residual urine before overflow incontinence occurs.

Typical causes of acontractile dysfunction are diabetes mellitus and other causes of a peripheral autonomic neuropathy but the same pattern is occasionally seen in spina bifida and spinal cord injury.

Treatment

If there is evidence of impaired renal function, treatment is urgent. If there is no evidence of impaired renal function, then it is not. If the patient's general condition, as alluded to above, does not warrant a selective approach, treatment is palliative and involves the use of catheterisation, external appliances (in males), or urinary diversion. If the patient has a significant residual urine, clean intermittent self-catheterisation [7] may correct any secondary upper tract problems by establishing adequate urinary drainage and also provide continence. If there is

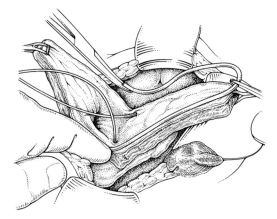

Fig. 18.4. "Clam" ileocystoplasty 1. The bladder is bisected in the coronal plane and the bladder circumference is measured. From [10].

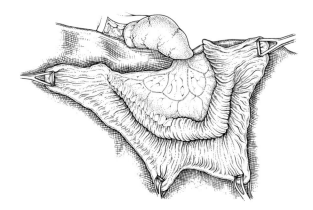

Fig. 18.5. "Clam" ileocystoplasty 2. A section of ileum equal in length to the measured bladder circumference is isolated on its vascular pedicle and opened to form a patch. From [10].

no significant residual urine volume, the patient will require indwelling catheterisation, an external appliance (preferable to indwelling catheterisation in most males but not applicable to females), or appropriate purpose-designed absorptive underwear. An alternative, if these are unsatisfactory, is an ileal conduit urinary diversion.

If the patient's general condition, inclinations and motivation makes him or her suitable for a selective approach to treatment, that treatment is decided on the basis of the objectively demonstrated urodynamic abnormality according to the three groups described in the last section.

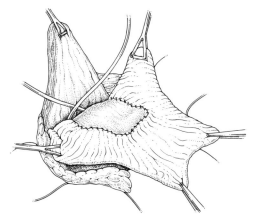

Fig. 18.6. "Clam" ileocystoplasty 3. The ileal patch has been sewn onto the posterior bladder wall.
From [10].

Contractile Dysfunction

The majority of patients with contractile dysfunction respond to anticholinergic
medication with oxybutynin 5 mg t.d.s. or q.d.s [8] with the exception of patients
with Parkinson's disease, which rarely responds to any form of medication. If
the patient does not respond to anticholinergic medication, the only option is
surgical and this option will not be appropriate in the majority of patients with
suprapontine lesions because of their general condition. In those with suprasacral
cord lesions (who tend to be younger and fitter), surgical correction should be
considered. Surgical treatment involves a "clam" ileocystoplasty [9] in which the
bladder is bisected in the coronal plane except for a short bridge around the
bladder neck, where continuity is maintained in order to preserve an adequate
blood supply to the bladder (Fig. 18.4). A segment of ileum, well away from
the ileocaecal valve (to avoid nutritional problems), is then mobilised and opened
on its antimesenteric border to form a patch (Fig. 18.5) which is then sewn into
the bisected bladder (Figs. 18.6 and 18.7). This is extremely effective at eliminating
involuntary bladder contractions but also makes voluntary contractile activity
relatively ineffective. This means that thereafter some patients will need to use
clean intermittent self-catheterisation (CISC) to achieve adequate bladder emptying and avoid the risk of recurrent urinary infection. All patients should be warned
of this possibility in advance.

Intermediate Dysfunction

In intermediate bladder dysfunction, the problems are, on the one hand, bladder
overactivity and poor compliance, and on the other hand, sphincteric obstruction
and incompetence. Bladder overactivity is treated in the same way as in the contractile group but anticholinergic medication is not nearly so effective and the requirement for cystoplasty is much greater. Sphincteric problems are treated according
to which is the predominant factor – obstruction or incompetence. If there is
predominantly obstruction, which is best assessed by whether or not there is a

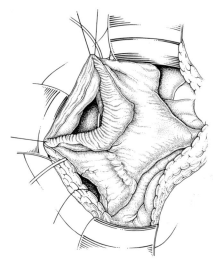

Fig. 18.7. "Clam" ileocystoplasty 4. The ileal patch has been flipped over and tacked to the anterior bladder wall with stay sutures prior to completing the anastomosis.

significant volume of residual urine, the patient can be treated by CISC, with a cystoplasty if necessary to give an adequate capacity and low pressure bladder. If on the other hand the sphincter is predominantly incompetent, or if incompetence is a major factor – as is usually the case – then the cystoplasty will need to be combined with implantation of an artificial sphincter [6]. As in the contractile group, CISC may be required postoperatively to achieve adequate bladder emptying and patients should be warned about the possibility of this.

Acontractile Dysfunction

In acontractile dysfunction the bladder does not require attention surgically, and nothing can be done medically to make an acontractile bladder contract [11]. Treatment is therefore directed towards the incompetent urethral sphincter mechanism. In theory the patient can be helped by a standard bladder neck suspension procedure as in simple stress incontinence, but this does not work nearly so well in neuropathic patients as in their non-neuropathic counterparts unless it produces complete bladder outflow obstruction [12]. Acontractile neuropathic bladder dysfunction usually requires implantation of an artificial sphincter (Figs. 18.8 and 18.9) [13,14]. Again patients should be warned that an artificial sphincter is extremely effective at holding urine in the bladder but does not guarantee effective bladder emptying and CISC may be required to achieve this. In practice, acontractile bladder dysfunction does not usually require surgical treatment with implantation of an artificial urinary sphincter except in patients with spina bifida and spinal cord injury, in whom acontractile dysfunction is in any case unusual [6]. In diabetes there is usually a much higher level of urethral resistance and therefore a much higher level of residual urine and these patients are best treated by intermittent self-catheterisation. Measures designed to lower the urethral resistance (such as urethrotomy or urethral overdilatation) and thereby improve

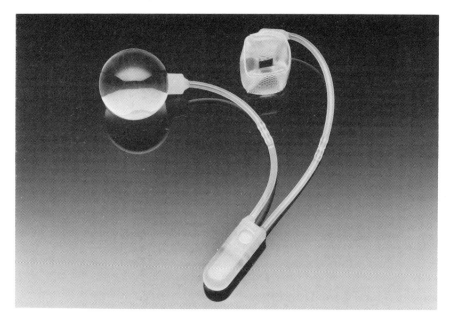

Fig. 18.8. The Brantley Scott artificial urinary sphincter (AUS) – the AS 800 model. This consists of a circumferential cuff that is placed around the bladder neck or (in males) the bulbar urethra, a pressure regulating balloon that lies extraperitoneally in the pelvis or iliac fossa, and a control pump which lies subcutaneously in either a labium majus or (in males) the scrotum, all of which are fluid filled and interconnected via the control pump. The pressure inside the system is controlled by the pressure regulating balloon and this is predetermined during manufacture. This pressure is transmitted to the cuff which thereby occludes the bladder neck (or bulbar urethra) constantly, unless the pump is squeezed. From [10].

bladder emptying should not be used (as a general rule) as bladder emptying is achieved at the expense of a degree of stress incontinence.

Special Problems

In general then, the mainstays of treatment of the neuropathic bladder are anticholinergic medication or "clam" ileocystoplasty to correct detrusor overactivity, CISC to provide adequate bladder emptying in the face of an obstructive sphincter mechanism, and artificial urinary sphincter implantation to correct sphincteric incompetence. These are applied to patients in whom such a scale of surgery is a realistic proposition. For those in whom this is not realistic, palliative measures such as urethral catheterisation, either indwelling or intermittent, purpose-designed underwear for containment, or urinary diversion are more appropriate. Each patient has to be judged on his or her own merits and it is the patient who should be treated not the urodynamic disorder.

Certain other categories of patients require special consideration.

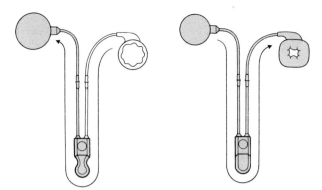

Fig. 18.9. The Brantley Scott artificial urinary sphincter. When the pump is squeezed 2–3 times, fluid is rapidly transmitted from the cuff through the control assembly part of the control pump to the balloon allowing the patient to void. The fluid then slowly returns from the balloon to the cuff through a series of delay-resistors in the control assembly until the occlusive pressure of the cuff is fully restored. This allows about 3–4 minutes for the patient to void. From [10].

Complete Spinal Cord Transection

If the spinal cord is completely transected but the spinal cord and nerve roots below the level of the lesion are preserved, as may be the case in spinal cord injury, the patient should be considered for implantation of a sacral anterior root stimulator as designed by Professor Brindley [15]. This treatment may be applicable, in theory, to patients with other neurological disturbances causing a complete spinal cord transection but other factors usually rule out this possibility.

Patients with Pre-existing Urinary Diversions

If a patient has a urinary diversion with which they are happy and which is working satisfactorily, it should be left alone. If there is a problem with the diversion requiring surgical correction, for example a retracted stoma or uretero-ileal obstruction, undiversion should be considered. This involves restoring urinary tract continuity and correcting the urodynamic abnormality along the lines discussed above according to the urodynamic diagnosis. A further discussion of the problems and details of urinary undiversion is beyond the scope of this chapter [16].

Parkinson's Disease

Although Parkinson's disease has a pattern of detrusor hyperreflexia on urodynamic evaluation, which makes it indistinguishable from other causes of detrusor hyperreflexia, such hyperreflexia rarely responds to anticholinergic (or other) medication and the patient's general condition usually prohibits surgical intervention. Such patients are best treated by containing the incontinence by means of appropriately designed absorptive underwear.

Brain Failure

Brain failure may be the result of old age, trauma, a birth defect such as hydrocephalus, or some other factor related to an underlying neurological problem. As with Parkinson's disease the problem of incontinence is best treated by containment with absorptive underwear. Such patients are not suitable candidates for surgery and they do not tolerate indwelling catheters.

Conclusions

There is a wide range of treatment options available to correct almost any urodynamic disturbance. Indeed it is theoretically possible to take a patient with no kidney or urinary tract, make a urinary tract out of available alternative tissues, transplant a kidney into this urinary tract and produce a perfectly satisfactory nephrourological system. The problem then is not how to treat the lower urinary tract dysfunction but how best to use the available treatments in the most economical and most effective way for the individual patient in the light of his overall neurological disability and with the fewest complications. With a young healthy individual with little or no problem outside the lower urinary tract a satisfactory solution can almost be guaranteed. In the elderly or more severely afflicted patient, the problem may end up being more of a philosophical and ethical one than a medical one.

References

1. Bors E, Comarr AE. Mortality (associated with neurogenic bladder dysfunction). In: Bors E, Comarr AE, eds. Neurological urology. Basel: S. Karger, 1971; 346–57.
2. Miller H, Simpson CA, Yeates WK. Bladder dysfunction in multiple sclerosis. Br Med J 1965; i:1265–9.
3. Rickwood AMK, Thomas DG, Philp NH, Spicer RD. Assessment of congenital neuropathic bladder by combined urodynamic and radiological studies. Br J Urol 1982; 54:512–18.
4. Mundy AR, Shah PJ, Borzyskowski M, Saxton HM. Sphincter behaviour in myelomeningocele. Br J Urol 1985; 57:647–51.
5. Mundy AR. The neuropathic bladder. In: Postlethwaite RJ, ed. Clinical paediatric nephrology. Bristol: John Wright, 1986; 312–28.
6. Parry JRW, Nurse DE, Boucaut HAP, Murray KHA, Mundy AR. The surgical management of the congenital neuropathic bladder. Br J Urol 1989; 64 (in press).
7. Lapides J, Diokno AC, Silber SJ, Lome BS. Clean intermittent self-catheterisation in the treatment of urinary tract disease. J Urol 1972; 107:458–61.
8. Moisey CU, Stephenson TP, Brendler CB. The urodynamic and subjective results of treatment of detrusor instability with oxybutynin chloride. Br J Urol 1980; 52:472–5.
9. Mundy AR. Cystoplasty. In: Mundy AR, ed. Current operative surgery – Urology. London: Bailliere Tindall, 1988; 140–59.
10. Mundy AR. Urodynamic and reconstructive surgery of the lower urinary tract. Edinburgh: Churchill Livingstone (in press).
11. Rickwood AMK. The neuropathic bladder in children. In: Mundy AR, Stephenson TP, Wein AJ, eds. Urodynamics: principles, practice and application. Edinburgh: Churchill Livingstone, 1984; 326–47.

12. Lawrence WT, Thomas DG. The Stamey bladder neck suspension operation for stress incontinence and neurovesical dysfunction. Br J Urol 1987; 59:305–10.
13. Mundy AR, Stephenson TP. Selection of patients for implantation of the Brantley Scott artificial urinary sphincter. Br J Urol 1984; 56:717–20.
14. Nurse DE, Mundy AR. One hundred artificial sphincters. Br J Urol 1988; 61:318–25.
15. Brindley GS, Polkey CE, Rushton DN, Cardozo L. Sacral anterior root stimulators for bladder control in paraplegia: the first fifty cases. J Neurol Neurosurg Psychiatry 1986; 49:1104–114.
16. Mundy AR. Refunctional urinary tract surgery with particular reference to undiversion. In: Hendry WF, ed. Recent advances in urology/andrology. Edinburgh: Churchill Livingstone, 1987; 147–68.

Discussion

DeLancey: I have a question about the sphincteric mechanism in the acontractile patients. The tracing of the radiographs appeared as if the proximal portion of the urethra was opened and the distal portion was closed. Is it a common finding in these people, that their distal mechanism is closed but the proximal portion is not?

Mundy: The full statement would be that in patients with the intermediate type or the acontractile, the bladder neck is always incompetent at normal bladder volumes. Some of these patients will have large residual urines and if all the residual urine is emptied and they are then filled, radiologically the bladder neck may be competent or be closed – not necessarily competent. But at normal bladder volumes in the intermediate and acontractile group they are always open. In both groups the sphincter active part of the urethra is closed to start off with. The level of resistance in these patients depends to a certain extent on their sex and on the level of the lesion, particularly where there is preservation of the sympathetic outflow. But there is always a degree of resistance, maybe only passive resistance, at the level of the urethral sphincter mechanism, which varies in degree from patient to patient and from level of lesion, cauda equina to peripheral. But basically the message is that in the intermediate and acontractile groups the behaviour of the bladder neck and the urethra is the same but varies in degree, with obstruction predominating in the intermediate, incompetence in the acontractile, and it must be expected to be present. If one operates on somebody with an intermediate bladder, for example, to drop their bladder pressure, what appeared to be an insignificant degree of sphincteric obstruction with an aggressive bladder may become a very potent cause of obstruction in a patient who has had a cystoplasty.

DeLancey: The patients with spinal cord injuries will be clearly recognised as a separate group. I am thinking about the diabetics who might present with symptoms of urinary incontinence. Did I hear right in that a regular urethral suspension does not cure their incontinence problem?

Mundy: I am talking about predictable results. We can guarantee to make these people dry if they are pulled up so tight that they will never again be able to pass water. But a standard suspension procedure hoping to give them continence and normal adequate voiding does not predictably follow.

Shah: In any discussion of the three groups – the contractile, the intermediate and acontractile – it is important to separate them from the spinal injury patients. I know that we have discussed this before, but the intermediate bladder never occurs in spinal injury patients unless their management has been neglected: I can quite categorically say that from my experience of spinal injury patients. It occurs in patients with hyperreflexic bladders which have not been treated either by anticholinergic agents and catheter drainage or sphincterotomy, because those contractions are high pressured.

Mundy: I would agree that it rarely if ever occurs in the average road traffic accident or riding accident causing spinal cord transection. But in the old-fashioned mining injuries – which we still get in Kent – with crush injuries to the thoracolumbar spine and extensive spinal cord damage, then I would beg to differ.

Shah: But to qualify that, the ones that I have seen it in, in other words the poorly compliant bladder with added hyperreflexia, have always been in patients with hyperreflexic bladders, contractile bladders, and they have occurred as a secondary feature as a consequence of trabeculation and then connective tissue replacement.

Mundy: We are not disagreeing about that.

Shah: No. But it may be that some of the patients described as intermediate are as a consequence of longstanding high-pressure behaviour, because one does not know that.

Mundy: Yes, that is true. Some of them are. If a hyperreflexic bladder is left untreated there can be all sorts of complications. But I am talking about the basic primary patterns. There are also the people who have paracentral lobule syndromes, who have got spastic pelvic floors. There may be a slightly different appearance in cerebral palsy. There is a different appearance in Shy–Drager syndrome, and a different appearance in those with partial lesions and preservation of sensation. But these only serve to modify one of those three patterns.

Shah: There was no mention of the use of indwelling catheters as part of the management of the female with severe disability. It is very important.

Mundy: I stressed, and would stress again, that these are the forms of treatment in patients in whom a selective approach to treatment is a realistic proposition. If the patient does not want it, if they are too immobile, if they have inadequate manipulative skills, if they are too unintelligent, or if there are any other of a number of associated factors, catheterisation has to be considered as a definitive option, either indwelling (suprapubic or urethral) or intermittent – or containment using underwear, or urinary diversion.

Andersson: Is there a place for α-receptor antagonists in modifying peripheral resistance?

Mundy: There is a group of patients following spinal cord injury who develop for some strange reason an acontractile bladder that has the typical appearance, but in whom the sphincter mechanism is peculiarly sensitive to a-blockade. In sympathetic preservation in a spinal cord injury patient with an acontractile bladder – not a common group – a-sympathetic blockade will often work and it is one of the reasons why people have proposed the so-called triple innervation of the somatic sphincter. In fact probably residual sympathetic innervation of the smooth muscle of the sphincter active urethra, and nothing else, is maintaining urethral tone. Indeed it may be that that produces most of the urethral tone in the acontractile bladder overall.

Also for some reason 7–9-year-old girls with spina bifida seem to respond to a-receptor blockade for sphincteric obstruction in both the acontractile and the intermediate group, whereas older women do not. I have no explanation.

Murray: When I was working in Cardiff we did voiding pressure profiles in spinal cord-injured patients, looking at the effect of intravenous a-blockade both on the tone between dyssynergic contractions in the sphincter active urethra and on the contractions, and in fact although phenoxybenzamine, which is what we were using at that time, reduced the pressure in the urethra between contractions, it had absolutely no effect on the peak pressures of the contractions themselves. So I would say that the answer is probably limited.

Hudson: On a slightly different tack, when there is a problem of sorting out the neuropathic component in a woman with grave micturition control problems following extensive pelvic surgery with or without radiotherapy, it is very uncertain as to how much the dysfunction should be ascribed to local neurological damage and how much to fibrosis and other problems immediately in the bladder wall. I would be glad to hear of ideas on how to proceed in this situation.

Mundy: There are two elements to that. There are those who have had radiotherapy and those who have not had radiotherapy to complicate issues.

The crucial factor in neuropathy is to look for evidence of sphincteric obstruction, evidence of poor bladder compliance and evidence of short duration low-amplitude detrusor contractile activity, because those three are all rare in the absence of neuropathy. The abnormal detrusor activity is very uncommon in the women described, and so the only two things that might commonly be found are poor compliance – and by that I mean not just marginally poor compliance but end-filling pressures in the region of 25 cm H_2O or more, three months after surgery, by which time the associated fibrosis will have settled – and any evidence of sphincteric obstruction on the voiding phase of urodynamic study with simultaneous fluoroscopy. Where there is poor compliance or evidence of sphincteric obstruction, a neurological aetiology can be invoked. If in addition to that they have reduced contractile activity, then it can be more or less guaranteed because poor compliance is sometimes a complication of bladder outflow obstruction and detrusor overactivity, but in the absence of either of those it only occurs in neuropathy.

Where radiotherapy is a complication, then almost certainly compliance will be poor. Detrusor instability is more likely than arreflexia; there will be reduced compliance, and there is a tendency to poor compliance and reduced capacity in the vagina and rectum as well (that is, if the patient has the ability to fill up the bladder, which any patient with any extensive vesicovaginal fistulation may not have).

Chapter 19

The Management of Sensory Urgency

A. B. Peattie

Definition

Sensory urgency describes patients complaining of urinary urgency but without demonstrable detrusor instability. The International Continence Society [1] has defined urgency as a strong desire to void accompanied by fear of leakage or fear of pain, which may be associated with two types of detrusor dysfunction: urgency with overactive detrusor dysfunction is motor urgency, whereas urgency with detrusor hypersensitivity is sensory urgency. The problem remains of defining what exactly is meant by detrusor hypersensitivity but many authors have investigated patients with urinary urgency unaccompanied by objective evidence of detrusor instability and a number of terms have been used – primary vesical sensory urgency [2], urge syndrome [3] and sensory urge incontinence [4].

Jarvis [2] defined his group of patients with frequency and painful urgency using urodynamic criteria – first sensation of filling at less than 75 ml saline and maximum desire to void at less than 400 ml with painful urgency and a stable detrusor. We selected patients with objectively demonstrable incontinence and complaints of urgency and frequency but no evidence of detrusor instability [4].

The diagnosis of sensory urgency rests on a combination of symptoms (urgency and frequency) and urodynamic parameters (detrusor hypersensitivity) after exclusion of other pathologies.

Incidence

The incidence of sensory urgency is unclear due to the difficulty in defining the condition. Many urodynamic units will include these patients in their normal population as objective testing fails to demonstrate abnormality, in particular detrusor instability, but others will treat the patients similarly to detrusor instability on the basis of symptoms. A tighter definition and positive diagnostic aid would enable this group to be readily identified, investigated and treated. In 558 patients complaining of incontinence who underwent routine cystometry in our urodynamic unit, sensory urgency was the final diagnosis in 6%, a small proportion by comparison with the 31% incidence of detrusor instability in the same group [4].

Aetiology

Frewen [5] has proposed that frequency and urgency may initiate detrusor instability rather than being symptoms due to the condition but Jarvis [2] notes that sensory urgency does not always progress to detrusor instability nor is detrusor instability invariably preceded by sensory urgency. Frewen [6,7] has stressed the psychosomatic nature of urgency and urgency incontinence in women and Hafner et al. [8] reported that psychotherapy resulted in considerable benefit to a third of their group of 26 patients. They also noted that during all the interviews, no patient left the room on account of urgency. This fact was noted by O'Boyle and Parsons [9] who recorded that all patients were able to refrain from voiding for 3 hours prior to urodynamic assessment despite complaints of severe urgency and frequency. In a study of a mixed group of patients with sensory urgency and detrusor instability Macaulay et al. [10] found that those patients with sensory urgency were more anxious than those with genuine stress incontinence whilst although those with detrusor instability were equally anxious they scored higher on the hysteria scale.

Investigations

History and examination

A detailed history is taken and an examination performed. Diuretic intake, previous pelvic surgery or irradiation, pelvic mass or pregnancy are noted and a mid-stream urine culture is performed.

Urinary Diary

A urinary diary is very useful as it gives a more objective measure of the frequency and nocturia that are part of this condition. The patient is requested to record her fluid intake and measure her urinary output over the course of a week, also noting any episodes of incontinence or urgency. The record gives information on frequency, volumes voided and the average daily intake and output. It is then a simple matter to detect excessive intake as the cause of frequency and urgency.

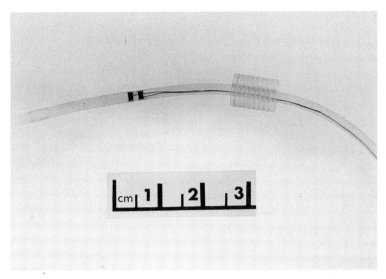

Fig. 19.1. BNEC catheter with electrodes mounted near the tip.

Other Tests

Other tests which may be relevant include blood sugar estimation if diabetes is suspected, urea and electrolyte sample for renal disease and a urethral swab if dysuria is present.

Cystoscopy is necessary to exclude interstitial cystitis, calculus or tumour within the bladder and may show urethral diverticulum, or other relevant urethral lesion.

Subtracted cystometry is essential to exclude detrusor instability. Where these investigations are negative bladder neck electric conductance studies may be informative.

Urethral electric conductance (UEC) is a concept which arose from the work of Plevnik et al. [11]. The test relies on urothelium and urine having different electric impedance: using a specially designed conductivity catheter, this difference can be used to detect opening of the bladder neck. During measurement of bladder neck electric conductance (BNEC), Holmes et al. [12] noted a highly significant correlation between the grading of symptoms of urgency and variations in the BNEC recording.

The conductivity catheter is a 7FG silastic catheter with two gold-plated brass electrodes 1 mm wide and 1 mm apart mounted near the tip (Fig.19.1). A non-stimulatory current of 20 mV is applied across the electrodes and the conductivity recorded in microamps (μA) on a UEC meter. The conductivity measurements are made with the patient lying supine with 250 ml normal saline in the bladder and the UEC catheter placed to record at the bladder neck mechanism. Using this technique we tested patients with sensory urgency and compared them to a group of asymptomatic patients. Fig. 19.2 shows the tracing obtained from an asymptomatic patient which contrasts sharply with Fig. 19.3 which is the recording from a patient with sensory urgency. The variable measured is the maximum deflection at rest (MDR) and comparing the two groups of patients the asymptomatic patients had a lower MDR (range 12–44 μA) than the symptomatic

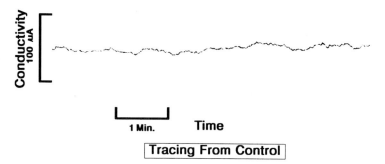

Fig. 19.2.   BNEC tracing from asymptomatic patient (MDR = 16 µA).

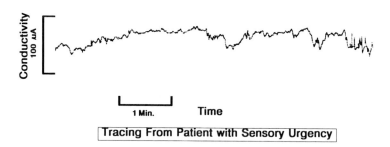

Fig. 19.3.   BNEC tracing from patient with sensory urgency (MDR = 56 µA).

patients, whose MDR was 36–108 µA. From the spread of results, a level of 36 µA distinguished the symptomatic from the asymptomatic group, with a highly significant difference between the value of MDR for the two groups (Fig. 19.4). Thus, with this difference between normal and asymptómatic patients, we have a test for positively diagnosing sensory urgency rather than the diagnosis of exclusion used previously.

Management

The variety of types of therapy applied in managing sensory urgency indicates our lack of knowledge on aetiology. Many classes of drugs have been used, mainly on the rationale that as the symptoms are the same as in detrusor instability it is appropriate to try medications that have shown benefit in that condition. Bladder drill has been used on a similar basis and psychotherapy because of the possible psychosomatic aetiology. Biofeedback has been reported to be successful as has electrical stimulation but many of the therapies have been used in combination making it difficult to determine which modality of therapy is most efficacious.

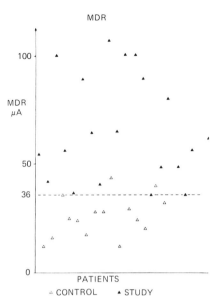

Fig. 19.4. Urethral electric conductance: maximum deflection at rest (MDR) of control patients and patients with urgency (study group).

Drug Therapy

Anticholinergic Drugs

Propantheline. Propantheline is an anticholinergic which has been in use for many years and produces its effect by competitive blockade at the ganglionic receptor site. In a study of a mixed group of patients with detrusor instability and sensory urgency, who were randomly allocated to three treatment groups, the group given propantheline 15 mg three times daily for 3 months showed a modest improvement in frequency of micturition [10]. The side effects of this therapy – dry mouth, visual upset and constipation – may limit the dosage that can be achieved when titrating the dose against symptomatic relief.

Terodiline. More recently, in an attempt to lessen the adverse side effects experienced, drugs which combine different modes of action have been introduced. Terodiline is one of these and combines anticholinergic action with calcium channel blockade. In a study of 20 female patients with sensory urgency terodiline and bladder drill were compared to placebo and bladder drill in a double-blind cross-over comparison [13]. Treatment was for 3 weeks with a 1 week washout before cross-over. A significant decrease was shown in urinary frequency and number of episodes of incontinence, while on urodynamic testing bladder capacity and first sensation of filling were increased. Both objectively and subjectively terodiline was significantly better than placebo with 50% more patients improved on terodiline than on placebo. After withdrawal of terodiline 30% of the patients relapsed.

In a multicentre study of 100 women with urgency/urge incontinence given 25 mg terodiline twice daily a statistically significant decrease of episodes of voluntary as well as involuntary micturition was seen [14]. The clinical benefit obtained after 3 months persisted at 6 months and about 75% of the patients considered themselves improved. Twelve patients withdrew due to side effects and about half the group reported dry mouth, blurred vision or nausea during the first 3 months of use.

This problem with a high incidence of side effects with the anticholinergic group of drugs led to a search for other types of drug therapy.

Bromocriptine

The use of bromocriptine was investigated after a report of its use in patients with detrusor instability had shown symptomatic relief although bladder instability was not abolished [15]. A double-blind, randomised crossover of bromocriptine against an inert placebo in 14 patients with primary vesical sensory urgency showed no therapeutic advantage [9]. This group also noted that despite distressing urgency all patients were able to go for prolonged periods without having to void. They went on to discuss whether the functional component noted in this syndrome was the cause or the effect of the symptomatology.

Sedation

Frewen [6] records that "treatment by sedation and anticholinergic drugs has been found to be very efficacious both in cases of urgency of micturition and urgency incontinence". He combined emepronium with diazepam or chlordiazepoxide and continued the sedative for at least six months in his 100 patients. At the end of one year 80 patients were still continent but half of these had some residual urgency. This was one of the earliest reports of bladder drill and prompted further work by Elder and Stephenson [16] who used the same regime. They also reported on the long-term results of this therapy with an overall 3-year response rate of about 50% [3] but felt that bladder drill must have an additional effect to the drugs as in some patients who relapsed this occurred many months after the withdrawal of drug treatment. In a mixed group of 65 females with detrusor instability and sensory urgency the Frewen technique was employed, combining sedation with anticholinergic treatment and bladder training, and in those with sensory urgency favourable results were reported prompting the authors to suggest that the Frewen regime may be indicated as primary treatment in sensory urgency [17].

Bladder Drill

Bladder retraining or bladder drill was popularised by Frewen [5] who described the basic concept as focusing the patient's attention on the adoption of a graduated negative response to the desire to micturate and overcoming by instruction her abnormal voiding routine. The patient is given an explanation of the rationale behind bladder retraining and keeps a voiding chart, recording the time interval between each micturition. The aim is to increase this interval, gradually, by timed voiding, until a 3–4 hourly voiding pattern is established. Frewen [5] reported an 80% subjective cure rate after 12 weeks treatment of a mixed group with detrusor instability and sensory urgency. A cystometric cure was only achieved in three of eight patients with proven detrusor instability and Frewen commented that patients with sensory urgency responded better to the retraining, though he also felt that these patients may be in an earlier phase of the disorder. He discussed the possibility that voluntary frequency may be an initiating factor in detrusor instability rather than simply a symptomatic consequence of it, but in a later paper reports that the symptomatic cure rate is uninfluenced by the presence or absence of detrusor instability and that such instability is irrelevant to the patients' progress and the eventual return to normal voiding [18]. With no objective measure of sensory urgency the assessment of cure rates and the length of follow-up are impossible to standardise.

In a study that assessed the long-term effect of bladder training on patients with the "urge syndrome" an overall cure/improvement rate of 85% was reported [3], patients with sensory urgency achieving the best results. The authors state that repeated bladder training after relapse is not as effective as on the first occasion and emphasise the need for careful follow-up and outpatient reinforcement of bladder drill by the individual physician. This is not substantiated in the article and would require confirmation in a controlled manner.

The question of whether bladder drill should be inpatient or outpatient therapy or whether to combine with drug therapy remains unresolved. Jarvis [2] reported on 30 females with sensory urgency who had inpatient bladder drill over a mean stay of 9.25 days. He achieved 54.5% of patients symptom free and dry on pad testing 6 months after treatment. Ferrie et al. [17] combined inpatient bladder drill with drug therapy, 100 mg emepronium bromide daily, and fluphenazine/ nortriptyline 30 mg daily in 65 females with frequency and urgency and urge incontinence. Those who had cystometry showed a mix of detrusor instability and sensory urgency. Fourteen days of inpatient treatment resulted in 88% improvement but this fell to 38% at six months, with a 37% default rate from follow-up. Few studies report use of outpatient bladder drill though the practice is fairly widespread. With a continence advisor or other specialised personnel showing an active interest in the treatment programme it should prove possible to conduct this, with regular review, on an outpatient basis . This would be less disrupting for the patient and should also prove cost effective for the health service. A comparison of inpatient and outpatient therapy is needed to allow assessment of efficacy and possibly the question of adjuvant drug therapy could be addressed.

Psychotherapy

Many authors refer to bladder drill as a form of psychotherapy. The fact that time is taken to explain the situation to the patient may indeed have an important role in her recovery. Ferrie et al. [17] found a good initial response in all of their introverted patients, a group who have previously been reported to respond well to psychological conditioning [19]. These patients had psychological investigation during the time in hospital with 60% showing a high neuroticism score in keeping with the findings of Hafner et al. [8] who showed a correlation between psychological disorder and symptoms of frequency, urgency and urge incontinence. Macaulay et al. [10] reported a study on the mental state of 211 women attending a urodynamic clinic and found that patients with sensory urgency and detrusor instability were more anxious than those with genuine stress incontinence and some of their patients, whose urinary symptoms rendered life intolerable, were as anxious, depressed and phobic as psychiatric inpatients. They went on to randomise patients with detrusor instability and sensory urgency into treatment comparing psychotherapy, bladder drill and propantheline. The psychotherapy group significantly improved on measures of urgency, incontinence and nocturia though not on frequency and there was no appreciable change in their psychological ratings. Interestingly patients having bladder drill became less anxious and depressed whilst also decreasing their frequency of micturition despite attempts to study the benefit of therapy in as "pure" form as possible and give no supportive element during bladder drill. From this it would appear that bladder drill may be acting on the psychosomatic component of the disorder.

Electrical Therapy

It has been shown previously that anal and pudendal stimulation can result in inhibition of reflex detrusor activity [20]. McGuire et al. [21] reported on the use of electrical stimulation to treat detrusor instability and during assessment noted an absence of urgency among the patients.

Biofeedback

Biofeedback is the process of providing visual or auditory evidence of the status of an autonomic bodily function, so that the patient may exert control over this function. Rises in the detrusor pressure can be demonstrated to the patient in the form of a bell ringing or by showing her the tracing of the pressure rise and asking the patient voluntarily to inhibit the detrusor contraction. In patients with sensory urgency we have shown that as they appreciated the sensation of urgency this was associated with a rise in the conductivity recording [4]. This allowed the conductivity recording to be used to teach patients how to control their symptoms [4].

In a group of 20 patients with sensory urgency, bladder neck electric conductance (BNEC) recordings were made with the patient lying supine, with 250 ml normal saline in the bladder. The conductivity catheter was placed to record at the bladder neck, located by using the urethral electric conductance profile, as described previously [4] (Fig. 19.5). A recording was obtained with the patients at rest and the maximum conductivity deflection (MDR) at rest was found to be significantly higher in our symptomatic group compared with the normal controls. The rise in conductivity is due to urine passing through the bladder neck. Thus, either the bladder neck is opening or the urethra is shortening around the catheter. Biofeedback could be used to teach the patient to control this movement.

The patients were shown the conductivity reading on a UEC meter and taught how to close the bladder neck which reduced the conductivity reading and was associated with abolition of the sensation of urgency. Whilst lying observing the UEC meter, patients were instructed to try to inhibit micturition and if no reduction in conductivity reading was achieved, they tried to imagine they were also controlling an attack of diarrhoea. After two or three sessions, most patients could at will reduce the conductivity reading. The patients attended for a minimum

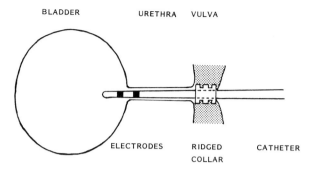

BLADDER   URETHRA   VULVA

ELECTRODES   RIDGED   CATHETER
                    COLLAR

Fig. 19.5.   Diagram of BNEC catheter in position.

of four half-hour sessions of biofeedback and practised the same movements at home for half an hour each day. At completion of treatment all patients showed a reduction in the maximum BNEC variation (MDR), most patients achieving a level within our normal range (Fig. 19.6).

The BNEC test allows positive diagnosis of the condition of sensory urgency and can be used as a successful alternative mode of treatment for sensory urge incontinence.

Summary

The condition of sensory urgency is probably much underdiagnosed, being either grouped with detrusor instability because of the similar symptomatology or classed as normal, as subtracted cystometry shows no abnormality. Further work with bladder neck electric conductance is needed to determine the incidence of the condition and may also throw light on the aetiology, which remains obscure. The optimal management of the condition will only be possible when treatment is orientated towards the cause and not, as is presently the case, a treatment of the symptoms only. Current management involves bladder drill, often combined with anticholinergic medication and sedation, with success rates in the region of 80%. There is a definite relationship with altered psychoneurotic profile though whether the disease process causes the psychological upset, or the reverse, is difficult to assess. Further work may determine the contribution of the psychological factor in the genesis of this complaint and may lead to valuable treatment options.

References

1. Abrams P, Blaivas JG, Stanton SL, Anderson JT. The standardisation of terminology of lower urinary tract function. Scand J Urol Nephrol 1988; Suppl 114.
2. Jarvis GJ. The management of urinary incontinence due to primary vesical sensory urgency by bladder drill. Br J Urol 1982; 54:374–6.
3. Holmes DM, Stone AR, Bary PR, Richards CJ, Stephenson TP. Bladder training – 3 years on. Br J Urol 1983; 55:660–4.

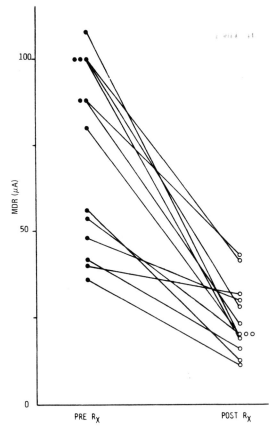

Fig. 19.6. Pre- and posttreatment MDR (μA) in a group having biofeedback therapy. Reproduced by kind permission of Editor, Journal of the Royal Society of Medicine.

4. Peattie AB, Plevnik S, Stanton SL. The use of bladder neck electric conductance (BNEC) in the investigation and management of sensory urge incontinence in the female. J R Soc Med 1988; 81:442–4.

5. Frewen WK. The management of urgency and frequency of micturition. Br J Urol 1980; 52:367–9.

6. Frewen WK. Urgency incontinence. J Obstet Gynaecol Br Commonw 1972; 79:77–9.

7. Frewen WK. Urgency incontinence. Br J Sex Med 1976; 3:21–4.

8. Hafner RJ, Stanton SL, Guy J. A psychiatric study of women with urgency and urgency incontinence. Br J Urol 1977; 49:211–14.

9. O'Boyle PJ, Parsons KF. Primary vesical sensory urgency. A clinical trial of bromocriptine. Br J Urol 1979; 51:200–3.

10. Macaulay AJ, Stern RS, Holmes DM, Stanton SL. Micturition and the mind: psychological factors in the aetiology and treatment of urinary symptoms in women. Br Med J 1987; 294:540–3.

11. Plevnik S, Brown M, Sutherst JR, Vrtacnik P. Tracking of fluid in the urethra by simultaneous electric impedance measurement at three sites. Urol Int 1983; 38:29–32.

12. Holmes DM, Plevnik S, Stanton SL. Bladder neck electric conductance test in the investigation and treatment of sensory urgency and detrusor instability. Proceedings of the fifteenth annual meeting of the International Continence Society, London, 1985; 96–7.

13. Klarskov P, Gerstenberg TC, Hald T. Bladder training and terodiline in females with idiopathic urge incontinence and stable detrusor function. Scand J Urol Nephrol 20:41–6.

14. Fischer-Rasmussen W and the Multicentre Study Group. Evaluation of long term safety and

clinical benefit of terodiline in women with urgency/urge incontinence. A multicentre study. Scand J Urol Nephrol Suppl 1984; 87:35–47.

15. Farrar DJ, Osborne JI. The use of bromocriptine in the treatment of the unstable bladder. Br J Urol 1976; 48:231–3.

16. Elder DD, Stephenson TP. An assessment of the Frewen regime in the treatment of detrusor dysfunction in females. Br J Urol 1980; 52:467–71.

17. Ferrie BG, Smith JS, Logan D, Lyle R, Paterson PJ. Experience with bladder training in 65 patients. Br J Urol 1984; 56:482–4.

18. Frewen WK. A reassessment of bladder training in detrusor dysfunction in the female. Br J Urol 1982; 54:372–3.

19. Eysenck HJ. The structure of human personality. London: Methuen, 1970; 436.

20. Godec C, Cass AS, Ayala GF. Bladder inhibition with functional electrical stimulation. Urology 1975; 6:663.

21. McGuire EJ, Shi-Chung Z, Horwinski ER, Lytton B. Treatment of motor and sensory detrusor instability by electrical stimulation. J Urol 1983; 129:78–9.

Discussion

Mundy: Do I take it then that a diagnosis of sensory urgency is made by doing a urodynamic study and failing to find unstable detrusor activity?

Peattie: Once other things have been excluded. Infection would be excluded. They would be cystoscoped to exclude interstitial cystitis or pathology within the bladder, and urgency and incontinence episodes would be objectively assessed and objective evidence of frequency ascertained. Obviously that could only be done with a urinary diary.

Mundy: I was wondering because there was no mention of bladder stimulants in drink and removing them, of *Chlamydia* and fastidious organisms, cystoscopy, or biopsy to exclude carcinoma in situ. Surely some specific parameter other than just everything else negative is used to make a diagnosis of idiopathic sensory urgency? In other words, if there is no detrusor instability, no cystoscopic evidence of abnormality, negative MSU, then the patient has sensory urgency.

Peattie: Yes.

Mundy: So that there is no distinction between those with an intense hypersensitivity to catheterisation and a very early first sensation of filling and those who have an entirely normal urodynamic study? They are both sensory urgency?

Peattie: No. These patients that we looked at were all patients with normal urodynamic assessment. We did not seem to have any of this group of patients who supposedly have this early first desire to void and a reduced bladder capacity with painful urgency, who are probably a different group. That is obviously an alteration in the sensitivity or the sensation from the bladder.

We did not see it in this group of patients and we find a very low incidence.

I know it is reported, but in our unit we really did not have much of that from our patients.

Mundy: So these are patients with symptoms who have absolutely no evidence whatsoever of any abnormality – bacteriologically, endoscopically or urodynamically?

Peattie: Right.

Stanton: Or by biopsy either.

Mundy: Why does that not worry anybody?

Warrell: What is being described is in my experience highly unusual. Almost all of these patients have cystometric abnormalities in the shape of an early first desire and a reduced capacity and a lot of them have endoscopic abnormalities. Whether that is called sensory urgency is how words are used. To have the symptom of urgency and everything else absolutely normal is really quite uncommon.

Versi: Is there a difference between the patients in whom UEC has been done and who have got sensory urgency as it was defined, and those who have detrusor instability in the UEC readings? In other words, is there an order of magnitude difference?

Peattie: No. There was no change at all. Basically there was a wide scatter. But they were all very different from the patients who were asymptomatic or the control group.

Versi: Is it possible that these patients have detrusor instability which is being missed on the first cystometry?

Peattie: It is entirely possible, yes. But then we are left with a group of patients in whom we do not find anything at first cystometry: either, as has been suggested earlier, we leave them for, say, six months and repeat the studies when we have found nothing, or we do a second test. Our second test was bladder neck electric conductance.
   If we are finding the same abnormality, sensory urgency or detrusor instability, we may then be justified in offering the same sort of treatment for these patients.

Sutherst: I am becoming confused by this. In the women whom I regard as having sensory urgency with a small capacity bladder and an early desire to void, an investigation like cystoscopy and biopsy is crucial to exclude bladder carcinoma in the older women in that group.

Stanton: We do not disagree. If a person has had longstanding symptoms of urgency and frequency I would not cystoscope them straight away, but if it was of recent onset I would be more inclined to do so on the basis that that could be a carcinoma. I would include in that category those that have sensory disturbance on catheterisation. But, from those investigations that Dr Peattie has detailed there are a number of patients who do not manifest any of those other signs or symptoms. If they have a small capacity then usually the bladder pressure has risen anyway, so I do not acknowledge seeing them with a small capacity with absolutely no pressure change whatsoever. I do not believe in the concept of urethrotrigonitis, and if we see inflammation or if we pick up chlamydia then as far as I am concerned they do not come into the category of sensory urgency.

Mundy: But surely what the group is doing is to exclude everybody with sensory urgency and treating a group of patients who happen to have a symptom but who are entirely normal to all objective assessment.

Peattie: No, they are not normal.

Mundy: But having excluded any urodynamic abnormality, any endoscopic abnormality, or any bacteriological abnormality, those who are being treated are objectively normal. Then we are told that because one test shows the same thing as another, it is probably the same condition; in other words, if someone were to do an intravenous pyelogram (IVP) and see a space-occupying lesion, that proves that carcinoma of the kidney is due to renal cyst formation.

Stanton: No. That is an incorrect extrapolation. If the patient has a urinary infection and complains of urgency then what she has is a urinary infection. It is not sensory urgency. If she has a stone in her bladder, she has a stone in her bladder, and I do not care whether she complains of urgency, or frequency, or whatever. If she has a small capacity bladder and we fill it and it cracks, she has urgency but she has interstitial cystitis.

We are saying that when a number of pathologies are excluded, one is left with the patient who complains of urgency, and there is nothing to be found apart from those features that we have already mentioned.

Mundy: I disagree. You are saying that if the woman has a urinary tract infection, that is the diagnosis. What you mean is if she has the symptom of sensory urgency and she has the diagnosis of urinary tract infection you treat that, or if she has the symptom of sensory urgency and a diagnosis of stone disease. Then you are using sensory urgency as a diagnostic category akin to urinary infection or interstitial cystitis, which it is not.

Stanton: No. If the symptoms still remain then we are in a different ballgame – after we have treated her complaint. In other words, if her stone has been removed or her urinary infection has been treated and she still has a complaint of urgency, then she would fall into my category of sensory urgency.

Shah: Dr Peattie has selected a group of patients to which a definition has been applied and she has discussed the management of those. I quite agree that there are other patients who have those very same symptoms who have other abnormalities and who are different.

Cardozo: Dr Peattie has described symptomatic urgency as opposed to sensory urgency.

Shah: In the absence of any other abnormality.

Cardozo: Sensory urgency being low first sensation, small capacity and hypersensitivity on catheterisation.

Stanton: But we have already said it has those characteristics. You are no further on.

Mundy: Of course you are further on. If someone puts up a paper that discusses the symptom of sensory urgency, and there is no mention of cystoscopy, biopsy, interstitial cystitis, and other abnormalities, obviously this is an entirely different disease group of problems.

Stanton: It was implied that those would be excluded.

Mundy: So objectively normal patients are undergoing treatment?

Stanton: No. These are patients who are complaining of urgency. They may not have early first sensation, hypersensitive urethra and a small capacity. You are no further on in terms of making a diagnostic label by those three factors.

Mundy: They are objectively normal by the tests that you yourself did.

Peattie: Not by all of them. Bladder neck electric conductance was abnormal, which means there is movement at the bladder neck which is also found in patients who have detrusor instability. So there is an objective abnormality in this group.

Quinn: I see this on the ultrasound from time to time whereby we see women who for no other reason have a twitchy bladder neck; they do not have objectively demonstrated detrusor instability. I think that is what this group sees with the bladder neck urethroelectric conductance. They see a little bit of this or that going on with a fixed catheter there. Whether that is a manifestation of detrusor instability that we have not detected by other methods may or may not be the case.

Versi: It is bladder neck instability.

Peattie: Yes. But it tends to be associated. As the conductivity rises, as the bladder neck opens, that is associated with them appreciating the sensation or urgency. So we have objectively demonstrated an abnormality.

Sutherst: There will be a whole range of symptoms and objective signs presumably. There are some people with "sensory urgency" with rather few objective signs on cystoscopy or urodynamic testing, and a biopsy of the bladder wall might find some more mast cells. Probably those that I regard as sensory urgency are at one end of a range with interstitial cystitis at the other end. But I would not accept that the entirely normal parameters that have been mentioned would come into my sensory urgency group.

Cardozo: What about oestrogens? Do women not have sensory urgency postmenopausally because they are oestrogen deprived? Certainly in our population of patients – and we use a definition for sensory urgency – a proportion of those women respond very well to oestrogens.

Peattie: As treatment of their symptoms?

Cardozo: As treatment of their symptoms.

Peattie: That is an entirely reasonable approach. It is the same sort of rationale as using them in the patients who have detrusor instability.

Stanton: This is, with great respect, a continuation of the oestrogen myth. If oestrogen really worked every postmenopausal patient would be cured, or 90% would be cured. And they are not.

Cardozo: No. I am talking about patients in whom all the other pathologies have been excluded.

Stanton: I agree. And it is presumed that one of the factors of causation might be a lack of oestrogen.

Cardozo: I am not just supposing. There is good evidence in the literature.

Stanton: Then why is the cure rate not better than the one that has been put forward?

Cardozo: For sensory urgency it is much better than for any of the other urodynamic abnormalities.

Murray: In the oestradiol study surely urgency was the only symptom that was not improved.

Cardozo: No. It was reduced. Also nocturia and frequency as well, not just urgency. Urgency is not cured in all patients but a proportion are significantly helped.

Stanton: What proportion? I doubt if it is 50%.

Versi: It went down from 20% of the sample to 12%, but that was not statistically significant because the sample was small. These were patients who were postmeno-pausal who were being treated with implants and we were looking at symptoms before and after. These are not the same patients as those who have sensory urgency urodynamically. By that we mean lowered first sensation and lowered bladder capacity in the absence of detrusor instability, who are being treated with oestrogen.

Cardozo: This is not from our data. This is from data from America and from other people's data in the UK. I am not talking about studies that we have done because we have not specifically used it in sensory urgency. It is probably useful for that particular indication.

Shah: On that note we should wind up the session, which has been very interesting. Good presentations, comprehensively presented and discussed, leaving some unanswered questions which there always are, implying that we need to do further work. We need to do more on the aetiology of bladder instability and certainly we need to find out more about sensory urgency and its related conditions and to look for new therapies and agents in the management of detrusor instability, and perhaps an alternative to phenol.

Prolapse and Alimentary Tract

Chapter 20

Aetiology of Pelvic Floor Prolapse and Its Relevance to Urinary and Faecal Control

C. N. Hudson and C. Spence-Jones

Traditionally a prolapse of the anterior vaginal wall (urethrocele or cystourethrocele) was regarded as the "cause" of stress urinary incontinence and nearly all these women were submitted to one, sometimes more, anterior vaginal repairs – often in association with other procedures for uterine prolapse. This simplistic approach was founded on false premises which accounts not only for the poor success rate but also for the multiplicity of operations which were devised.

Another problem is that the description of uterovaginal prolapse has always been based on clinical assessment, most frequently in the left lateral position with the patient lying down. This may not demonstrate the full extent of abnormality and has the drawback of being subjective. Radiological tests have helped to define prolapse [1] but cannot be used in every patient because of the high dose of radiation. Ultrasound can be used to assess the bladder neck [2] and will give dynamic information, but does not enable uterovaginal descent to be defined relative to the bony pelvis. The use of magnetic resonance imaging (MRI) to visualise the whole pelvis is still only available for research, but may provide a means of non-invasive objective investigation of women with prolapse.

The significance of some pertinent observations on prolapse was perhaps overlooked. First, it was observed that the worst cases of stress urinary incontinence were commonly associated with only minor vaginal wall prolapse rather than major cystocele. Second, patients with major uterovaginal prolapse were unlikely to have apparent stress urinary incontinence. Third, regrettably, correction of major uterovaginal prolapse rarely precipitated for the first time the onset of the symptom of stress urinary incontinence. Fourth, although the most severe degree of uterovaginal prolapse (procidentia) may be associated with incontinence, it is usually of a totally different variety, that is, the overflow incontinence caused by urethral obstruction due to kinking. In a rather more sinister situation, relatively symptomless uterine procidentia may be associated with obstructive uropathy due to a ureteric kinking, and this is one of the few potentially life-threatening complications of genital prolapse.

Aetiology

Theories of a presumed cause-and-effect relationship between prolapse and defective control of micturition have not stood the test of time and the association seems largely to be one of coincidence. Nevertheless, the fact that there is still a certain overlap between the sufferers of these conditions suggests that some may share a common factor in their aetiology. Moreover, it remains true that mechanical correction of uterovaginal prolapse in some instances is capable of restoring defective control of micturition without prejudice to whether this is considered to be the best method of achieving this objective.

Types of Prolapse

The derivation and spelling of the suffix "cele" is from a Greek word meaning hernia. Although uterine descent is more akin to intussusception than hernia, the commonly associated posterior peritoneal sac is in fact a true hernia or enterocele. It might just as easily be called an epiplocele if the omentum were long enough to reach to this position. The protrusions of bladder or rectum below the peritoneum correspond therefore to extraperitoneal hernia formation (hernia en glissade): it is not surprising therefore that most of the factors recognised as having an aetiological role in hernia in other sites play an important part in determining the onset of genital prolapse and also to a certain extent of the independent symptoms of defective control of micturition. The factors include obesity, chronic cough, chronic constipation and occupational activity, e.g. heavy lifting. Attention to these may be as important for therapy for defective control of micturition as it is for the repair of uterovaginal prolapse, or indeed hernia in any other site. In addition, infantile or adolescent hernia of different aetiology can occur at most sites and prolapse of the female genital tract is no exception, although it is exceptionally rare in the prepubertal girl. Babies born with spina bifida may have congenital uterovaginal prolapse [3]. There are also reports of prolapse present at birth not associated with spina bifida [4].

Mechanism of Prolapse

It is necessary to consider how these causative mechanisms bring about prolapse and also play a role in defective control of micturition. Such a role is likely to be facilitatory rather than directly causative.

For prolapse to occur, the structural supports of the genital tract have to become stretched and attenuated. There is a phylogenetic basis for the occurrence of genital prolapse in the human. One factor is the need to give birth to an infant with a relatively greater head size than occurs in many similar mammals. Another is the adoption of the plantigrade posture as this alters the resultant forces acting on the genital tract from within the abdomen. Studies of comparative anatomy have shown that the ewe is more likely to develop uterovaginal prolapse if constipated and if the animal lies with its rump downhill! [5]. Ethnic anatomical variations cause racial differences in the prevalence of genital prolapse [6].

In nulliparous individuals, even the quite young, an exceptionally deep pouch of Douglas may predispose to genital prolapse.

Pathology

The morbid anatomical changes found in cases of utcrovaginal prolapse are:

1. Attenuation of the ligamentary supports as a result of periodic physical stretching.
2. Attenuation and weakness of the pelvic floor muscles for a variety of reasons, one of which may be traction neuropathy.
3. Often the presence of an enlarging hernial sac (congenital, traction or pulsion variety).
4. Supravaginal cervical elongation.

Anatomical Changes

It has been customary to describe the supporting mechanisms of the pelvic viscera and the pelvic floor in terms of static structures. We are, however, dealing with a very dynamic situation and the anatomy has to be considered in dynamic terms. If there is failure of the dynamic support, the static anatomical structures may well be unable to sustain the position. Some alteration in the anatomical relation occurs which immediately aggravates the displacement of early genital prolapse, setting the stage for a vicious circle and almost inevitable progression. For instance, axial displacement of the uterus is a prerequisite for descent or intussusception into the vagina and this is most commonly a sequel to retroversion. Similarly, as soon as a cystocele is large enough to fill the introitus it receives no support during the valsalva manoeuvre and therefore has a much greater tendency to enlarge. Studies using proctography have shown that a small defect in the anterior rectal wall just above the anorectal margin, i.e. a rectocele, is a normal finding in 50% of women [7].

What then are the supports for the genital tract and what part do they play in the poor control of micturition? As far as the uterus is concerned, it is the fascial condensation known as the cardinal ligaments which are critical. The posterior limbs of the cardinal or uterosacral ligaments are subjected to stress in the erect posture and may be damaged in disorders of defaecation. Certainly, posterior displacement of the cervix over the levator plate rather than indirect apposition to the genital hiatus is a very important feature in the maintenance of normal anatomy and uterosacral attenuation could be one of the early factors in this chain of events. The positioning of the cervix and vagina towards the posterior part of the pelvis also facilitates uterine anteversion, in itself an important factor, prophylactic against uterovaginal intussusception. The anterior horns of the cardinal ligament in its butterfly shape are termed the pubocervical ligaments. In women with vaginal prolapse they are commonly grossly attenuated and scarcely identifiable. Under normal circumstances they provide support but do not embrace closely the urinary hiatus.

The urethra itself passes through a ligamentous structure recognised in the male as the perineal membrane. In the female this anterior triangle is divided into three parts by the vagina, which is normally almost adherent to the inferior pubic ramus, producing two lateral membranes and the pubourethral ligaments. The anterior triangular ligament supports the distal urethra, fanning out laterally to the inferior pubic rami, with a central gap which transmits the clitoral vessels. The two halves of this structure are probably what Zacharin has displayed in his anatomical dissections and termed the posterior pubourethral ligaments. There is an anterior pubourethral ligament which supports the short female urethra anterior or inferior to the membrane. Attenuation of the pubourethral or triangular ligaments merely allows the urethra to be dislocated in a rotating movement under the pubic arch when stressed from above rather than producing a bulge. This movement, termed "cartwheeling" by Chassar Moir, is characteristically associated with genuine stress urinary incontinence, although it may well not be the only anatomical cause. Certainly, laxity sufficient to allow cartwheeling may be enough to prevent abdominal pressure transmission to the proximal urethra with preservation of the urethrovesical pressure differential, so essential to continence.

The vagina itself is normally fairly firmly attached to the medial aspects of the pubococcygeus/puborectalis muscles. Under normal circumstances the vagina is collapsed with a transverse slit and without any inherent tendency for the vault to intussuscept. In the erect posture under normal conditions the apex of the vagina lies posteriorly over the levator plate and contraction of the pelvic floor muscles in the valsalva manoeuvre will accentuate this position without providing any tendency for intussusception to occur. Further down the vagina, the anterior wall is supported against the displacement of straining by the posterior vaginal wall, in turn supported by the perineal body below the levator ani complex.

The Effects of Childbirth

There is such an obvious association between childbirth and the subsequent genital hernia or prolapse and to a certain extent defective control of micturition that the anatomical changes induced need to be considered in some detail. At various levels, supporting structures are damaged.

1. The anterior horns of the cardinal ligament (pubocervical ligaments) are inevitably forced apart by the descent of the fetal head. Resulting damage to the support of the bladder base is the reason why a measure of cystocele is so common in parous women.

2. Distraction of the margins of the genital hiatus formed by the pubococcygeus and the puborectalis muscles. In other words, a big head is forced through a small gap.
3. Disruption of the perineal body, resulting in gaping of the introitus with exposure of the lowest part of the anterior vaginal wall and sometimes with exposure of the posterior vaginal wall, above the level of the partly separated perineal body which allows the formation of a rectocele.

Some of these anatomical changes are associated with the alterations in ligaments which occur during pregnancy. As has been stated, quite commonly the symptom of stress urinary incontinence develops during pregnancy, only to improve for a while thereafter.

Neurological Damage

There is an increasing amount of evidence that damage to the nerves supplying the pelvis may be an important factor associated with the subsequent development of prolapse. The striated muscles of the pelvic floor are tonically active at rest, and also contract reflexly to protect against sudden rises in abdominal pressure with coughing etc. This reflex is present in paraplegic patients, as long as the cord is not damaged below S2. If, however, there is damage to the sensory nerves, motor nerves or the sacral segment of this reflex, pelvic floor muscle activity will be compromised.

The pudendal nerve innervates the external anal sphincter, the pubococcygeus and the external urethral sphincter. The remainder of the puborectalis and the intramural urethral rhabdosphincter are supplied by autonomic nerves.

So what is the evidence that denervation is important in pelvic floor prolapse?

1. Studies of biopsies of the histology/histochemistry of the pelvic floor muscles have shown the changes characteristic of denervation, both in women with rectal prolapse [8] and in women with uterovaginal prolapse [9].
2. Electromyography of the pubococcygeus shows the changes consistent with denervation and reinnervation in women with prolapse [10].
3. Studies of the pudendal nerve itself, measuring the speed of conduction along the nerve (i.e. the latency) have demonstrated a neuropathy in patients with rectal prolapse.

   The results from patients with uterovaginal prolapse do not agree: some show evidence of a pudendal neuropathy [10] and others do not [11].

What, therefore, are the events which cause neurological damage in the pelvis?

There is considerable evidence that chronic straining induces a traction neuropathy towards the posterior part of the pelvis with impairment of function of the anal sphincter [12]. It is apparent that the single major episode of straining due to parturition may contribute to this state of affairs as has been demonstrated by Snooks et al. [13]. In this study, vaginal delivery was shown to be the cause of a pudendal neuropathy, particularly when associated with forceps delivery. There was no evidence of a pudendal neuropathy in patients delivered by Caesarean section. It is interesting to note that some women still have evidence of a pudendal neuropathy five years later [14].

The relative importance of this isolated contribution to chronic pelvic floor weakness is not entirely clear. The late Sir Alan Parks showed the nerves to the anal sphincter would be exposed to the greatest distraction during forced pelvic floor descent. In more severe cases, puborectalis and pubococcygeus are affected. This sets the stage for defective control of defaecation and rectal prolapse.

Although there is an association between rectal prolapse and genital prolapse it is by no means universal in either direction, and would appear to be a situation of overlap of common factors rather than direct linkage.

Conclusion

We are left with the hypothesis that childbirth, as the principal cause of genital prolapse, produces this effect by stretching the urogenital hiatus and allowing expulsive forces of the uterus to be directed down the vagina rather than against the levator plate. Chronic straining at stool with pelvic floor inhibition is the major factor in rectal prolapse.

The contribution of genital prolapse to defective control of micturition would appear to be stretching and weakness of the anterior perineal compartment, in particular the so-called posterior pubourethral ligaments, allowing the proximal urethra to be dislocated from the protective effects of the intra-abdominal pressure zone. Chronic disruption of the perineal body with gaping of the introitus removes a second line of defence in this situation, as is more clearly seen after removal of the perineal body with rectal excision. A second common theme for all the above is pelvic floor nerve damage from both childbirth and chronic straining. The relative importance of these factors is not yet clear.

References

1. Berglas B, Rubin IC. Study of the supportive structures of the uterus by levator myography. Surg Gynaecol Obstet 1933; 97:677–92.
2. Quinn MJ, Beynon J, Mortensen NJMMcC, Smith PJB. Transvaginal endosonography: a new method to study the anatomy of the lower urinary tract in urinary stress incontinence. Br J Urol 1988; 62:414–18.
3. Lee A, McComb G. Neurogenic perineal prolapse in neonates. Radiology 1983; 148:433–5.
4. Cottom D, Williams E. Procidentia in the newborn. J Obstet Gynaecol Br Commonw 1965; 72:131–6.
5. Zacharin RF. Genital prolapse in ruminants. Aust NZ J Obstet Gynaecol 1969; 9:236–9.
6. Zacharin RF. "A Chinese anatomy" – the pelvic supporting tissues of the Chinese and occidental female compared and contrasted. Aust NZ J Obstet Gynaecol 1977; 17:1–11.
7. Bartram C, Turnbull GK, Leonard-Jones JE. Evacuation proctography: an investigation of rectal expulsion in 20 subjects without defaecatory disturbance. Gastrointest Radiol 1988; 13:72–80.
8. Parks AG, Swash M, Urich H. Sphincter denervation in anorectal incontinence and rectal prolapse. Gut 1977; 18:656–65.
9. Gilpin SA, Gosling JA, Smith ARB, Warrell DW. The pathogenesis of genitourinary prolapse and stress incontinence of urine. A histological and histochemical study. Br J Obstet Gynaecol 1989; 96:15–23.
10. Smith ARB, Hosker GL, Warrell DW. The role of partial denervation of the pelvic floor in the aetiology of genitourinary prolapse and stress incontinence of urine. A neurophysiological study. Br J Obstet Gynaecol 1989; 96:24–8.

11. King DW, Lubowski Beevors M. Pelvic floor function in uterovaginal prolapse (Abstract). Proceedings of the Tripartite Surgical Meeting, 1989.
12. Henry MM, Parks AG, Swash M. The pelvic floor musculature in the descending perineum syndrome. Br J Surg 1982; 69:470–2.
13. Snooks SJ, Swash M, Henry MM, Setchell M. Injury to innervation of pelvic floor sphincter musculature in childbirth. Lancet 1984; ii:546–50.
14. Snooks SJ, Henry MM, Swash M. Five-year follow-up of changes in pelvic floor innervation after childbirth. Br J Surg 1989; 76:636.

Chapter 21

Lower Alimentary Tract Disorder

M. M. Henry

Pelvic floor failure may be responsible for a variety of disorders (Table 21.1) which cross the boundaries of differing specialties, sometimes to the detriment of the patient. For the purposes of this account, only those conditions affecting the anorectum will be considered.

Anorectal Incontinence

Patients with the inadvertent passage of faecal material per anum exist in a state of social alienation which is frequently intensified by an unsympathetic approach to management from attendant clinicians. Positive help can be provided, sometimes by the provision of relatively simple methods.

Anorectal Continence

A certain degree of dispute still exists concerning the mechanisms which maintain normal control. The various factors which are considered to play a role are listed in Table 21.2. The dispute lies as to which of these plays the principal part. The internal anal sphincter is responsible for a high pressure zone in the anal canal which is maintained at rest and is beyond voluntary control. Various surgical procedures which abolish internal anal sphincter function and hence resting tone (e.g. manual dilation, sphincterotomy) rarely cause a major loss of function. The deficit is usually restricted to loss of control to flatus and soiling in the presence

Table 21.1. Disorders associated with pelvic floor failure

Anorectal incontinence
Urinary incontinence
Rectal prolapse
Genital prolapse
Solitary rectal ulcer syndrome
Descending perineum syndrome

of severe diarrhoea. The external anal sphincter is responsible for a further rise in intra-anal pressure during periods of voluntary contraction. Similarly, there is only a minor degree of faecal incontinence if this muscle ring is divided surgically (e.g. during anal fistula surgery). The puborectalis, however, would appear to play a major role in anorectal continence since damage to this muscle usually results in major incontinence [1]. The contraction of the puborectalis muscle is responsible for the maintenance of an angle between the lower rectum and upper anal canal (the anorectal angle). The true significance of this anatomical entity is in dispute. Parks [2] believed that the angle permitted a flap-valve to operate. He believed that intra-abdominal pressure was conducted via the anterior rectal wall. Any rise in pressure caused by such acts as coughing or sneezing would force this part of the rectum down onto the upper anal canal so effectively excluding the anus from intrarectal contents. Bartolo [3] found no evidence of this action using radiological studies in subjects undergoing Valsalva manoeuvre. It can be argued that the latter does not physiologically reproduce the physical forces operating when continence mechanisms are threatened.

Table 21.2. Factors responsible for normal anorectal continence

Anal sphincters
   Internal sphincter innervated by hypogastric and sacral parasympathetic nerves
   External sphincter innervated by pudendal nerves
Pelvic floor
   Anorectal angle (flap valve) innervated by direct branches of sacral plexus (above pelvic floor)
Sensation
   Receptors in pelvic floor
   Recto-sphincteric inhibitory reflex (sampling)
Miscellaneous
   Valves of Houston
   Anal cushions
   Force vectors acting in a cephalad direction

The sensory receptors responsible for the sensation of rectal filling probably reside in the pelvic floor muscles and not in the rectum itself [4]. As a consequence of a reflex whereby the internal anal sphincter is inhibited by distension of the rectum, a small sample of rectal contents enters the proximal anal canal and comes into direct contact with sensory receptors at the dentate line. In this way the nature of the rectal contents (i.e. flatus or faeces) is perceived and sensory discrimination can occur at cortical level.

Minor Anorectal Incontinence

Minor incontinence is defined as the inadvertent loss of flatus or the occasional faecal soiling usually in the presence of diarrhoea. Hence any disorder responsible for creating liquid stool, such as infection with salmonella or proctitis, may cause soiling in the presence of normal function of the sphincters and pelvic floor. The internal sphincter may be rendered deficient by previous anal surgery (e.g. haemorrhoidectomy) and as a result a minor degree of incontinence may result.

Treatment in these groups is usually by non-surgical methods. Hence the diarrhoea will require management according to the underlying cause; there is no treatment of flatus incontinence.

Major Anorectal Incontinence

Major incontinence is defined as incontinence of formed stool and clearly represents a more serious functional disorder often requiring surgery to correct. It is this group in whom denervation of the pelvic floor and external anal sphincter has been found to play an important role in pathogenesis [5]. Nerve conduction studies have provided evidence to suggest that the site of the neurogenic injury is peripheral (pudendal nerves) rather than central (cauda equina) [6]. The cause of such injury is probably multifactorial but the role of childbirth seems to be of principal importance. In a study of the effects of childbirth on the pelvic floor, it was shown that the external anal sphincter and its innervation can be damaged during vaginal delivery but not if the fetus was delivered by Caesarean section [7]. The abnormalities were most marked in multiparae and correlated strongly with a prolonged second stage of labour and with forceps-assisted delivery. Substantial recovery occurred within 2 months after delivery but the recovery was least complete in the multiparae.

Excessive straining at defaecation can also lead to pudendal nerve damage by inducing stretch damage to these nerves [8]. This is particularly pronounced in the presence of abnormal perineal descent (see below).

Treatment

Wherever the degree of functional loss is severe thereby giving rise to major incapacity to the patient, the management is usually surgical. Conservative measures which include Faradism, biofeedback and physiotherapy, have not been generally found of long-term value.

If incontinence is the consequence of simple division of the external sphincter ring (e.g. third degree perineal tear) then sphincter repair using a non-absorbable suture material will usually restore full continence provided that there has been no co-incidental damage to the nerve supply [9]. Where the incontinence results from denervation of the pelvic floor, the operation of post-anal repair [2] will restore reasonable control in about 60% of patients. Parks originally believed that function was recovered as a direct consequence of restoration of the anorectal angle. In practice there is very little evidence to support this theory but there does seem to be strong evidence that the anal canal is lengthened by the procedure and this may explain its success [10].

Descending Perineum Syndrome

This is descent of the perineum below the level of the bony outlet of the pelvis during a straining effort [8]. These patients strain excessively and often experience a sense of incomplete evacuation at the completion of the defaecatory act. The latter is caused by prolapse of the anterior rectal wall into the lumen of the anal canal. At the completion of defaecation the prolapse remains in the anal canal where it comes into contact with the sensory receptors at the dentate line. The prolapse is thereby perceived as faecal matter and further futile attempts at defaecation are made.

The true significance of the condition lies in its direct relationship to denervation [11]. With increasing descent, increasing damage is inflicted on the pudendal nerves and anorectal incontinence may become the more serious sequel.

Solitary Rectal Ulcer Syndrome

Excessive straining may lead to the development of a shallow ulcer in the anterior part of the mid rectum. The defaecation disorder is then accompanied by rectal bleeding which can be profuse and by mucus discharge. These patients may similarly exhibit denervation of the pelvic floor and may ultimately develop incontinence [12].

Rectal Prolapse

Although rectal prolapse can occur at any age, it is most common at the extremes of life. In children, this may be associated with mucoviscidosis and in the remainder it is usually transient and can be managed by simple conservative measures.

In adults, the condition is potentially serious since the prolapsing bowel wall causes increasing traumatic damage to the anal sphincters and pelvic floor. Management is usually surgery to correct the prolapse in the first instance. Where incontinence persists after successful correction of the prolapse, a small proportion of patients will require pelvic floor surgery as a secondary procedure to restore continence.

References

1. Milligan ETC, Morgan CN. Surgical anatomy of the anal canal with special reference to anal fistulae. Lancet 1934; ii:1150–6.
2. Parks AG. Anorectal incontinence. Proc R Soc Med 1975; 68:681–90.

3. Bartolo DCC. Flap-valve theory of anorectal incontinence. Br J Surg 1986; 73:1012–14.
4. Lane RHS, Parks AG. Function of the anal sphincters following colo-anal anastomosis. Br J Surg 1977; 64:596–9.
5. Parks AG, Swash M, Urich H. Sphincter denervation in anorectal incontinence and rectal prolapse. Gut 1977; 18:656–65.
6. Snooks SJ, Swash M, Henry MM. Abnormalities in central and peripheral nerve conduction in patients with anorectal incontinence. J R Soc Med 1985; 78:294–300.
7. Snooks SJ, Swash M, Henry MM, Setchell ME. Injury to innervation of pelvic floor sphincter musculature in childbirth. Lancet 1984; ii:546–50.
8. Henry MM, Parks AG, Swash M. The pelvic floor muscle in the descending perineum syndrome. Br J Surg 1982; 62:470–2.
9. Laurberg S, Swash M, Henry MM. Delayed external sphincter repair for obstetric tear. Br J Surg 1988; 75:786–8.
10. Womack NR, Morrison JFB, Williams NS. Prospective study of the effects of postanal repair in neurogenic faecal incontinence. Br J Surg 1988; 75:48–52.
11. Jones PN, Lubowski DZ, Swash M, Henry MM. Relation between perineal descent and pudendal nerve damage in idiopathic faecal incontinence. Int J Color Dis1987; 2:93–5.
12. Snooks SJ, Nicholls RJ, Henry MM, Swash M. Electrophysiological and manometric assessment of the pelvic floor in solitary rectal ulcer syndrome. Br J Surg 1985; 72:131–3.

Discussion

Warrell: The concept of pelvic damage, of which bladder and rectum are elements of the same spectrum, is an important consideration in how we manage patients and in the training of rectal surgeons and gynaecologists. But that is a philosophic aside. Why should straining for a short period of time change the conduction time in the pudendal nerve? No patient is squeezing out myelin like toothpaste from a tube.

Henry: No, but they are causing undoubted temporary damage to that nerve. In the environment of a clinic patients are rarely asked to strain, but if patients who have pelvic floor descent are asked to strain, the whole pelvic floor can be seen to balloon downwards. The hypothesis is that the pelvic floor may not balloon downwards in the resting state, but when they strain the pelvic floor drops down very dramatically and it is pulling on the nerve because the nerve is fixed at the ischial spine. That is the hypothesis: as they strain, the pelvic floor descends, stretching the nerve, and we can demonstrate an increase in latency in the nerve.

Warrell: I thought this was dependent on the myelin sheath. I do not see how myelin can be lost and recovered quickly.

Henry: Permanent neurological damage is picked up in this way. It is undoubtedly true that temporary neurogenic injury will still cause slowing of conduction. If the myelin sheath becomes hypoxic, if the blood supply to the myelin sheath is cut – which can be done as an agonal event – then delay in conduction can be demonstrated immediately; absolutely immediately.

Peattie: Is it normal for the pelvic floor to descend to that extent?

Henry: No. The pelvic floor descends up to 3 cm in the normal individual. By using radiographic means at least 3 cm of descent can be easily demonstrated. But anything more than 3 cm descent is definitely in the realms of the abnormal. And in patients who have this syndrome, descent of up to 7 cm can occur, 4 cm over and above the normal.

Peattie: But there was neurological damage in some even up to 3 cm.

Henry: Yes. But that is a heterogeneous group. Some of them may do but then there will be other factors. They may have had childbirth problems. They are not all nulliparous patients that form that group. It is very difficult to get a pure group for studies.

Hudson: As part of this vicious circle that we developed, so many women describe the onset of their subsequent constipation as an event which has coincided with or followed the first pregnancy. So it is sometimes difficult to sort out which is the chicken and which is the egg in the subsequent events.

Henry: I agree. The dilemma is: is the neuropathy due to perineal descent or just associated with it? It may be that the amount of perineal descent mirrors very nicely the amount of neurogenic injury just because the pelvic floor descent occurs pari passu with the denervation damage.

I think that it actually occurs secondary to pelvic floor descent, because of that study showing that as they strain we can demonstrate a definite neurogenic change taking place. So I think it is the secondary event.

Stanton: What causes the primary straining?

Henry: Childbirth, I think. And then this intensifies it.

DeLancey: Men do not have the problem?

Henry: Very rarely. Men can get incontinence, but there are other factors: diabetes, alcohol, and AIDS now. We are seeing a number of peripheral pudendal neuropathies in AIDS patients right at the beginning of the illness, almost before diagnosis is made, which suggests to us that the virus is entering the central nervous system through the pudendal nerves.

Incontinence is an early stage of AIDS. So if a healthy male presents with incontinence, I really would say that AIDS is the first thing one should consider.

Stanton: What are the effects of pregnancy following a successful treatment of female incontinence? Are such women told not to get pregnant, or that they may get pregnant but that they will need a caesarean section?

Henry: The second.

Stanton: We have some evidence that denervation may well be initiated by the pelvic mass which is enveloping the fetus, and therefore one might have to be very firm with the patient and tell her that she really must have conservative treatment until she has completed her family because even getting pregnant may initiate it.

DeLancey: The mass is abdominal, up until the very late stages.

Stanton: It is still a mass on the pelvic floor.

Sutherst: Taking that a step further, is this evidence telling us that we should be changing our obstetric practice quite radically?

Henry: Yes. I think it probably is. Only in the sense that the threshold for caesarean sections should perhaps be a little lower. I realise this is not much help to you.

Where we can help is when there has been a difficult delivery and the patient remains continent, but the gynaecologist is not quite sure whether any damage has been done. We can help enormously by doing these studies, and if we say there is definite evidence of denervation, it means that in the event of any second insult or onslaught on that pelvis, she may not get away with it the second time. Possibly in that situation it does help to be able to show that the threshold perhaps should be that much lower for the consideration of caesarean section.

Hilton: Does this open up the whole episiotomy debate again?

Henry: It does indeed. I was hoping that this would be something that the profession would go on to study in greater detail, if they have not done so already.

I think it does open up the episiotomy debate. When we looked at a much bigger study of more than 100 women studied pre- and post-delivery – because that was the big criticism here – then episiotomy seemed to have some kind of protective effect, but this was not statistically shown. But certainly those women who had had episiotomies came into the low-risk group.

Stanton: What about the role of pelvic floor exercises in ameliorating it?

Henry: We had a physiotherapist at St Mark's who was very keen on physiotherapy and really she lost enthusiasm after 12 months.

Our experience has not been a very happy one, but I know the American experience has been better. But I fear that once muscle has been denervated it is very difficult to re-educate the surviving muscle fibres to take over and provide sufficient hypertrophy to give a significant degree of control afterwards.

Stanton: That is interesting because I have the belief that physiotherapy for the elderly is little joy, especially based on the 65 year cut off. I am also unimpressed by the sight of physiotherapists in the postnatal ward teaching the old routines which they have taught for decades. No one has ever assessed them and one wonders.

I wonder whether the group would agree that there is not much joy in teaching a woman over 65? On the other hand Ms Shepherd says there is always some hope. How do we reconcile the two views?

Shepherd: Are we talking about the same thing? Are we discussing bladder control or is it the pelvic floor? If we are talking about pelvic floor I would agree.

It is only circumstantial evidence, but we have experience that people who have sufficient motivation will get quite satisfactory results from pelvic floor re-education in any age group, and it should be looked into more thoroughly.

DeLancey: I wonder if Mr Henry is dealing with the end stage of the worst of the denervations rather than the other forms of pelvic floor dysfunction that may have less denervation.

Henry: We are, I think. Obviously we are not seeing the patients who have only minor soiling and they may be the patients who do extremely well. We are seeing patients who really are in desperate trouble by the time they come to us, and we are often the final common pathway through a whole scatter of specialists, GPs etc., who have all told them that it has a psychological basis.

I am afraid that is probably true, and by that time they have got established atrophy of the muscle and there are very few surviving motor units left which can take over active support.

I wish we could get the patients earlier, then probably we could avoid surgery.

Hudson: Surely one of the most important considerations is to try to correct the abnormal defaecation habit. The longer that an elderly person has been constipated and straining at stool, the more difficult it will be to overcome. Surely this would do as much good as concentrating on the physiotherapy. Physiotherapy will be undone if they continue to strain two or three times a week or every day.

Henry: That is certainly true. The trouble is we see two different categories of patients. We see those with incontinence, and very often those with incontinence do not have defaecation disorders. And then we see those with defaecation disorders who do not necessarily have incontinence.

I would rather deal with the incontinent patients because I feel I can help those. The ones who strain with defaecation and cannot empty their rectum are a misery to treat because there really is no form of treatment that is very effective.

Shepherd: I would agree with Mr Stanton to a large extent that having physiotherapists or midwives standing at the ends of patients' beds in the early postnatal stage is probably a total waste of time. The time to teach pelvic floor exercises if they are to be used for prevention is at the antenatal stage.

Warrell: One of the things that it seems differs between urinary control and faecal control is something that was mentioned although we did not go into detail, and that is rectal sensation. It is most extraordinary to me that people can distinguish between flatus and fluid and solid material and that they can adapt their social behaviour, as we heard today, to combat that.

What is the role of rectal sensation and how is it lost?

Henry: Rectal sensation is interesting. I wanted to join in the earlier debate when the problems of detrusor instability and what it meant were discussed. I have been trying to think whether we have parallels in colorectal surgery, and the answer is that yes, we have to deal with urgency of defaecation. The situation arises when there is decreased sensory awareness of rectal filling, in the event of pelvic sepsis, particularly if the surgeon has done a very low anterior resection and technically there have been problems and there has been major pelvic sepsis occurring as a result. These patients have marked urgency of defaecation, tenesmus, etc., because they have a small capacity rectum. They also have diminished sensory awareness, because there has been a barrier created between the pelvic floor, where sensation is thought to arise, and the rectum. It is very important that there should be an intact segment of tissue – I cannot think of a better way to put it – between the rectum and the pelvic floor, because we think the sensation of rectal fullness arises from the pelvic floor and not from the rectum itself. Otherwise we would not be able to do low anterior resection and these patients have a normal sensation. So the intact pelvis is very important for rectal sensation.

The sensation of discrimination between flatus and the stool is a different mechanism which is a feature of the rectosphincteric reflex. When the rectum fills up, there is rectal distention with a reflex operating through the internal sphincter. The internal sphincter relaxes, allowing a small sample of rectal contents to enter the proximal anal canal where there are a profusion of sensory nerve endings, and it is the contact between the rectal content and the sensory receptors that allows one to discriminate. So sensation may be lost if there has been pudendal neuropathy, because the pudendal nerve is a mixed nerve, motor and sensory, and not only is there a loss of motor function but there is unquestionably a loss of sensory function, and that sensory loss may be felt in the loss of discrimination.

Warrell: And that is important.

Henry: It is important, but not of overriding importance. I maintain that if one were to lose sensation but keep motor function intact, one would probably be all right. One might have difficulty because one might not know that one had a full rectum, but if one were to work into a daily routine for example – the gut can be trained to work on a routine basis – then probably one would have reasonable control.

Subject Index